DIHLM

BI 3271903 5

D0344115

Topics in
COLORECTAL
SURGERY

Topics in
COLORECTAL
SURGERY

editor

Francis Seow-Choen
Singapore General Hospital

SGH
PGMI

SGH Postgraduate Medical Institute

World Scientific

NEW JERSEY • LONDON • SINGAPORE • SHANGHAI • HONG KONG • TAIPEI • BANGALORE

Published by:

World Scientific Publishing Co. Pte. Ltd.

P O Box 128, Farrer Road, Singapore 912805

USA office: Suite 1B, 1060 Main Street, River Edge, NJ 07661

UK office: 57 Shelton Street, Covent Garden, London WC2H 9HE

Singapore General Hospital Pte. Ltd.

Outram Road, Singapore 169608

British Library Cataloguing-in-Publication Date
A catalogue record for this book is available from the British Library.

Topics in Colorectal Surgery

ISBN   981-238-373-5
ISBN   981-238-374-3 (pbk)

Typeset by Stallion Press
Printed in Singapore by World Scientific Printers

Preface

Colorectal surgery is a very ancient art that has, over the last few decades, found a sound basis in science. Amongst its very famous ancient practitioners was Hippocrates (5th Century BC) himself. Nevertheless, it has taken many years for the science of colorectal surgery to be recognized by modern day academics as a specialty in its own right. Colorectal-surgical departments have been springing up all over the world and many of the surgical colleges and academies are only now beginning to see the importance of this branch of medicine. After rising from humble beginnings, the specialty of colorectal surgery is now a much-sought-after career amongst young doctors all over the world. Indeed, Shit is the Star now. At St Mark's Hospital the slogan was "Tops for Bottoms" for many years, and we may rightly say that "Bottoms are Tops" now! This worldwide phenomenon owes its impact to the strength and brotherhood of its practitioners and the support that the members of the fraternity gave one another in the face of opposition and resistance. The Department of Colorectal Surgery at the Singapore General Hospital has grown from strength to strength as well. Since the First Annual Colorectal Week, held in 1996, we have had a series of very successful annual colorectal-surgical weeks. This book is a collection of some of the best lectures, which we have gathered together in order that more people may share in the wisdom that may be obtained from them.

These meetings owe their success in no small part to the many experts who have visited with us during the week and shared their expertise, wisdom and wit with us and our many other visitors. We wish to record here our thanks to Professors Russell Stitz, Joe Tjandra, Victor Fazio, David Schoetz, Herand Abcarian, Wang Jeng Yi and Patricia Roberts.

We hope that you will share with us in this development and be a part of it!

Francis Seow-Choen
Head, Department of Colorectal Surgery
Singapore General Hospital

December 2002

Contributors

List of Principal Authors:

Christopher Paul **Barben**
MBBS, FRCS (London), BSc (Anatomy)
Registrar
4 Oast Cottages
Plum Pudding Lane
Dargate, Faversham
Kent ME13 9EY
UK
E-mail: cbarben@hotmail.com

Registrar with the Department of Colorectal Surgery,
Singapore General Hospital,
from December 2001 to October 2002

Steven Ross **Brown**
Consultant Surgeon
Sheffield 310–3QN
UK
E-mail: stevenbrown@doctors.org.uk

Registrar with the Department of Colorectal Surgery,
Singapore General Hospital,
from 1 October 1999 to 30 September 2000

Cheah Peh Yean
PhD
Senior Scientist
Colorectal Cancer Research Laboratory
Department of Colorectal Surgery
Singapore General Hospital
Outram Road
Singapore 169608
E-mail: gcscpy@sgh.com.sg

Eu Kong Weng
MBBS, FRCS (Ed), MMed (Surgery)
FICS (USA), FAMS (General Surgery)
Senior Consultant Surgeon
Director, Cancer Research Laboratory
Department of Colorectal Surgery
Singapore General Hospital
Outram Road
Singapore 169608

Visiting Senior Consultant
Surgical Oncology
National Cancer Centre

Visiting Senior Consultant
Gynaecologic Oncology
KK Women's and Children's Hospital

Clinical Senior Lecturer
National University of Singapore
E-mail: gcsekw@sgh.com.sg

Richard John **Guy**
MD, FRCS (Gen)
Consultant General & Colorectal Surgeon
Peterborough District Hospital
Thorpe Road, Peterborough

Cambridgeshire, PE3 6DA
UK
Registrar with the Department of Colorectal Surgery,
Singapore General Hospital,
from October 2000 to October 2001

Heah Sieu Min
MB BCH, FRCS (Ed), FAMS
Consultant Surgeon
Director, Transanal Ultrasound Laboratory
Director, Endoscopy Centre
Department of Colorectal Surgery
Singapore General Hospital
Outram Road
Singapore 166608

Visiting Staff Specialist, Surgical Oncology
National Cancer Centre
E-mail: gcshsm@sgh.com.sg

Ho Kok Sun
MBBS, FRCS (Ed), MMED (Surg)
Associate Consultant
Department of Colorectal Surgery
Singapore General Hospital
Outram Road
Singapore 169608
E-mail: gcshks@sgh.com.sg

David George **Jayne**
BSc (Anatomy), MB BCh, MD FRCS
Senior Lecturer & Honorary Consultant Surgeon
Academic Surgical Unit
Level 8, Clinical Sciences Building
St James's University Hospital
Leeds, LS9 7TF
UK
E-mail: dgjayne@hotmail.com

Registrar with the Department of Colorectal Surgery,
Singapore General Hospital,
from April 2001 to April 2002

Kam Ming Hian
MBBS
Registrar
Department of Colorectal Surgery
Singapore General Hospital
Outram Road
Singapore 169608
E-mail: kam.ming.hian@singhealth.com.sg

Lim Jit Fong
MBBS, FRCS (Glasg)
Registrar
Department of Colorectal Surgery
Singapore General Hospital
Outram Road
Singapore 169608
E-mail: gcsljf@sgh.com.sg

David **Lloyd**
MBBS, FRACS
Consultant Surgeon
St Vincent's Hospital
5 Frederick Street, Launceston
Tasmania, 7250 Australia
E-mail: lloydied@hotmail.com
Registrar with the Department of Colorectal Surgery,
Singapore General Hospital,
from October 2000 to September 2001

Loi Tien Tau, Carol
RN, MSC (Healthcare Management)
Programme Coordinator
Singapore Polyposis Registry
Department of Colorectal Surgery
Singapore General Hospital

Outram Road
Singapore 169608
E-mail: gcsltt@sgh.com.sg

Ng Kheng Hong
MBBS, MRCS (Ed)
Registrar
Department of Colorectal Surgery
Singapore General Hospital
Outram Road
Singapore 169608
E-mail: ng.kheng.hong@singhealth.com.sg

Ooi Boon Swee
MBBS (S'pore), FRCS (Ed), FRCS (Glasg), FRCS (I)
FAMS (General Surgery)
Consultant Surgeon
Department of Colorectal Surgery
Director, Anorectal & Pelvic Floor Physiology Laboratory
Singapore General Hospital
Outram Road
Singapore 169608

Visiting Staff Specialist, Surgical Oncology
National Cancer Centre
E-mail: gcsobs@sgh.com.sg

Patricia L **Roberts**
MD
Consultant Surgeon
Colon and Rectal Surgery
Lahey Clinic
41 Mail Road, Burlington
MA 01805
USA

Francis **Seow-Choen**
MBBS, FRCS (Ed), FAMS, FRES
Head & Senior Consultant Surgeon
Department of Colorectal Surgery

Singapore General Hospital
Outram Road
Singapore 169608

Director, Surgical Oncology
National Cancer Centre

Associate Clinical Professor
National University of Singapore

Adjunct Associate Professor
Natural Sciences
Nanyang Technological University
E-mail: gcsscf@sgh.com.sg

Paul Gerard **Skaife**
MB ChB, FRCS
Consultant Surgeon
University Hospital Aintree
Longmoor Lane, Liverpool
L9 7AL, Liverpool
UK
E-mail: PAUL.SKAIFE@aht.nwest.nhs.uk
*Registrar with the Department of Colorectal Surgery,
Singapore General Hospital,
from August 2000 to September 2001*

Tang Choong Leong
MBBS, MMED (Surgery), FRCS (Ed), FAMS
Consultant Surgeon
Director, Singapore Polyposis Registry
Department of Colorectal Surgery
Singapore General Hospital
Outram Road
Singapore 169608

Visiting Consultant, Surgical Oncology
National Cancer Centre

Joe J **Tjandra**
MBBS, MD, FRACS, FRCS, FRCPS, FASCRS
Associate Professor of Colorectal Surgery

Royal Melbourne Hospital
University of Melbourne
Suites 15 & 16, Private Medical Centre
Royal Parade, Parkville
Victoria 3050
Australia

Quah Hak Mien
MB ChB, MRCS (Ed), MMed (Surgery)
Registrar
Department of Colorectal Surgery
Singapore General Hospital
Outram Road
Singapore 169608
E-mail: quah.hak.mien@singhealth.com.sg

Contents

CHAPTER 1

Anatomical Insights into Common Anal Diseases

F Seow-Choen

Introduction

Anatomy is the basis upon which all surgical art is built. Without an appreciation of normal anatomy, surgery is but another form of butchery. The pathoanatomy of surgical disease, therefore, must be clearly understood if proper diagnosis and therapy are to be arrived at.[1–4] Nonetheless, despite the learning of anatomy in both the undergraduate and postgraduate curricula, too much surgery is being performed without clear anatomical insight, resulting in excessive morbidity and non-healing.

In this paper, the anatomical basis of several important perianal conditions is discussed. It is hoped that this will result in better care of such afflicted patients.

Anatomy of the Anal Canal

The perianal surgeon must possess a skilled and well-trained finger for accurate perianal examination and diagnosis. The anal canal is formed by the embryonic fusion of the hind gut tube with the invaginating procto-derm. This line of fusion of endoderm with proctoderm is represented by the dentate line with a varying zone of transitional cell epithelium. The anal canal between the dentate line and the anal verge is non-hair-bearing squa-mous cell epithelium and is richly supplied by nerve endings and fibres. It is therefore capable of sensing heat and cold as well as somatic pain. The haemorrhoidal plexuses lie within the submucosal and subepidermal plane below this. At the level of the anorectal junction lies the internal haemorrhoidal plexus within this submucosal plane. This internal haem-orrhoidal plexus, otherwise known as anal cushions, is present from early embryonic life. There are usually three columns but only about 29% are present at the classical 3, 7 and 11 o'clock positions. The internal haemor-rhoidal plexus is made up of arteriovenous "erectile" channels capable of swelling in response to parasympathetic stimulation. The external haem-orrhoidal plexus is a venous plexus situated circumferentially around the anal verge and draining the latter within the subepidermal layer. Deep to the haemorrhoidal plexuses and subepithelial layer lie the internal anal sphincters.

The circular internal anal sphincters are traversed by the longitudinal fibres of the internal anal sphincter. Fibres of the latter perforate the for-mer to insert into the dentate line as the suspensory ligaments of Parks at the dentate line. Other fibres penetrate the external anal sphincter as the corrugator ani to insert into the perianal skin. Between the longitu-dinal internal anal sphincter and the external anal sphincter is a potential space. The external anal sphincter complex is a complex group of muscles. Superiorly, the puborectalis and levator ani lie at the level of the anorectal junction. Inferior to this lie the deep, superficial and subcutaneous external anal sphincters respectively. External to the external anal sphincter lies the ischiorectal fossa filled with fat and traversing nerves and vessels.

At the level of the dentate line is a series of crypts. From the crypts arise the anal glands. Recent work due in the department showed that there are 6 (range 3–10) glands in each anus.[1,3] Eighty per cent of these are submucosal and are of no surgical importance. Only 20% of anal glands penetrate the anal sphincters to any degree at all.

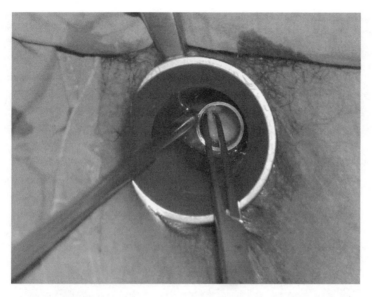

Figure 1. The right technique for rubber band ligation draws rectal mucosa and the haemorrhoidal plexus above the dentate line back into the anal canal.

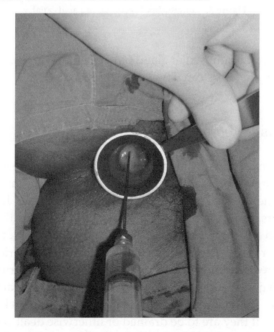

Figure 2. Sclerosing agents must be injected above the dentate line to avoid the severe pain of a subcutaneous injection.

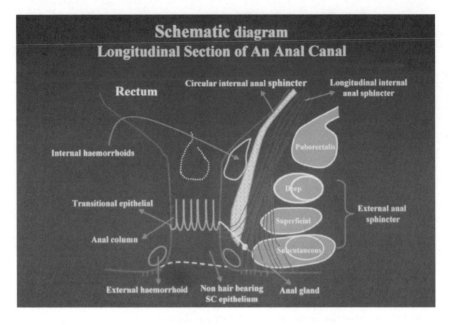

Figure 3. Longitudinal section of an anal canal.

Furthermore, intramuscular glands are only found in 60% of all patients. Not all persons therefore can develop anal sepsis.

Anal Sepsis

A sound understanding of the perianal anatomy is a necessary prerequisite before a surgeon can understand perianal sepsis. A primary anal fistula passes from the external opening to the internal opening. In such a situation, an intersphincteric track normally opens very near the anal verge, usually within a few centimetres. The transphincteric track tends to open slightly further away. Suprasphincteric and extrasphincteric tracks open more than three centimetres away generally. Goodsall's rule also holds good in the majority of cases. Secondary tracks are blind extensions of the primary track. The anatomy of such tracks has to be accurately appreciated by the surgeon if they are to be drained or otherwise dealt with appropriately. Tracks are most often felt as a rock-hard asymmetry within the anal canal.

The skilled perianal surgeon must also be able to assess the amount of anal sphincters to divide or to save, as maintenance of anal continence is an important aspect of fistula surgery. Accuracy of such an assessment is critical, especially in patients with previous anal surgery and where sphincter function is suboptimal due to scarring, neuropathy or injury.

Haemorrhoids

The thrombosed perianal haematoma is exactly that and is a thrombus occurring at the external haemorrhoidal plexus. Such an occurrence is easily treated by an incision and drainage under local bupivacaine/lignocaine infiltration, with immediate relief. The internal haemorrhoidal plexus, on the other hand, may cause symptoms by displacement of engorged anal cushions due to fragmentation of the subepithelial connective tissues.[4] Increasing severity of prolapse leads to an increasingly severe degree of haemorrhoidal prolapse. The internal haemorrhoidal plexus is held in place by surrounding supporting tissues and suspensory ligaments. Early incomplete breakage of some of these ligaments allows the haemorrhoids to prolapse on defecation. Following stoppage of the defecating force, elastic tissues recoil, pulling the haemorrhoids back into the anal canal. A more complete disruption of these supporting tissues causes more permanent haemorrhoidal prolapse. Further shearing force following this will drag perianal skin with it, forming skin tags. The arteriovenous nature of internal haemorrhoids is evidenced by the fact that more than 90% of haemorrhoidal bleeding is bright red and spurting or dripping in nature.

The treatment of fourth and severe third degree piles may involve surgical ablation. However, a lesser degree of prolapse may be efficaciously treated by methods which draw the prolapse back into the anal canal as well as decreasing the amount of vascular distension. Such therapy may include venotonic agents like Daflon 500, sclerotherapy, rubber band ligation, infrared photocoagulation as well as toilet retraining. Ligation and sclerotherapy should therefore not be aimed at the prolapsed aspect of the piles. These latter therapies should be applied superiorly to the excess tissue at the anorectal ring, seeking to ultimately pull the prolapse back to its original place as healing occurs. The most current method of haemorrhoidectomy using PPH-01 (Ethicon Endosurgery, Cincinnati, Ohio, USA) is also based on a correction of this pathology, unlike more conventional haemorrhoidectomy methods.[4]

Idiopathic Anal Fissure

Idiopathic anal fissure is a common cause of anal pain. The pain is often described as tearing and lasts throughout defecation to minutes or hours after the bowel movement is over. This is understandable as the fissure typically occurs in the midline of the sensitive anoderm.

What was confusing in the past was why anal fissure occurred in the anal midline and why it healed following lateral sphincterotomy. A post-mortem angiographic study has shown that the terminal branches of the inferior rectal artery decussate in the midline and this connection is especially tenuous in the posterior midline.[2] Spasm of the internal anal sphincter will hence stop blood flow, resulting in an ischaemic anal fissure or ulcer. Lateral sphincterotomy performed correctly will relax the internal anal sphincter and re-establish anodermal blood flow, with fissure healing resulting.

References

1. Seow Choen F and Ho JMS. New insights into anal glands, *Dis Colon Rectum* 1994; 37: 24.
2. Schouten WR, Briel JW, Anwerda JJA and De Graaf EJR. Ischaemic nature of anal fissure, *Br J Surg* 1996; 83: 63–5.
3. Seow Choen F and Jean Ho. Histoanatomy of the anal glands, *Dis Colon Rectum* 1994; 37: 1315–18.
4. Seow Choen F. Surgery for haemorrhoids: ablation or correction, *Asian J Surg* 2002; 25: 265–6.

CHAPTER 2

The Art of Proctoscopy

F Seow-Choen

Introduction

Surgery is as much art as science. In both art and science, tools of the trade are essential for getting the job done. Indeed, although a poor workman may blame his tools, without the right tools no great work can be accomplished. The proctoscope is to the proctologist what the paintbrush is to the painter, the guitar to the guitarist or the piano to the pianist. Without such exact tools, no great artist can show his skill. The great pianist cannot make music or show his skill to any extent with an inferior-grade or untuned piano. However, the proctologist more often than not has no idea what proctoscope he will be given to use and, worse, he often does not even know the differences between the various proctoscopes. Of necessity, foremost is the fact that the proctoscopic obturator must be close-setting and have a smooth rounded end for easy insertion during use.

Types of Proctoscopes

The proctoscope (or anoscope in the USA) comes in various diameters, lengths and "ends". Disposable proctoscopes are ideal as far as infection prevention is concerned but proper sterilization of used scopes should be effective in preventing cross-contamination in all cases. Self-illuminating proctoscopes using wall electricity are not as commonly used but are excellent if available. Battery-powered illuminated proctoscopes need very regular maintenance and change of batteries. I find that a good wall-mounted angle-poise lamp is sufficient to provide visual clarity for proctoscopy. The proctoscopic handle should be obtuse to the scope as right-angled handles may be obstructive to the proper use of the instrument.

However, the most important differentiating features in modern proctoscopes are the length, bore and "ends".

Proctoscopic lengths vary from 50 to 100 mm. The anal canal and pathology that are treatable or identifiable via the proctoscope are located up to about 5 cm from the anal verge. Therefore, proctoscopic lengths should be about 5–7 cm and no longer. Shorter proctoscopes may be frustrating to use if the anal canal is long. If a lesion deeper in the rectum is present, it is better to proceed to sigmoidoscopy; hence a long proctoscope does not serve any routine purpose.

The proctoscopic bore also varies from instrument to instrument and ranges from 10 to 30 mm in diameter. Extremely wide bore ones are very useful for specialized surgical work but are not acceptable for routine office use. Small bore ones may seem beneficial for patient comfort but may hinder proper proctoscopic therapy. The most suitable for routine use appear to be those with a bore of 20–30 mm. Split-sided or split-tipped proctoscopes as well as bevel-ended proctoscopes are the most useful for routine use, as they enable proctoscopic therapy to be carried out efficaciously. Straight-ended proctoscopes are useless for therapy and diagnosis, and should not be used. Bevel-ended proctoscopes like the Graeme Anderson proctoscope allow one aspect of the anorectal wall to be carefully inspected and treated at one time. A straight-ended proctoscope like the Kelly proctoscope either looks into empty space of the rectum or else the entire wall of the anus (plus the three haemorrhoidal masses) obstructs the view entirely, hence precluding proper examination and therapy.

The best proctoscopes for routine use are the ones which have a bore of about 20–30 mm, a length of about 5 cm and an angled end.

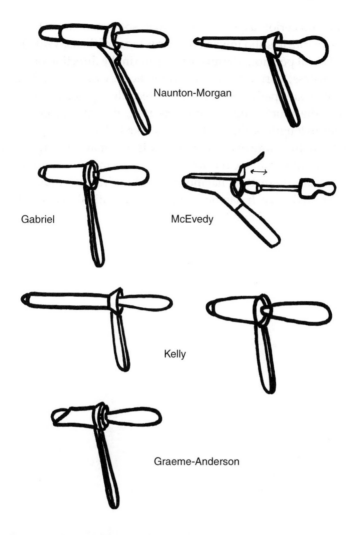

Naunton-Morgan

Gabriel

McEvedy

Kelly

Graeme-Anderson

Conducting a Proctoscopic Examination

Instruments and medication for therapy of haemorrhoids, biopsy, etc should be routinely available before proctoscopy, to prevent the repeated insertion of the proctoscopy if an additional proctoscopic procedure is needed, e.g. rubber band ligation. An assistant must be available to help with instrumentation or to fetch additional instruments or medications.

Adequate lubrication of the proctoscope is necessary before insertion. The proctoscope should be pressed firmly but gently with its obturator against the posterior aspect of the anal sphincters to relax the anal sphincters, before it is slid inwards towards the umbilicus. With the patient in the left lateral position, the anal canal runs in the direction of the umbilicus. Nonetheless, a prior per rectal examination is essential for determining this as well as any pathology that may preclude a proctoscopic examination. Once the proctoscope is fully inserted, the introducer is removed and the entire length of the anal canal is noted. Making a special note of abnormal structures and of the dentate line is essential. The procedure to be performed should be above the dentate line, as skin below this is extremely sensitive to pain. In treating haemorrhoids, the Graeme-Anderson proctoscope is directed at each haemorrhoid in turn, until all haemorrhoids are appropriately assessed and treated.

CHAPTER 3

Aetiology of Anal Fistulas

F Seow-Choen

Introduction

Anal sepsis may cause considerable discomfort and disability, especially in economically active adults in the third to fifth decades of life. Nonetheless, although anorectal sepsis has been recognized for thousands of years, the treatment of difficult or recurrent anal sepsis and fistula continues to challenge surgeons.[1] The relation of anal sepsis to fistula has been discussed by this author previously, but the aetiology of anal sepsis and fistula still remains relatively unknown.[2]

Aetiology of Anal Sepsis

Anal glands

Anal intramuscular glands were first reported as a cause of anal abscess and fistula in 1880.[3,4] This was forgotten until 1929, when anal glands were again blamed for anal sepsis.[5] The usual surgical opinion of that time blamed anal cryptitis as the principal cause of anal fistula.[6] However, microscopic examination of more than 400 anal specimens showed that anal sepsis originated in anal ducts which opened into crypts and which allowed a ready path for infection to ascend from the intestinal lumen into the wall of the anal canal.[5] They showed without exception that the pathological process was confined to anal ducts and not to the crypts of Morgagni.[7]

There are two types of anal glands arising from the lower part of the rectal sinuses or crypts of Morgagni.[8] Submucosal glands are the commonest (80%) and lie completely within the submucosa. About 20% are intramuscular glands which pierce the muscular layers of the anal canal. There are usually six to eight of these glands in the anus. However, these intramuscular glands are found in only 60% of all patients.[7] Of the intramuscular anal glands, 41% reach the circular internal sphincter only, 41% penetrate the longitudinal internal sphincter only, 12% lie within the intersphincteric space and only 6% penetrate the external anal sphincter. These anal glands are lined by stratified columnar epithelium capable of secreting mucus and are often surrounded by a small to moderate amount of lymphoid tissue. India ink injected into the anal ducts passes readily into lymphatic vessels, suggesting that ascending infection from the anal canal may also follow a similar path easily.

When infection occurs in a submucous gland, it forms a small abscess which rapidly bursts into the anal canal to heal spontaneously. When glands deep to muscles become infected, however, the muscle acts as a barrier and prevents the abscess from rupturing into the lumen. Pus, however, may spread in other directions, following the paths of least resistance. Cystic dilation of anal glands may occur first and infection sets in later as a secondary phenomenon in a dilated mucus-filled cavity.

There are quite wide individual variations in the number, depth and shape of anal glands, and this variation has been postulated as the reason for the individual susceptibility to anorectal sepsis.[8] Only people with susceptible glands can develop an anal fistula of cryptoglandular origin.

Apocrine gland infection

Apocrine glands can cause perianal abscesses which can grow skin-associated micro-organism sepsis. These have also been blamed as the causative factor in 30% of patients with anal abscesses.[9] However, such infection does not have a demonstrable internal fistulous opening. Only abscesses with a demonstrable internal opening are due to glandular infection.

Breach of anal mucosa

Enterogeneous organisms have been thought to cause infection by invading the submucosal space by ulceration, injury, faecal abrasion or "pure" penetration. The anal mucosa is especially susceptible to faecal trauma, because the anal lining is inelastic and rigid and tethered to the underlying tissues. Ingested sharp foreign objects may perforate the anal sphincters and result in anal abscess.[10]

Anal mucosal breaches, however, cannot be the commonest cause of anal sepsis, as minor anal surgery, including haemorrhoidectomy, does not always result in anal sepsis or fistula.

Longitudinal layer of the internal anal sphincter

Another theory postulates that infection spreads from the anal canal into perianorectal tissue to form abscesses and fistulas by tracking along the fibres of the longitudinal anal muscle which transverses the internal and external anal sphincters. This may explain how an ischiorectal abscess may track along the fibres of the longitudinal muscle in between fasciculi of both the external and internal sphincters to burst into the anal canal. Intermuscular abscess may result by infection spreading along the main portion of the longitudinal muscle. This abscess may then enter the anal canal at any level by extending through the internal sphincter along a fasciculus of the longitudinal muscle.

The central space

Shafik described the central space as the seat of all anal sepsis and fistulas.[11] Shafik's central space lies circumferentially around the lower part of the anal canal bounded superiorly by the termination of the longitudinal muscle and inferiorly by the lowermost loop of the external sphincter. The central space is occupied by the central tendon of the longitudinal muscle. The central tendon was described as giving rise to multiple fibres medially, laterally and inferiorly. The central space therefore communicates with the submucous space medially, the ischiorectal space laterally, the subcutaneous space inferiorly and the intersphincteric and pelvirectal spaces superiorly. Infection within the central space may therefore spread in various directions along the septa of the central tendon. Dissemination of infection was said to be caused by repeated contraction of the anal musculature.

Perivascular space

Another theory describes infection reaching the poorly vascularized fatty areas of the ischiorectal triangle by following the perivascular spaces. This has been said to explain the "constant" location of the internal openings of anal fistulae at 5 or 7 o'clock.[12] Dissemination of sepsis via the longitudinal muscle or perivascular spaces was evoked to explain the origin of the more complicated suppurative disease and fistulas as their existence cannot be explained fully by the cryptoglandular theory.

Submucosal epithelial debris

Sequested embryonic debris in the subanoderm has been held responsible for the perpetuation of anal sepsis and fistula.[10] In this view, anal glands are actually developmental vestiges remaining from embryonic fusion of the proctoderm with the hindgut. This epithelial debris is buried in the anal submucosa and acts as sequestra that harbour and maintain infection. However, the constant occurrence of anal crypts and anal intramuscular glands contradicts this epithelial debris theory. Anal developmental vestiges are not the cause of anal sepsis.

Bacterial colonization

An anal fistula might reasonably be induced or perpetuated by the chronic presence of large numbers or virulent strains of micro-organisms. However, although pus from anorectal abscesses contains very large numbers of organisms, chronic anal fistulas contain very much smaller numbers of micro-organisms. An excess number of micro-organisms was not found in anal fistulas and bacteria could only be grown from enriched bacteria cultures in one study.[13] Furthermore, specially virulent organisms were not found in chronic fistulas and bacteria culture was of normal commensals of the lower gastrointestinal tract. Chronicity of anal fistulas is not linked either to excessive numbers of organisms or to organisms of an unusual type or virulence.

Animal fistula

McColl[14] dissected the ani of 80 animals of 20 different species and concluded that only animals with anal intramuscular glands can develop anal fistulas; dogs have anal intramuscular glands and develop anal fistulas, whereas cats do not have anal intramuscular glands and do not suffer from anal fistulas. Middle-aged German shepherds and Irish setters are particularly prone to anal fistulas compared to other breeds of dogs.

Gender

The question why there is a difference in the incidence of anal sepsis and fistula between the sexes may be important in helping to elucidate the aetiology of anal suppurative disease. Certainly, in the adult population, anal fistula and sepsis occur two to seven times as commonly in males as in females.[1] Sex hormones have been investigated but do not seem to be involved in the causation of anal sepsis or fistula.

Other aetiological factors

Specific causes of anal sepsis and fistula, such as pelvic or intra-abdominal sepsis, fungal infection, mycobacterium infection, Crohn's disease and cancer, are not uncommon but are not related to idiopathic cryptoglandular sepsis.

A Personal View

This author believes that the available evidence shows that the initial event in the pathogenesis of anal sepsis and fistula begins in the anal gland and ducts. Ducts of anal glands are initially blocked by excessively viscid secretions which may be related to an abnormal function of the sex hormones. Cystic dilatation of the anal intramuscular glands occurs and accumulates within the dilating anal intramuscular gland. The dilated gland is prone then to infection arising from ascending bacterial infection via the anal ducts which open at the lower parts of the anal crypts of Morgagni. An intramuscular glandular abscess forms. The infection may then track in several directions, following the fibres of the longitudinal layer of the internal anal sphincter. Chronic nonspecific anal fistulas, therefore, are always the consequence of an intramuscular anal gland abscess. A primary anal abscess is defined as the anal abscess that occurs in a patient who has not had any previous episode of an anal abscess or fistula. Patients with an anal abscess or fistula who have undergone previous surgery for anal sepsis or fistula are more prone to recurrence compared to patients who never had a previous episode of anorectal sepsis.[15] This is because the natural barrier to infective complications is destroyed and the presence of a chronic internal opening into the anorectum may perpetuate chronic inflammation and persistence of the septic process.

Do acute primary anal abscesses treated by incision and drainage lead invariably to chronic anal fistulas? A permanent cure for an acute anal abscess was believed to be possible only when the offending anal gland was excised and the internal opening or the related anal duct laid open in addition to simple drainage of the abscess alone. But does this dogma hold good in actual practice?

About two-thirds of all patients with anal abscesses do not have demonstrable internal openings during examination for drainage of the abscess.[15] Although it is possible that the low incidence of demonstrable internal openings may be due in some series to the tyro being afraid to probe deep cavities, it is equally plausible that the experienced surgeon may too readily diagnose internal openings by enthusiastic probing.

No reasonable explanation has yet been offered for the formation of an internal opening during the course of an intersphincteric abscess. The pathogenetic mechanisms are especially puzzling where chronic anal fistulas with external openings are concerned, as back pressure and pus bursting back through the internal sphincter to form the internal opening cannot be acceptable theoretically, since the path of least resistance must be through the external opening.

Conclusion

Idiopathic chronic anal fistulas are always the result of an intramuscular anal gland abscess. But an acute intramuscular anal gland abscess, especially a primary abscess, does not lead inevitably to a chronic anal fistula or to a recurrent anal abscess. The initial treatment of an anal abscess should consist of simple but thorough drainage of pus under adequate anaesthesia.

References

1. Seow-Choen F and Nicholls RJ. Anal fistula, *Br J Surg* 1992; 79: 197–205.
2. Seow-Choen F. Relation of abscess to fistula in anal fistula. Phillips RK and Lunnis PJ (eds.), Chapman & Hall, 1996.
3. Chiari H. *Uber die Naten Divertikelder Recttumschleimhaut und ihre Beziehung zu den Anal fisteln, Med Jahrbucher Wien* 1880; 8: 419–27.
4. Herrmann G and Desfossess L. *Sur la muquese de la region cloacale du rectum, Comptes Rend Acad Sci (III)* 1880; 90: 1301–2.
5. Lockhart-Mummery JP. Discussion on fistula-in-ano, *Proc R Soc Med* 1929; 22: 1331–41.
6. Rankin FW, Bergen JA and Buie LA. The colon, rectum and anus. Philadelphia, WB Saunders, 1932.
7. Tucker CC and Hellwig CA. Histopathology of anal glands, *Surg Gynecol Obstet* 1933; 58: 145–9.
8. Seow-Choen F and Ho JMS. Recent insights into anal glands, *Dis Colon Rectum* 1994; 37: 24.
9. Grace RH, Harper IA and Thompson RG. Anorectal sepsis; microbiology in relation to fistula-in-ano, *Br J Surg* 1982; 69: 401–3.
10. Seow-Choen F, Leong AFPK and Goh HS. Acute anal pain due to ingested bone, *Int J Colorectal Dis* 1991; 6: 21–3.
11. Shafik A. A new concept of the anatomy of the anal sphincter mechanism and physiology of defecation. VI. The central abscess: a new clinopathological entity in the genesis of anorectal suppuration, *Dis Colon Rectum* 1979; 22: 336–41.
12. Hiller RJ. The anal sphincter and the pathogenesis of anal fissure and fistula, *Surg Gynecol Obstet* 1931; 52: 921–40.
13. Seow-Choen F, Hay AJ, Heard S and Phillips RKS. Bacteriology of anal fistula, *Br J Surg* 1992; 79: 27–8.
14. McColl I. The comparative anatomy and pathology of anal glands, *Ann R Coll Surg Engl* 1967; 40: 36–67.
15. Seow-Choen F, Leong AFPK and Goh HS. Results of a policy of selective immediate fistulotomy for primary anal abscess, *Aust NZJ Surg* 1993; 63: 485–9.

Management of Anal Sepsis

F Seow-Choen

Introduction

Although much has been written about anal fistulas,[1] a great deal remains uncertain and controversial and the ailment continues to be troublesome to both surgeons and patients. This review deals with some of those issues and is limited to idiopathic or nonspecific anal fistulas and abscesses.

Epidemiology of Anal Fistulas

The majority of studies of anal fistulas involve small groups of selected patients. The male–female ratio varies from 2 : 1 to 7 : 1.[1] The age distribution is spread throughout adult life, with the maximal incidence between the third and fifth decades. The incidence for men is about 12.3 per 100 000, and that for women, 5.6 per 100 000.[2]

Classification of Anal Fistulas

Accurate and meaningful description of complex fistulas is difficult. Many systems of classification have been used throughout the world: most are complex, and impractical for routine clinical use. The most widely used system is probably that of Parks *et al.*,[3] and subsequent discussion will be based on this system.

Parks *et al.*[3] related their system both to the cryptoglandular origin of the fistula and to the anal sphincters and levator ani. Superficial fistulas were not included in their classification as these were considered to be of different aetiological origin. They divided anal fistulas into four major groups:

1. Intersphincteric fistulas were subdivided into: simple; with high blind track; with high track opening into the rectum; without a perineal opening; with pelvic extension; those due to pelvic disease.
2. Trans-sphincteric fistulas have tracks that may penetrate the external sphincter at varying levels, i.e. high or low, and could be subdivided into: uncomplicated; those with a high blind track.
3. Suprasphincteric fistulas pass upwards in the intersphincteric plane to loop over the top of the puborectalis and emerge through the levator ani to reach the skin.
4. The fourth group consists of the extrasphincteric fistulas.

Fistulas are classified according to the course taken by the main or primary track, which is the track linking the internal and external openings. Secondary tracks are defined by qualifying the primary tracks, e.g. a trans-sphincteric track with a supralevator extension. The term "secondary track" or "extension" is usually used for important extensions from the main or primary tracks. An important type of secondary track is that due to circumferential spread or horseshoeing; it takes place mainly in the intersphincteric, ischiorectal or supralevator planes.

Evaluation of Anal Fistulas

Accurate preoperative delineation of the anatomy of an anal fistula is important if recurrence or incontinence after operation is to be avoided. The five essential points to be obtained from a clinical examination are the location of the internal opening, the external opening, the primary track and the secondary track, and the presence or absence of underlying disease. The external opening is usually obvious, so that the pathoanatomy of most fistulas can be delineated clinically by locating the internal orifice and defining the presence and type of secondary extension. Poor resting tone before operation and poor voluntary anal contraction respectively indicate an already compromised internal or external anal sphincter function, and mean that conservative surgery may be necessary to avoid anal incontinence.

Systematic and careful examination is important and will give the clinician useful data about the pathoanatomy of the fistula. Intersphincteric tracks tend to open externally close to the anal verge, while transsphincteric and more complicated fistulas tend to open further away. The major problem is in locating the internal opening. Edward[4] was the first to point out what has now come to be known as Goodsall's rule. He stated in 1887 that fistulas which have their external opening behind a plane passing transversely through the centre of the anus usually have their internal aperture in the midline posteriorly, while those with an external orifice anterior to this plane have their internal opening immediately opposite.

Internal openings may be felt as indurated nodules or pits leading to an indurated track, or they may be seen to exude pus when the tracks or abscesses are gently massaged. Fibrosis is a frequent pointer to the site. Gentle use of probes along the dentate line or through the external opening may be useful in locating internal openings. Besides the use of probes, intraoperative injection of methylene blue, saline or other solutions has been advocated. The injection of 0.5–2 ml of hydrogen peroxide through the track may help locate the internal orifice by producing a stream of white bubbles at the latter site. If the internal opening cannot be found but the probe tip is in the immediate vicinity of the dentate line, a direct association may be presumed. When the internal opening cannot be found and the probe tip is remote from the dentate line, it is probably safer to leave the search to another day. Intraoperative traction on the external opening or track may sometimes show a dimple at the site of the internal opening. Granulation tissue that will not curette away is a helpful marker of and guide to the presence of secondary tracks.

Fistulography may be advantageous in some patients with recurrent fistulas.[5] More recently, anal endosonography has been shown to be useful in the evaluation of an anal fistulous abscess.[6]

Secondary tracks are often diagnosed when induration or asymmetry between the right and left sides of the anorectum is palpated. Careful bidigital palpation will also define the relationship of the track to the anal sphincters and levators, and help determine the correct surgical technique. Sigmoidoscopy should be performed as part of the clinical routine to uncover associated underlying pathology. Barium enema or colonoscopy, however, need not be routinely carried out as their diagnostic yield is low in relation to anal fistulas; they should be performed only when specially indicated. In selected cases (e.g. women with suspected previous obstetric trauma, patients with multiple previous laying open of anal fistulas, the very elderly, or patients with a high fistula), preoperative anal manometry may be useful in helping the surgeon to decide which surgical technique should be employed to prevent postoperative incontinence.

Acute Anorectal Abscess

The term "fistulous abscess" was introduced in 1954 to stress that anal abscesses and fistulas are parts of a spectrum of the same disease process.[7] Traditionally, an anorectal abscess has been treated by drainage, via either a stab incision or sucerization. With the wide acceptance of the cryptoglandular aetiology of anal suppuration, primary or delayed fistulotomy with excision of the offending anal gland has been advocated.[8] An anorectal abscess is said to be cured permanently only when crypts and ducts are removed in addition to providing adequate drainage.

Complicated Forms of Anorectal Fistulous Abscess

Three factors in complicated fistulae tend to perpetuate the disease process: first, the presence of a disease focus within the anal intramuscular gland or elsewhere within the anal canal; second, the constant contamination resulting from a high intrarectal pressure forcing intraluminal contents through the internal opening; and third, repeated surgery, which may create complicated tracks if not performed correctly. Complicated anorectal fistulous abscesses include supralevator abscesses and intralevator horseshoe extensions. Although complicated fistulous abscesses are viewed with anxiety by many nonspecialist surgeons, proper treatment should result in a low recurrence rate. Incision and drainage of primary fistulotomy may be used for the primary fistulous abscess.[9–12] Setons can be used whenever laying open might interfere with anal continence. Secondary extensions may be drained by counter-incision, complete laying open, insertion drained of various types of surgical drains, or by setons. Generous skin incisions are helpful during surgery, and skin conservation although well-meaning, may delay discovery of secondary tracks and hinder drainage and healing. Defunctioning colostomy may be required occasionally, either because adequate fistulotomy will cause anal incontinence or because of severe anal sepsis.

Sometimes patients with problematic fistulae after multiple operations may prefer a permanent colostomy. Indeed, some patients may require proctectomy because of chronic disability if all else fails.

Massive Anorectal Suppuration

An anorectal abscess can precipitate extensive and severe infection, which may lead to death, especially in the obese diabetic. Surgeons must be especially careful when treating diabetics with anorectal suppuration. These patients may be septic or moribund on presentation or they may rapidly become so if not adequately treated. Spreading soft tissue infection of the perineum can be classified broadly into two groups. The first group includes anorectal sepsis wherein the infection extends superficially around the perineum, causing necrosis of the skin, subcutaneous tissue, fascia or muscle. Affected patients may be recognized by perianal crepitation, erythematous indurate perianal skin, blistering or gangrene. The second group includes sepsis wherein the preperitoneal or retroperitoneal spaces are also involved. Affected patients may have quite subtle signs, such as abdominal wall induration, tenderness or a vague mass. Plain abdominal radiographs may show soft tissue gas in both groups, and leucocytosis with a marked shift to the left may also be present in both. These two groups of patients require radical debridement of infected or necrotic tissue, and the latter group may require laparotomy if intra-abdominal sepsis is suspected. The use of a defunctioning colostomy alone is neither curative nor palliative; it is grossly inadequate and may expose the already compromised patient to an insurmountable bacterial load.

Broad-spectrum antibiotics should always be used while awaiting sensitivity results. Mixed pathogens are usually grown, including gram-negative aerobes such as *Escherichia coli* and gram-negative anaerobes such as *Bacteroides fragilis*.

Common gas-forming organisms include clostridial species and anaerobic gram-positive organisms such as *Peptococcus* and *Peptostreptococcus*.

Chronic Anal Fistulas

Approximately 85–95% of all anal fistulas are easy to treat. Superficial, intersphincteric and low trans-sphincteric fistulas are readily managed either by classical laying open (fistulotomy) or by excision (fistulotomy), with a low recurrence rate and with minimal risk of postoperative incontinence. The 5–15% of anal fistulas that are difficult to manage must be dealt with differently.

Setons in the Management of Difficult Fistulas

The use of setons in the treatment of anal fistulas is not new. Setons may be used in patients with complex fistulas, high fistulas, or difficult fistulas where the landmarks have been so distorted that continence cannot be guaranteed if fistulotomy is performed (or if the surgeon opts to be cautious). They may be used in several ways. First, they may be applied loosely when used as drains, or as a stimulant to fibrosis around the track, or as markers to enable better postoperative assessment by outlining the track. Secondly, they may be applied tightly if the intention is to cut slowly through the track.

When used to promote fibrosis, setons act by holding the muscle ends together, thereby preventing separation of the anal sphincter muscle when fistulotomy is performed.

Seton material may be any type of foreign substances, which can be inserted through the fistula track. Ayurvedic treatment of fistulae in ano using the insertion of a thread impregnated with a caustic solution to destroy the fistula track and therefore performing chemical fistulotomy does not appear to be as promising as it was originally made out to be.[13]

Closure of the Internal Opening in the Management of Chronic High Fistulas

High anal fistulas may sometimes be treated using the rectal mucosal advancement flap technique. The advantages include a reduction in the duration of the healing, no additional damage to the anal sphincter, no risk of deformity to the anal canal, and it is a one-stage procedure if primary healing is achieved. The technique involves a total fistulectomy or coring out of the primary and secondary tracks, excision of the internal opening, and closure of the rectal defect with a mucosal advancement. The mucosal suture line must be at a different level from the muscular suture line, as disruption of the latter is common. Although called a "mucosal" flap, the raised flap should include at least partial thickness of the rectal wall for added strength. The width of the proximally placed flap base should be at least twice as long as the widths of the apex, to ensure an adequate blood supply. A more cautious approach uses at least half the circumference of the rectal wall in forming the flap to reduce necrosis.

Defunctioning colostomy or ileostomy is not a necessary prerequisite in the mucosal advancement flap technique.

Other Techniques for Difficult Anal Fistulas

Polymethylmethacrylate copolymer beads have been used to prevent post-operative infection and enhance rapid wound healing after high fistulotomy and primary wound closure.

Conclusion

An anal fistula is a common cause of chronic irritation. A good appreciation of normal anorectal anatomy and fistula pathoanatomy, as well as a wide and practical knowledge of the possible treatment regimens, may decrease treatment failure rates.

References

1. Seow-Choen F and Nicholls RJ. Anal fistula, *Br J Surg* 1992; 79: 197–205.
2. Sainio P. Fistula-in-ano in a defined population: incidence and epidemiological aspects, *Ann Chir Gynaecol* 1984; 73: 219–24.
3. Parks AG, Gordon PH and Hardcastle JD. A classification of fistula-in-ano, *Br J Surg* 1976; 63: 1–12.

4. Edward S. On some of the rarer forms of rectal fistulae, *Lancet* 1887; i: 1089.

5. Weisman RI, Orsay CP, Pearl RK and Abcarian H. The role of fistulography in fistula-in-ano, *Dis Colon Rectum* 1991; 34: 181–4.

6. Law PJ, Talbot RW, Bartram CI and Northover JMA. Anal endosonography in the evaluation of perianal sepsis and fistula-in-ano, *Br J Surg* 1989; 76: 752–5.

7. Eisenhammer S. Advances in anorectal surgery with special reference to amulatory treatment, *S Afr Med J* 1954; 28: 264.

8. Seow-Choen F. Relation of abscess to fistula in anal fistula. Phillips RKS and Lunnis PI (eds.), Chapman and Hall, 1996.

9. Seow-Choen F, Leong AFPK and Goh HS. Result of a policy of selective immediate fistulotomy for primary anal abscess, *Aust NZ J Surg* 1993; 63: 485–9.

10. Tang CL, Chew SP and Seow-Choen F. Prospective randomised trial of drainage alone vs drainage and fistulotomy for acute perianal abscesses with proven internal opening, *Dis Colon Rectum* 1996; 39: 1415–17.

11. Seow-Choen F. Fistulotomy in the management of acute anorectal sepsis, *Dis Colon Rectum* 1997; 40: 1130–1.

12. Ho YH, Tan M, Chui C, Leong A, Eu KW and Seow-Choen F. Controlled trial of primary fistulotomy with drainage alone for perianal abscesses, *Dis Colon Rectum* 1997; 40: 1435–38.

13. Ho KS, Tsang C, Seow-Choen F, Ho YH, Tang CL, Heah SM and Eu KW. Prospective randomized trial comparing ayurvedic cutting seton and fistulotomy for low fistula-in-ano, *Tech Coloproct* 2001; 5: 137–41.

CHAPTER 5

Chronic Anal Fissure

JF Lim

Introduction

An anal fissure is a common complaint commonly affecting healthy young adults and makes up about 10% of new referrals to our colorectal clinic. The majority of patients have acute fissures which respond well to local and oral painkillers aided by increased dietary fibre. They classically present with anal pain which begins during defecation and lasts from a few minutes to a few hours after that. This may be associated with a modest amount of fresh rectal blood. Patients usually give a history of abnormal bowel habits which may be constipatory or diarrhoea-like. If there is concurrent haemorrhoidal disease (which is common), the blood loss may be more significant.

However, some of these patients present with chronic fissures. Strictly speaking, chronic fissures are defined as those which do not heal within six weeks despite adequate medical treatment.[1,2] Personally, patients who have signs of chronicity on examination but symptoms for less than six weeks should be classified as having chronic fissures, because these anatomical changes could not have happened over such a short time.

Clinical Findings

Pain may not be the predominant symptom in chronic fissures. Bleeding, which may be from concurrent haemorrhoids, or the presence of a perianal skin tag may be more prominent to the patient. It is important in history taking to document symptoms of the altered bowel habit and defecatory pattern. If there is a suspicion, a proximal colonic lesion should be excluded first.

Abdominal examination is usually not fruitful. The main abnormalities are found during perianal and digital rectal examination. There is usually a skin tag (sentinel pile) overlying the external edge of the fissure. To the untrained, a fissure may be missed if the sentinel pile is not exposed to reveal it. The fissure is usually single, located at either the 6 or 12 o'clock position. The majority are in the 6 o'clock position, with 2.5–10% in the 12 o'clock position.[3,4] If the fissure is multiple in number or abnormally located, the surgeon must be wary of underlying inflammatory bowel disease, tuberculosis, syphilis or HIV infection.

If the pain is minimal, a gentle digital examination and proctoscopy may be done. This will show a fibrotic ulcer with the white, transverse internal sphincter fibres exposed. There may be a hypertrophic papilla at the internal edge of the fissure. The presence of rectal mucosal prolapse or haemorrhoids is not unusual.

Aetiology

Historically, fissures were thought to be due to passage of a hard bolus of faeces causing a tear of the anal mucosa. However, not all patients report constipation and 4–7% actually report a bout of diarrhoea preceding the symptoms.[5,6] A recent review by Hananel and Gordon[7] showed that only 10% of patients complained of constipation and 30% needed to strain during defecation. Another 10% developed fissures after childbirth. I have found that the majority of my patients admit to an episode or period of altered defecation (either a bout of hard stool evacuation which often entails straining or explosive watery diarrhoea) prior to or during the initial painful presentation. Their bowel habits are otherwise normal.

Internal anal sphincter hypertonia is another theory which partially explains the aetiology. The resting pressure in the anal canal is largely a function of the internal sphincter, which is in a continuous state of partial contraction. This is mediated through α-adrenergic pathways. Relaxation occurs automatically in response to rectal distension (the recto-anal inhibitory reflex). Patients with chronic anal fissures commonly have a raised resting anal pressure from internal anal sphincter hypertonia, the cause of which is unknown.[8] Administration of pharmacological agents to relax the internal sphincter has been shown to lead to fissure healing but the resting anal pressure returns to pretreatment levels once the fissure has healed and treatment stopped.[9] These findings suggested that internal sphincter hypertonia and anal spasm predate the onset of the fissure. However, the anal spasm does not appear to be a response to pain because application of topical local anaesthetics relieves pain but does not reduce the anal spasm.[8,10]

Over the past decade, the theory of local ischaemia has gained credence as a significant event in the aetiology of chronic anal fissures. Klosterhalfen *et al.*[11] showed a paucity of arterioles in the posterior commissure of the anal canal in 85% of cadaveric cases, site of predilection of fissures. Schouten *et al.*[12] measured the microvascular perfusion of the anoderm in patients with chronic anal fissure and controls. They found raised resting anal pressures and reduced anodermal blood flow at the posterior commissure in patients with chronic anal fissures when compared with controls.

Another theory suggests that the weak areas of the anal canal are in the anterior and posterior midline where the external sphincter muscles decussate. During the passage of firm/hard stools, lateral force is distributed anteriorly and posteriorly due to the weakness, leading to a tear in these locations.[13]

Yet another theory suggests that partial eversion of the anal canal during stool evacuation is inhibited anteriorly and posteriorly because the skin is tethered to the sphincter in these locations, leading to more tension and stretch. As a result tearing is most likely in these locations.[14]

Brown *et al.*[15] studied the biopsy specimens of the internal anal sphincter taken from the base of the chronic fissures and at sites remote from it, and found fibrosis in all areas. They postulated an inflammatory process in which myositis occurs early in the condition, with subsequent fibrosis.

Postpartum anal fissures appear to be a separate group, as they are more commonly anterior. The risk is increased in traumatic deliveries. Shearing forces from the passage of the foetal head may be significant, and the tethering of the anal mucosal to the skin is another component which is cited as a possible causative factor. Postpartum patients do not appear to have a raised internal anal sphincter resting pressure but commonly complain of constipation.

As you can see from the multitude of theories presented, the actual cause or causes of chronic anal fissures are still debatable. As in most other medical conditions, the cause in each patient could be different or multifactorial. As such, treatment would require the surgeon to address several issues concurrently to achieve optimal results.

Medical Treatment

Dietary modification is an important step in management. A high-fibre diet with high water intake alone may be sufficient for acute fissures but are still an important component when treating patients with chronic anal fissures. Topical anaesthetic gels like 1% Lignocaine or lubricated anal dilators can be tried in acute fissures but results have been poor, with a high recurrence rate. I prescribe 1% Lignocaine gel for patients with chronic fissures to provide symptomatic relief only.

The recognition of nitric oxide as a neurotransmitter mediating the relaxation of the internal sphincter[16] has led to many studies looking at the use of isosorbide dinitrate (ISDN) and glyceryl trinitrate (GTN) in the treatment of chronic fissures. Different authors have tried oral, patch, sprayed and topical GTN, and 0.2% GTN topical ointment has become the standard as it achieves optimal healing in up to 70% of cases, with minimal side effects (mainly headache).[17,18]

Two recent trials have compared topical GTN to lateral sphincterotomy in treating chronic fissures. Oettle *et al.*[19] randomized 24 patients to either sphincterotomy or 0.2% GTN three times a day. All 12 patients with sphincterotomy healed, whereas 10 of 12 in the GTN group healed. There were no side effects or recurrences in both groups. The 2 who failed on GTN had no pain relief after a week and sphincterotomy led to good healing. The Canadian Colorectal Surgical Trials Group[20] randomized 82 patients to receive either sphincterotomy or 0.25% GTN tds. At 6 weeks, 34 (89.5%) in the sphincterotomy group, compared with 13 (29.5%) in the GTN group, had achieved complete healing. Five of the 13 patients in the GTN group then relapsed. Eleven (28.9%) in the sphincterotomy group and 37 (84%) in the GTN group developed side effects. These contrasting results have not dampened the enthusiasm of surgeons for trying GTN as the first-line treatment for chronic fissures, as one can avoid the theoretical complication of delayed faecal incontinence from sphincterotomy. In Singapore, the manufacturer has withdrawn GTN ointment from the market and we have had to resort to other drugs for medical treatment.

Calcium channel blockers such as nifedipine and diltiazem have been shown to reduce resting anal pressure in patients with chronic fissures.[21,22] Both oral and topical preparations have shown healing in up to 67% of patients. Patients who are already on these drugs for hypertension and ischaemic heart disease are unsuitable for this form of treatment.

Bethanecol (a parasympathomimetic) has been shown to lower resting anal pressure and has been useful usually in conjunction with other topical medications. Indoramin, an α-adrenoceptor blocker, and salbutamol, a β-adrenoceptor agonist, are being studied as alternatives.

Botulinum toxin A (Botox) has been shown to reduce resting anal pressure and healing of anal fissures in up to 96%.[23] The mode of action of the botulinum toxin remains unclear. The toxin binds to presynaptic cholinergic nerve terminals and inhibits the release of acetylcholine at the neuromuscular junction. This will lead to relaxation of the external sphincter but there are no corresponding acetylcholine receptors in the smooth muscle of the internal sphincter. Its action is unlikely to be due purely to its effect on the external sphincter, as Brisinda *et al.*[23] showed that maximal squeeze pressures in patients receiving botulinum toxin were not significantly different from pretreatment levels at one and two months post-injection. The site of optimal injection is still unclear and complications include transient faecal incontinence, perianal haematoma, pain and sepsis.

Surgical Treatment

Anal dilatation, in all its varied manifestations in the literature, should be banned, as it is a form of uncontrolled fracturing of the internal sphincter. While studies have shown good rates of healing, the incidence of incontinence is unacceptably high, with unknown long-term consequences.

Posterior midline sphincterotomy is also shunned nowadays as its results are not superior to lateral sphincterotomy but produce a gutter (keyhole) defect, which leads to soilage.

Patients who have failed medical treatment and patients with physical features of chronicity such as a sentinel pile should be offered lateral sphincterotomy. This can be done either closed or open, with the current literature showing similar results. The current debate is on the length of optimal internal sphincter division.[24,25] Classically, sphincterotomy is done with division of the internal sphincter up to the depth of the dentate line. In tailored sphincterotomy, the sphincter is divided up to the depth of the fissure only. In practice, it is difficult to measure the exact length of division and, therefore, difficult to study and compare the results between the two groups.

There are many variations as to the actual technique of operation, which will not be discussed here. None has been shown to be superior and, therefore, the technique chosen should be tailored to the surgeon and case at hand. Most authors have described healing rates in the range of 85–95% after lateral sphincterotomy.

Recurrent or Atypical Fissures

If a patient presents with an anal fissure which is not in either the anterior or the posterior midline, the surgeon should be wary of concomitant Crohn's disease or any other immunosuppressed conditions, such as Aids. A careful history and physical examination will often elucidate the condition. These patients should not be offered surgery at the first consultation, and anal manometry with anal sphincter mapping (with either endoanal ultrasound or MRI) should be carried out. Still, Fleschner *et al.*[26] showed that in their series, 88% of patients with Crohn's associated fissures healed after lateral sphincterotomy, compared with 49% after medical treatment. No significant increase in complications was noted in the sphincterotomy group.

For patients with recurrence after lateral sphincterotomy, anal manometry and anal sphincter mapping is essential as it separates patients with low resting anal pressures from patients with persistently raised resting pressures who might benefit from a repeat lateral sphincterotomy in the opposite lateral quadrant.

Patients with low resting sphincter pressures should be offered anal advancement flaps with fissurectomy, as it is believed these patients would not have improved blood flow to the fissure even after sphincterotomy as sphincter hypertonia was probably not a causative factor in the first place. As such, further sphincterotomy will only increase the risk of incontinence. Nyam *et al.*[27] and Leong *et al.*[4] have shown that an island advancement flap from the perianal skin healed most fissures.

Summary

Anal fissures are common and their aetiology is multifactorial in most patients. There are many options for chemical sphincterotomy with good results but lateral sphincterotomy remains the gold standard in the treatment of chronic anal fissures.

References

1. Goligher J. Surgery of the anus, rectum and colon. London, Bialliere Tindall.
2. Keighley M and Williams N. Surgery of the anus, rectum and colon. London, WB Saunders.
3. Notaras MJ. Anal fissure and stenosis, *Surg Clin North Am* 1988; 68: 1427.
4. Leong AFPK and Seow-Choen F. Lateral sphincterotomy compared with anal advancement flap for chronic anal fissure, *Dis Colon Rectum* 1995; 38: 69.
5. Lock MR and Thomson JP. Fissure-in-ano; the initial management and prognosis, *Br J Surg* 1977; 64: 355.
6. Mazier WP. Haemorrhoids, fissures and pruritis ani, *Surg Clin North Am* 1994; 74: 1277.
7. Hananel N and Gordon PH. Re-examination of clinical manifestations and response to treatment of fissure-in-ano, *Dis Colon Rectum* 1977; 40: 229.
8. Keck JO *et al.* Computer-generated profiles of the anal canal in patients with anal fissure, *Dis Colon Rectum* 1995; 38: 72.
9. Lund JN, Parsons JL and Scholefield JH. Spasm of the internal anal sphincter in anal fissure—cause or effect? *Gastroenterology* 1996; 110: A711.
10. Minguez M *et al.* Pressure of the anal canal in patients with haemorrhoids or anal fissure, effect of the topical application of an anaesthetic gel, *Rev Esp Enfirm Dig* 1992; 81: 103.
11. Klosterhalfen B *et al.* Topography of the inferior rectal artery: a possible cause of chronic, primary anal fissure, *Dis Colon Rectum* 1989; 32: 43.
12. Schouten WR *et al.* Relationship between anal pressure and anodermal blood flow: the vascular pathogenesis of anal fissures, *Dis Colon Rectum* 1994; 37: 664.

13. Smith LE. Anal fissure, *Neth J Med* 1990; 37: S33.
14. Schouten WR *et al.* Ischaemic nature of anal fissure, *Br J Surg* 1996; 83: 63.
15. Brown AC *et al.* Histopathology of the internal anal sphincter in chronic anal fissure, *Dis Colon Rectum* 1989; 32: 680.
16. Chakder S and Rattan S. Release of nitric oxide by activation of nora-drenergic noncholinergic neurons of internal anal sphincter, *Am J Physiol* 1993; 264: G7.
17. Lund JN and Scholefield JH. A randomized, prospective, double-blind, placebo-controlled trial of glycerin trinitrate ointment in the treatment of anal fissure, *Lancet* 1997; 349: 11.
18. Carapeti EA, Kamm MA *et al.* Randomized controlled trial shows that glyceryl trinitrate heal anal fissures, higher doses are not more effective, and there is a high recurrence rate, *Gut* 1999; 44: 727.
19. Oettle GJ *et al.* Glyceryl trinitrate versus sphincterotomy for treatment of chronic fissure-in-ano: a randomized controlled trial, *Dis Colon Rectum* 1997; 40: 1318.
20. Richard CS *et al.* Internal sphincterotomy is superior to topical nitro-glycerin in the treatment of chronic anal fissure: results of a random-ized controlled trial by the Canadian Colorectal Surgical Trials Group, *Dis Colon Rectum* 2000; 43: 1048.
21. Chrysos E *et al.* Effect of nifedipine on rectoanal motility, *Dis Colon Rectum* 1996; 39: 212.
22. Jonas M, Neal KR, Abercrombie JF and Scholefield JH. A randomized trial of oral vs. topical diltiazem for chronic anal fissure, *Dis Colon Rectum* 2001; 44: 1074.
23. Brisinda G *et al.* A comparison of injections of botulinum toxin and top-ical nitroglycerin ointment for the treatment of chronic anal fissures, *N Engl J Med* 1999; 341: 65.
24. Khubchandani IT and Reed JF. Sequelae of internal sphincterotomy for chronic fissure-in-ano, *Br J Surg* 1989; 76: 431.
25. Littlejohn DR and Newstead GL. Tailored lateral sphincterotomy for anal fissure, *Dis Colon Rectum* 1997; 40: 1439.
26. Fleschner PR, Schoetz DJ *et al.* Anal fissure in Crohn's disease: a plea for aggressive management, *Dis Colon Rectum* 1995; 38: 1137.
27. Nyam DCNK, Bartolo DC *et al.* Island advancement flaps in the man-agement of anal fissures, *Br J Surg* 1995; 82: 326.

CHAPTER 6

Dealing with the Recurrent Fistula

RJ Guy

Introduction

Surgical treatments for fistulas-in-ano have been recorded since Hippo-crates in the 5th century BC,[1] and fistulas are still commonly encountered in modern colorectal practice. Fortunately, most are simple and low and can be dealt with safely by laying open (fistulotomy), with a high likelihood of a cure and a low risk of incontinence. Higher and more complex tracks pose a surgical challenge, treatment failure presenting as persistent or recurrent sepsis and fistulas. This article will address the causes and assessment of recurrence and discuss some of the surgical techniques.

Recurrence Versus Incontinence

A balance must be reached between elimination of the fistula track and risk of anal sphincter damage. Large series over the last 30–40 years have reported some degree of incontinence following fistula surgery in up to about a third of patients with recurrence rates up to 8%[2–9] (Table 1). These figures, however, take no account of the type of surgery, case mix, data acquisition or definitions of incontinence, in particular the distinction between minor and major episodes. Nevertheless, they illustrate that the integrity of the sphincter mechanism should be maintained as far as possible, but that a compromise may be necessary in order to reduce the recurrence rate. Previous fistula surgery is itself a risk factor for incontinence and further recurrence,[9] but many patients may be willing to accept a minor degree of incontinence in order to be cured of their troublesome symptoms.

In one questionnaire-based study addressing satisfaction in 375 patients undergoing fistula surgery over a five-year period, the recurrence rate was 8%, with 46% reporting some degree of incontinence.[10] Patients with recurrence reported a higher dissatisfaction rate (61%) than did those with incontinence (24%), but the attributable fractions indicated that 33% and 84% of dissatisfaction, respectively, were due to recurrence and incontinence.

Causes of Recurrence

Treatment failure may be attributed to one or more of the following:

- Failure to appreciate the anatomy (of the fistula and the anorectum)

Table 1. Fistula surgery results.

Author	Year	Patients	Recurrence (%)	Incontinence (%)
Bennett[2]	1962	108	2.0	36.0
Hill[3]	1967	626	1.0	4.0
Lilius[4]	1968	150	5.5	13.5
Mazier[5]	1971	1000	3.9	0.001
Marks & Ritchie[6]	1977	793	NS	25
Vasilevsky & Gordon[7]	1984	160	6.3	3.3
Sangwan et al.[8]	1994	461	6.5	2.8
Garcia-Aguilar et al.[9]	1996	375	8.0 (16*)	45 (67*)

NS = Not stated
* Previous fistula surgery

- Failure to control the primary track
- Overlooked secondary sepsis and tracks
- Iatrogenic tracks
- Unusual pathology

Fistula Anatomy and Classification

Safe and successful treatment of a fistula-in-ano requires an adequate knowledge of pelvic anatomy in order to determine the course of the primary track and the location of secondary tracks and sepsis. An appreciation of the complexity of the sphincter mechanism and an understanding of the existence of potential anorectal spaces[11] are fundamental for effectively tackling a recurrent fistula.

Sir Alan Parks' classification of fistulas-in-ano, devised from a personal series of 400 patients, remains the most useful.[12] Based on the cryptoglandular theory, it comprises four main fistula types, according to the relationship of the primary track to the sphincter complex: intersphincteric, trans-sphincteric, suprasphincteric and extrasphincetric, although the latter are rarely of cryptoglandular origin and more likely to result from pelvic pathology or iatrogenic injury.

Erroneous Assessment and Iatrogenic Fistulas

Inaccurate assessment is likely to lead to incorrect treatment and a greater likelihood of recurrence. An analysis of 24 patients with problematical anal fistulas treated at St Mark's Hospital revealed that, in 5 patients, failure could be attributed to wrongly diagnosed primary tracks or missed secondary tracks.[13]

Iatrogenic injury may result from erroneous assessment and inadvertent entry into the rectum during careless probing. Supralevator sepsis must be accurately defined and its origin determined. If an intersphincteric extension is drained via the ischiorectal fossa rather than the rectum, a suprasphincteric fistula will result. Conversely, a supralevator ischiorectal extension drained into the rectum, rather than via the ischiorectal fossa, will produce an extrasphincteric fistula.[12]

Unusual Pathology

Persistence or recurrence of anal fistulas must alert the clinician to the possibility of unusual pathology. The most likely conditions to be considered are Crohn's disease, tuberculosis and malignancy, although other conditions, such as actinomycosis and lymphogranuloma venereum, with geographical variation, may be responsible. Curettings from all persistent or recurrent fistula tracks should be examined to exclude these conditions.

Assessment

Clinical

Accurate clinical assessment in an awake patient and under anaesthetic is mandatory, particularly for recurrent fistulas. Inspection of the anus and perineum may reveal one or more external openings. Normal anatomical landmarks may be distorted following multiple attempts at fistula eradication, but the distribution of scarring may give some indication of the likely integrity of the sphincter mechanism. Goodsall's rule should be applied but is more likely to be broken by recurrent fistulas and by fistulas which have an anterior external opening, especially if it lies more than 3 cm from the anal margin.[14]

The perineum should be examined with the lubricated gloved finger when a cord-like fistula track may be felt, although distinguishing this from scar tissue may be difficult. Induration suggesting secondary sepsis may be apparent and often more easily assessed between index finger and thumb. The integrity of the sphincter complex and perineal body should be estimated, particularly for anterior fistulas in females, in whom previous obstetric injury may be apparent. An internal fistula opening may be felt as an indurated nodule or pit,[15] and supralevator induration, which may only be suggested by anal canal asymmetry, should be sought with the index finger. Clinical examination by an experienced coloproctologist may be extremely accurate and, in comparison with endosonography, is more likely to define primary superficial, suprasphincteric and extrasphincteric tracks or secondary supra- and infralevator sepsis.[16]

Imaging

Ultrasound

The accuracy and understanding of 2D ultrasound imaging have improved since its first use for fistulas.[17] It is simple, rapid, well tolerated and may be useful in the assessment of complex fistulae.[18] Intersphincteric and horse-shoe abscesses can be defined, trans-sphincteric tracks can be seen and the position of the internal opening can be inferred by various criteria.[16,17] However, the technique is limited by insufficient penetration beyond the external sphincter and an inability to distinguish infection from fibrosis. Hydrogen peroxide injected into the external opening may enhance sono-graphic reflectivity of the track,[19] and 3D reconstruction of the images may further improve sensitivity by permitting visualization in sagittal and coro-nal planes. Endosonography is useful in assessing sphincter integrity, par-ticularly following extensive surgery for fistulas.

Magnetic Resonance Imaging (MRI)

MRI has become the gold standard imaging investigation for anorectal sep-sis and fistulas since its proposal for this indication almost 10 years ago.[20] Its advantages include noninvasiveness (using a body coil), an ability to contrast granulation tissue and pus against pelvic floor anatomy, and mul-tiplanar imaging. Axial scans best relate the primary track to the sphincter complex and coronal scans best visualize the levator plate for diagnosis of supralevator sepsis. Most published studies report sensitivities and speci-ficities of 80–100% for fistula evaluation,[20–22] with superior accuracies in comparison with endosonography[23] and clinical examination[24] (Table 2).

Fistulography

Contrast fistulography is generally unreliable for anal fistulas, with a reported accuracy of only 16% and a 12% incidence of false openings and high extensions.[25] It has gained little popularity and cannot be advocated, although in one study of recurrent fistulas, unexpected pathology was dis-covered in 13/27 (48%) patients.[26] The pelvic source of an extrasphincteric fistula may sometimes be revealed by this technique.[27]

Table 2. Results of MRI for fistulas.

Author	Year	Patients	Sens (%)	Spec (%)	PPV (%)
Lunniss et al.[20]	1992	16	88	NS	
Lunniss et al.[23]	1994	20	NS	NS	100 (MRI)
					50 (AES*)
Barker et al.[21]	1994	35	94	NS	NS
Beckingham et al.[22]	1996	42	97	100	NS
Chapple et al.[24]	2000	52	81	73	75 (MRI)
			77	46	59 (CE†)

NS = Not stated
*AES = Anal endosonography
†CE = Clinical examination

Manometry

Fistulotomy for intersphincteric and trans-sphincteric fistulas causes a reduction in resting and squeeze pressures.[28,29] In selected cases, particularly recurrent fistulas, preoperative anal manometry may help to determine the most appropriate surgical procedure to employ in order to preserve maximum continence.[30]

Surgical Treatment

Thorough examination under anaesthesia allows planning of surgery in the light of preoperative assessment and imaging. Probing of fistulous openings should be done carefully using grooved Lockhart–Mummery probes, avoiding the creation of false tracks or inadvertent entry into the rectum. Fine lacrimal probes may detect narrower tracks but their use requires experience. Hydrogen peroxide injected into the external opening may reveal an otherwise elusive internal opening.

In the presence of sepsis the priorities are to drain pus and control the primary track. Hanley's procedure is effective for dealing with horseshoe abscesses arising from the deep postanal space in association with a midline fistula.[31] In this procedure the internal opening is located through a posterior drainage incision. Internal sphincterotomy to the level of the internal opening drains the intersphincteric space and a loose seton is inserted through the track. Counter-incisions are made over each ischiorectal fossa to drain the anterior extensions. Rubber drains (e.g. Penrose) may be used to assist drainage and irrigation as necessary. This method avoids large wounds which are slow to heal and definitive management of the primary track can be subsequently addressed following the resolution of sepsis.

Fistulotomy

Laying open of the fistula track remains the mainstay of treatment for primary fistulas and is most likely to result in a cure. However, impairment of function becomes more likely if, in achieving eradication, a significant proportion of the sphincter mechanism is divided. Recurrent fistulas, particularly following previous fistulotomy, demand extra caution. An appreciation of how much muscle can safely be divided is acquired through experience but will vary individually with gender, parity, continence and previous surgery. Preservation of puborectalis is paramount, and division of this muscle will inevitably result in total incontinence.[32]

If fistulotomy is performed, larger wounds should be marsupialized in order to reduce the size of the wound and encourage faster healing.[33]

Use of Setons

Various materials are available for insertion through the primary track, but most surgeons use nylon, silk or rubber. Their use can be tailored to the individual circumstances but they broadly serve one or more of the following functions:

- Drain for the primary track
- Marker for the primary track
- Stimulator of fibrosis
- Cutting action

Loose Setons

Placement of a loose seton is the safest treatment for fistulas, especially for the inexperienced surgeon, and particularly in the presence of acute sepsis, when anatomy and function may be less easily assessed. A loose seton allows time for maturation of the primary track and an informed decision on subsequent management. Some fistulas (44–78%) may heal following seton removal after a few weeks or months, provided that drainage of the

Table 3. Results of staged fistulotomy.

Author	Year	Patients	Recurrence (%)	Incontinence (%)
Ramanujam et al.[37]	1983	45	2	2
Kuijpers[36]	1984	10	0	10
Christensen et al.[38]	1986	21	0	29
Williams et al.[39]	1991	28	8	4
Pearl et al.[40]	1993	116	3	5
Graf et al.[41]	1995	25	8	44
Garcia-Aguilar et al.[9]	1996	63	9	64

intersphincteric space has been achieved by internal sphincterotomy to the level of the internal opening.[34,35] Minor incontinence may occur in up to half of these patients, presumably related to the degree of internal sphincter division.

Maturation by fibrosis of the primary track in the presence of a seton may create a situation in which fistulotomy becomes safer. In some cases this may be further assisted by spontaneous migration of the seton through the muscle. Prior to staged fistulotomy the patient should be examined awake, at which time the amount of incorporated muscle can be more accurately assessed. At fistulotomy the fibrosed muscle does not retract to the same extent, theoretically allowing better preservation of function.[36] Despite these arguments in favour of a staged procedure, incontinence rates of 2–64% have been reported, with recurrence rates of up to 9%[36–41] (Table 3). Use of a long-term loose seton can be useful in perianal Crohn's disease but has not been described for idiopathic fistulae. At Singapore General Hospital there are currently 12 patients, all male, who have had a seton in place for a median period of 24.5 months (Table 4). These patients have difficult recurrent fistulas for which no further surgery is planned and their quality of life remains good.

Cutting Setons

Tight setons, with the aim of producing a controlled fistulotomy, have not gained wide popularity. As divided muscle heals by fibrosis behind the advancing seton, sphincter function should be less impaired. Cutting setons require tightening every few weeks to be effective, which may be painful and require general anaesthesia. Several outpatient tightening

Table 4. Long-term setons: SGH experience.

Number of patients	12
Sex	All males
Median age (y)	50
Fistula types:	
– Trans-sphincteric	4
– Suprasphincteric	4
– Extrasphincteric	4
Median number of procedures	4
Median time with seton (mth)	24.5

Table 5. Results of cutting setons.

Author	Year	Patients	Recurrence (%)	Minor Incontinence (%)	Major Incontinence (%)
Culp[43]	1984	20	0	15	0
Christensen et al.[38]	1986	21	0	29	39
Ustynoski et al.[44]	1990	11	18	NS	NS
Williams et al.[39]	1991	13	0	54	7

NS = Not stated

methods have been described, one of the simplest being the use of a haemorrhoid bander.[42]

Most published series contain few cases but major incontinence may still occur in up to a third of patients and recurrence in almost a fifth[38,39,43,44] (Table 5).

Endorectal Advancement Flaps

Healthy tissue may be advanced in a cephalad direction from the anus or, more commonly, from proximally to cover the internal fistula opening. Anal advancement procedures are well described[45,46] and will not be discussed further.

Endorectal advancement flaps may be indicated in the following circumstances:

- Recurrent fistulas
- High/multiple/complex fistulas

Table 6. Results of endorectal advancement flaps.

Author	Year	Patients	Healing (%)	Minor Incontinence (%)	Major Incontinence (%)
Oh et al.[47]	1983	15*	87	NS	NS
Aguilar et al.[48]	1985	189	98.5	10	0
Wedell et al.[49]	1987	27	100	30	0
Kodner et al.[50]	1993	107	94	NS	NS
Miller & Finan[51]	1998	26	77	0	0

NS = Not stated
*All recurrent fistulas

- Anterior fistulas in females
- In the presence of impaired continence

Anterior fistulas are best tackled with the patient in the prone-jackknife position. The primary track is first excised by fistulectomy starting at the external opening and proceeding as far as possible through the sphincter complex to the internal opening, which is excised or curetted. An incision is made 1 cm distal to the internal opening and a flap containing mucosa, submucosa and circular muscle is raised, and developed proximally, with the end trimmed. The flap should be broad-based to ensure adequate vascularity and mobilized sufficiently to allow distal advancement and coverage of the defect without tension once sutured.

Several reasonable series testify to the generally good results with this procedure for difficult fistulas, including recurrent cases, with preservation of continence[47–51] (Table 6).

Tissue Adhesive

The injection of autologous or commercial fibrin sealant along the fistula track is an attractive concept as it is simple and avoids damage to the sphincter complex. The initial enthusiasm for this technique following impressive short-term results[52–54] has waned somewhat, with reports of later failures.[55] Success for recurrent fistulas is only around 50%, compared with 60–70% for those with no previous surgery (Table 7).

Finally, surgical management of anal fistulas, which may be prolonged, requires accurate documentation, preferably using reproducible multiplanar diagrams, such as in the St Mark's Hospital fistula sheet.

Table 7. Results for fibrin glue.

Author	Year	Patients	Follow-up (mth)	Healing (%)
Abel et al.[52]	1993	10	7	60
Cintron et al.[53]	1999	26	4	81
Park et al.[54]	2000	29	6	68
Cintron et al.[55]	2000	26*	18	54
		53†	18	64
		22§	18	55

*Autologous
†Commercial
§Recurrent fistulas

Conclusions

Management of a recurrent fistula-in-ano can present a significant challenge to even the most experienced colorectal surgeon. The management goals are to eradicate all tracks and associated sepsis whilst preserving function. The suggested logical approach to this problem comprises the following steps:

- Drain sepsis and control the primary track
- Delineate the anatomy
- Determine sphincter function
- Deal with the primary track
- If continent, either:

  • Staged fistulotomy, or
  • Cutting seton

- If continence impaired:

  • Endorectal advancement flap, or
  • Long-term seton

References

1. Adams F. On fistulae. In: Adams F (ed.), *The Genuine Work of Hippocrates*. Baltimore: Williams and Wilkins, 1939: 337–42.

2. Bennett RC. A review of orthodox treatment for anal fistula, *Proc R Soc Med* 1962; 55: 756–7.
3. Hill JR. Fistulas and fistulous abscesses in the anorectal region: a personal experience in management, *Dis Colon Rectum* 1967; 10: 421–34.
4. Lilius HG. Fistula-in-ano: a clinical study of 150 patients, *Acta Chir Scand* 1968; 383: 3–88.
5. Mazier WP. The treatment and care of anal fistulas: a study of 1000 patients, *Dis Colon Rectum* 1971; 14: 134–44.
6. Marks CG and Ritchie JK. Anal fistulas at St Mark's Hospital, *Br J Surg* 1977; 64: 84–91.
7. Vasilevsky C-A and Gordon PH. Results of treatment of fistula-in-ano, *Dis Colon Rectum* 1984; 28: 225–31.
8. Sangwan YP, Rosen L and Riether RD. Is simple fistula-in-ano simple? *Dis Colon Rectum* 1994; 37: 885–9.
9. Garcia-Aguilar J, Belmonte C, Wong WD, Goldberg SM and Madoff RD. Anal fistula surgery: factors associated with recurrence and incontinence, *Dis Colon Rectum* 1996; 39: 723–9.
10. Garcia-Aguilar J, Davey CS, Le CT, Lowry AC and Rothenberger DA. Patient satisfaction after surgical treatment for fistula-in-ano, *Dis Colon Rectum* 2000; 43: 1206–12.
11. Hanley PH. Reflections on anorectal abscess fistula: 1984, *Dis Colon Rectum* 1985; 28: 528–33.
12. Parks AG, Gordon PH and Hardcastle JD. A classification of fistula-in-ano, *Br J Surg* 1976; 63: 1–12.
13. Seow-Choen F and Phillips RKS. Insights gained from the management of problematical anal fistulae at St Mark's Hospital, 1984–88, *Br J Surg* 1991; 78: 539–41.
14. Cirocco WC and Reilly JC. Challenging the predictive accuracy of Goodsall's rule for anal fistulas, *Dis Colon Rectum* 1992; 35: 537–42.
15. Kuypers JHC. Diagnosis and treatment of fistula-in-ano, *Neth J Surg* 1982; 34: 147–52.
16. Seow-Choen S, Burnett S, Bartram CI *et al.* Comparison between anal endosonography and digital examination in the evaluation of anal fistulae, *Br J Surg* 1991.
17. Law PJ, Talbot RW, Bartram CI *et al.* Anal endosonography in the evaluation of perianal sepsis and fistula-in-ano, *Br J Surg* 1989; 76: 752–5.
18. Deen KI, Williams JG, Hutchinson R *et al.* Fistulas in ano: endoanal ultrasonographic assessment assists decision making for surgery, *Gut* 1994; 35: 391–4.

19. Cheong DMO, Nogueras JJ, Wexner SD and Jagelman DG. Anal endosonography for recurrent anal fistulas: image enhancement with hydrogen peroxide, *Dis Colon Rectum* 1993; 36: 1158–60.

20. Lunniss PJ, Armstrong P, Barker PG *et al*. Magnetic resonance imaging of anal fistulae, *Lancet* 1992; 340: 394–6.

21. Barker PG, Lunniss PJ, Armstrong P *et al*. Magnetic resonance imaging of fistula-in-ano: technique, interpretation and accuracy, *Clin Radiol* 1994; 49: 7–13.

22. Beckingham IJ, Spencer JA, Ward J *et al*. Prospective evaluation of dynamic contrast-enhanced magnetic resonance imaging in the evaluation of fistula-in-ano, *Br J Surg* 1996; 83: 1396–8.

23. Lunniss PJ, Barker PG, Sultan AH *et al*. Magnetic resonance imaging of fistula-in-ano, *Dis Colon Rectum* 1994; 37: 708–18.

24. Chapple KS, Spencer JA, Windsor ACJ *et al*. Prognostic value of magnetic resonance imaging in the management of fistula-in-ano, *Dis Colon Rectum* 2000; 43: 511–16.

25. Kuijpers HC and Schulpen T. Fistulography for fistula-in-ano: is it useful? *Dis Colon Rectum* 1985; 28: 103–4.

26. Weisman RI, Orsay CP, Pearl RK *et al*. The role of fistulography in fistula-in-ano: report of five cases, *Dis Colon Rectum* 1991; 34: 181–4.

27. Halligan S. Imaging fistula-in-ano, *Clin Radiol* 1998; 53: 85–95.

28. Sainio P. A manometric study of anorectal function after surgery for anal fistula, with special reference to incontinence, *Acta Chir Scand* 1985; 151: 695–700.

29. Lunniss PJ, Kamm MA and Phillips RKS. Factors affecting continence after surgery for anal fistula, *Br J Surg* 1994; 81: 1382–5.

30. Pescatori M, Marin G, Anastasio G and Rinallo L. Anal manometry improves the outcome of surgery for fistula-in-ano, *Dis Colon Rectum* 1989; 32: 588–92.

31. Hanley PH. Conservative surgical correction of horseshoe abscess and fistula, *Dis Colon Rectum* 1965; 8: 364–8.

32. Milligan ETC and Morgan CN. Surgical anatomy of the anal canal with special reference to anorectal fistulae, *Lancet* 1934; ii: 1213–17.

33. Ho YH, Tan M, Leong AFPK and Seow-Choen F. Marsupialization of fistulotomy wounds improves healing: a randomized controlled trial, *Br J Surg* 1998; 85: 105–7.

34. Thomson JPS and Ross AHMCL. Can the external anal sphincter be preserved in the treatment of trans-sphincteric fistula-in-ano? *Int J Colorect Dis* 1989; 4: 247–50.

35. Kennedy HL and Zegarra JP. Fistulotomy without external sphincter division for high anal fistulae, *Br J Surg* 1990; 77: 898–901.

36. Kuypers HC. Use of the seton in the treatment of extrasphincteric anal fistula, *Dis Colon Rectum* 1984; 27: 109–10.

37. Ramanujam PS, Prasad ML and Abcarian H. The role of seton in fistulotomy of the anus, *Surg Gynecol Obstet* 1983; 157: 419–22.

38. Christensen A, Miles J and Christiansen J. Treatment of transsphincteric anal fistulas by the seton technique, *Dis Colon Rectum* 1986: 454–5.

39. Williams JG, Macleod CA, Rothenberger DA and Goldberg SM. Seton treatment of high anal fistulae, *Br J Surg* 1991; 78: 1159–61.

40. Pearl RK, Andrews JR, Orsay CP *et al.* Role of the seton in the management of anorectal fistulas, *Dis Colon Rectum* 1993; 36: 573–9.

41. Graf W, Pahlman L and Egerbald S. Functional results after seton treatment of hightranssphincteric anal fistulas, *Eur J Surg* 1995; 161: 289–91.

42. Cirocco WC and Rusin LC. Simplified seton management for complex anal fistulas: a novel use for the rubber band ligator, *Dis Colon Rectum* 1991; 34: 1135–7.

43. Culp CE. Use of Penrose drains to treat certain anal fistulas: a primary operative seton, *Mayo Clin Proc* 1984; 59: 613–17.

44. Ustynoski K, Rosen L, Stasik J *et al.* Horseshoe abscess fistula. Seton treatment, *Dis Colon Rectum* 1990; 33: 602–5.

45. Del Pino A, Nelson RL, Pearl RK and Abcarian H. Island flap anoplasty for treatment of transsphincteric fistula-in-ano, *Dis Colon Rectum* 1996; 39: 224–6.

46. Jun SH and Choi GS. Anocutaneous advancement flap closure of high anal fistulas, *Br J Surg* 1999; 86: 490–2.

47. Oh C. Management of high recurrent anal fistula, *Surgery* 1983; 93: 330–2.

48. Aguilar PS, Plasencia G, Hardy TG *et al.* Mucosal advancement in the treatment of anal fistula, *Dis Colon Rectum* 1985; 28: 496–8.

49. Wedell J, Meier zu Eissen P, Banzhaf G and Kleine L. Sliding flap advancement for the treatment of high level fistulae, *Br J Surg* 1987; 74: 390–1.

50. Kodner IJ, Mazor A, Shemesh EI *et al.* Endorectal advancement flap repair of rectovaginal and other complicated anorectal fistulas, *Surgery* 1993; 114: 682–90.

51. Miller GV and Finan PJ. Flap advancement and core fistulectomy for complex rectal fistula, *Br J Surg* 1998; 85: 108–10.

52. Abel ME, Chiu YS, Russell TR and Volpe PA. Autologous fibrin glue in the treatment of rectovaginal and complex fistulas, *Dis Colon Rectum* 1993; 36: 447–9.

53. Cintron JR, Park JJ, Orsay CP *et al*. Repair of fistulas-in-ano using autologous fibrin tissue adhesive, *Dis Colon Rectum* 1999; 42: 607–13.

54. Park JJ, Cintron JR, Orsay CP *et al*. Repair of anorectal fistulae using commercial fibrin sealant, *Arch Surg* 2000; 135: 166–9.

55. Cintron JR, Park JJ, Orsay CP *et al*. Repair of fistulas-in-ano using fibrin adhesive, *Dis Colon Rectum* 2000; 43: 944–50.

CHAPTER 7

The Difficult Internal Opening of an Anal Fistula: Current Management

PL Roberts

"Friday morning was obliged to submit to a cruel operation, and the cutting out root and branch of a disease caused by working over much, which has been gathering it seems for years. Thank God it's all over and I am on the sofa again."

— Charles Dickens, 1841[1]

Anorectal abscess/fistula may be viewed as a continuum of disease, with "abscess" representing the acute phase and "fistula" representing the chronic form of infection. The incidence of abscess is 12.3/100 000 in men and 5.6/100 000 in women,[2] with a peak incidence in the third and fourth decades.[3] In 90% of patients, the abscess is cryptoglandular in origin, arising from a nonspecific infection in the anal glands which results in obstruction of the gland and duct. Other aetiologies of abscess/fistula include inflammatory bowel disease (particularly Crohn's disease), infections such as actinomycoses, tuberculosis, lymphogranuloma venereum, HIV, trauma, prior surgery, malignancy and prior radiation therapy. After drainage of an abscess, 30–50% of patients form a fistula.   A fistula is an abnormal communication between two epithelium-lined surfaces. Classified by their relationship to the sphincter muscle, fistulas include intersphincteric, trans-sphincteric, extrasphincteric and suprasphincteric fistulas.[4]

A fistula is suspected by persistent chronic drainage and/or bleeding, especially with a history of an abscess which has been surgically drained or which has spontaneously drained. The external opening is easily seen and a palpable cord may be present. Conversely, the internal opening, while suspected, is often not demonstrated in the office.   Examination under anaesthesia in the operating room is performed, and with gentle probing and knowledge of Goodsall's rule the internal opening can usually be demonstrated.

According to Goodsall's rule, an external opening found in the posterior hemi-circumference of the perianal skin usually communicates with the posterior midline, and an anterior external opening generally communicates in a radial fashion with the closest crypt. Goodsall's rule was recently re-examined in 216 patients (155 male) who underwent fistula surgery.[5] Ninety per cent of the patients with a posterior external opening had an internal opening in the posterior midline but only 49% of anterior external openings followed Goodsall's rule; furthermore, in women 90% of anterior external openings tracked to the anterior midline.

In some patients, the internal opening is not readily identified; injection of the external opening with hydrogen peroxide (my preference), methylene blue, or even milk may facilitate demonstration of the tract. If the tract still cannot be identified, it is probably best to core out the external opening and return to the operating room on another day, thus avoiding making a false internal opening.

Other radiographic studies, such as fistulography, anal endosonography and MRI fistulography, may assist in demonstrating the internal opening. The test selected is largely dependent on the experience and expertise at one's institution. Whatever test is selected must be combined with clinical expertise (as the best "tool" for locating the internal opening of a fistula is the "educated" index finger). Fistulography is easily performed in the operating room by injection of contrast material into the external opening. A small catheter, such as a pediatric feeding tube, is used and contrast injected slowly as overflow of contrast material may spuriously be interpreted as contrast in the rectal lumen.   In a series of 27 patients who underwent fistulography, management was changed in 13 patients.[6]

There were 7 unexpected findings and surgery was altered in 6. It was most useful in patients who had recurrent fistulas or inflammatory bowel disease. Endosonography is generally safe, quick and well tolerated. The internal sphincter is seen as a hypoechogenic ring, the external sphincter is of mixed echogenicity and fistula tracts are seen as hypoechoic defects. Unfortunately, endosonography cannot distinguish fibrosis from infection. Using hydrogen-peroxide-enhanced ultrasound and comparing it to conventional ultrasound and physical examination, Poen and colleagues were able to correctly identify the tract in 20 of 21 patients with the use of hydrogen-peroxide-enhanced ultrasound.[7] The concordance with the findings at surgery was 95%.

MRI has also been used and has the advantage of noninvasive multiplanar capabilities, operator independence, high inherent soft tissue contrast and the ability to contrast pus and granulation tissue. Thus MRI may identify both the tract and the relationship to the sphincter muscle. One drawback is that epithelialized tracts may not be visualized. In one study of MRI compared with endosonography, MRI had an accuracy of 89% compared to a 61% accuracy with ultrasound.[8]

Finally, if an internal opening is not found, it may indeed be because no internal opening exists. Anal abscesses may result from infection of the skin or skin appendages in up to one-third of patients. If an abscess cultures for skin flora, it is unlikely to be of cryptoglandular origin. In addition, other pathologic entities, such as hidradenitis, an infection of the apocrine sweat glands may occasionally be confused with anal abscess/fistula. Patients with perianal hidradenitis often have axillary disease also.

In conclusion, the majority of internal openings of anal fistulas are readily demonstrated intraoperatively by the experienced surgeon. If gentle probing and knowledge of Goodsall's rule fail to demonstrate the internal opening, the tract may be injected with hydrogen peroxide. Additional imaging modalities such as fistulography, endosonography and MRI may be helpful in selected patients with complex fistulas, recurrent fistulas and fistulas associated with inflammatory bowel disease.

References

1. Bowen WH. Charles Dickens and his family. W. Heffer and Sons: Cambridge, 1956, 38.

2. Saino P. Fistula-in-ano in a defined population: incidence and epidemiological aspects, *Annales Chirurgiue et Gynaecologiae* 1984; 73: 219–24.

3. Ramanujam PS, Prasad ML and Abcarian H. Perianal abscesses and fistulas. A study of 1023 patients, *Dis Colon Rectum* 1984; 27: 593–7.

4. Paks AG, Gordon PH and Hardcastle JD. A classification of fistula-in-ano, *Br J Surg* 1976; 63: 1–12.

5. Cirocco WC and Reilly JC. Challenging the predictive accuracy of Goodsall's rule for anal fistulas, *Dis Colon Rectum* 1992; 35: 537–42.

6. Weisman RI, Orsay Cp, Pearl RK *et al.* The role of fistulography in fistula-in-ano, *Dis Colon Rectum* 1991; 34: 181–4.

7. Poen AC, Felt-Bersma RJ, Eijsbouts QA *et al.* Hydrogen peroxide-enhanced transanal ultrasound in the assessment of fistula-in-ano, *Dis Colon Rectum* 1998; 41: 1147–52.

8. Hussain SM, Stoker J, Schouten WR *et al.* Fistula-in-ano: endoanal sonography versus endoanal MR imaging in classification, *Radiology* 1996; 200: 475–81.

Update on the Surgical and Nonsurgical Management of Haemorrhoids

F Seow-Choen

Aetiology of Piles

It has been widely accepted that piles derive from anal cushions.[1] Anal cushions are normal structures which are found in the left lateral, right posterior and right anterior positions of the anal canal. They consist of mucosa, submucosal fibroelastic connective tissues, smooth muscle, and blood vessels. The blood vessels include venous plexuses devoid of smooth muscles,[1,2] which form part of an arteriovenous fistula system.[2,3] These arteriovenous channels control the size of the anal cushions by regulating the volume of blood flowing through.[3] Anal cushions are normal structures, demonstrable in children, foetuses and even in the embryo.[1] It is possible that they complement the anal sphincter function, by changing in size to provide fine control over the continence of liquids and gases.[1,4]

Anal cushions function normally when they are in their proper position in the anal canal.[1] This fixation is by submucosal smooth muscle and elastic fibres (Treitz's muscle), which anchor the anal cushion to the anal sphincters. These fibres may be fragmented by prolonged downward stress related to straining to defecate hard stools.[1,2,5] There is some relationship between haemorrhoidal prolapse, symptoms and irregular bowel habits. It is quite common for patients with piles to have some constipation.[6,7] In addition, the bleeding and pain from haemorrhoids often settle through correction of bowel function with dietary supplements alone.[8] When the supporting submucosal fibres fragment, the anal cushions are no longer restrained from engorging excessively with blood. This results in bleeding and, later on, prolapse. Reading whilst on the toilet bowl aggravates this situation. Veins which traverse the anal sphincter are blocked whereas arterial flow continues, leading to massive haemorrhoidal congestion.

Principles of Managing Piles

Firstly, it must be recognized that haemorrhoids are very common and may therefore coexist with other more dangerous colorectal diseases.[10]

Conditions such as rectal cancer may give much the same symptoms as haemorrhoids. Indeed, there have been patients with bleeding piles for years (although sometimes with a recent change in the bleeding pattern) who were found on colonoscopy to have rectal cancer as well. Patients who have symptoms, including blood or mucus mixed in the stools, change in bowel habits, abdominal symptoms and a family history of colorectal cancer, should have a further evaluation of the colon and rectum.

Secondly, it should be recognized that anal cushions are normal functional anatomical structures. They do not require treatment unless they become symptomatic. The therapeutic strategies would then depend upon the amount of haemorrhoidal tissue prolapsing beyond the anal verge.

Management of Non- or Minimally Prolapsing Haemorrhoids

As discussed above, haemorrhoids have an important function in helping to maintain anal continence.[10] Therefore, if the piles have not permanently prolapsed, it would be sensible to resort first to nonoperative methods. The primary problem of inadequate dietary fibre and straining at stools needs to be addressed. Thus, dietary fibre intake should be increased and fibre supplements prescribed. A randomized controlled trial showed that fibre supplements were more effective in treating bleeding and discomfort from internal piles than placebos.[8] However, the fibre supplements took six weeks before significant symptomatic improvements were reported. In the meantime, it may be useful to add other forms of treatment, which can give more immediate symptomatic relief. These would include rubber band ligation, injection sclerotherapy, medications such as Daflon 500, and toilet re-education.

Rubber Band Ligation

In this technique, a small rubber band is applied at the base of the haemorrhoidal tissue. As the feeding vessels become strangulated, the blood flow is reduced and the bulk of the piles shrink. The strangulated tissue may become necrotic and slough in a few days. Subsequently, the wound undergoes fibrosis, resulting in fixation of the mucosa.[11] The pile tissue is thus prevented from engorging and prolapsing. Up to three haemorrhoids can be banded on the same occasion. It is relatively painless if the bands are placed above the dentate line, where the mucosa is innervated mainly by the pelvic splanchnic nerves.[12] Banding is usually 60–80% effective, depending on proper selection of cases.[13] There is a 2–5% risk of secondary haemorrhage, for which the patient should be warned to return for medical advice. It has been shown that a high fibre diet is important in maintaining the long-term cure rate after rubber band ligation.[14]

Injection Sclerotherapy

Sclerosant agents used include phenol (5%) in almond oil or sodium tetradecate.[11] These are injected into the submucosa around the pedicle of the pile, at the level of the anorectal ring. The sclerosant is likely to cause inflammation, leading to reduction of the blood flow into the haemorrhoid. This technique is about 70% effective.[13] Secondary haemorrhage is rare.

Other Methods

Daflon 500 is micronized diosmin and hesperidin, which belong to the hydroxyethylrutoside group of drugs.[15] Its pharmacological properties include noradrenalin-mediated venous contraction,[16] reduction in blood extravasation from capillaries[17] and inhibition of prostaglandin (PGE_2, PGF_2) inflammatory response.[18] These properties have a proven therapeutic action in the symptomatic relief of haemorrhoidal symptoms.[19] Side-effects have been very minimal.[20,21] Such drugs may therefore be an important alternative to rubber band ligation and sclerosant therapy, especially when the latter are not readily available.

Various other methods are also available. These include infrared photocoagulation, which requires elaborate equipment, and cryotherapy, which results in unpleasant discharge. For such reasons, these methods have not been as popular. Topical preparations which may contain local anaesthetics or steroids are also available, often without prescription. To date, there is no evidence that such agents are any more effective than spontaneous remissions.[11] Moreover, patient self-treatment may delay the diagnosis of serious diseases such as cancer, and can therefore be potentially harmful.

Management of Irreducible Prolapsed Piles

When anal cushions have prolapsed or thrombosed, they no longer function effectively to help maintain continence. In fact, the sensory function may be impaired[21] and this may partially account for the complaints of minor incontinence by some patients. Conventional haemorrhoidectomy removes these cushions. More recent methods of stapling haemorrhoidopexy preserve these cushions by returning them to their proper place in the anal canal.

There are variations to the technique of haemorrhoidectomy, particularly pertaining as to whether the wound after excision should be left open to granulate or primarily closed with sutures.[13,22–25] The main problems encountered are similar. These are mainly postoperative pain, anal incontinence and haemorrhage. Open haemorrhoidectomy may lead to faster and more reliable wound healing where three large prolapsed irreducible piles are excised.[22] These problems may worry patients so much that they would rather suffer the discomfort of large prolapsing haemorrhoids for years, than submit to surgery. Some have described haemorrhoidectomy pain as passing pieces of sharp glass fragments. Stapled haemorrhoidectomy is much less painful.

Since 1989, more than 13 000 surgical haemorrhoidectomies have been performed in the department. An even larger number, of course, perhaps

10 times more, have been treated by rubber band ligation, or injection sclerotherapy without need for actual surgery.

Most patients with symptomatic haemorrhoids do not require surgical intervention and are adequately treated without having to excise haemorrhoidal tissue. The remainder will need surgical management due to severity of prolapse. Thus third and fourth degree haemorrhoids are more appropriately treated by surgery, which is usually performed by excision of the three primary piles. Some patients nonetheless will have severe circumferential prolapse with massive engorgement of both external and internal haemorrhoidal plexuses. Such large haemorrhoids require extensive ablation to ensure adequate treatment in order to prevent residual or recurrent symptoms.

In the past such haemorrhoids had been dealt with by either standard haemorrhoidectomy plus excision of the largest secondary pile with subsequent mucocutaneous reconstitution, or a modification of the whitehead or radical haemorrhoidectomy.[26,27]

These techniques however, are not entirely satisfactory. Patients with large third or fourth degree circumferential prolapsed haemorrhoids deemed not suitable for conventional three-pile haemorrhoidectomy, admitted between January 1992 and June 1993 under the care of one surgeon, were prospectively randomized to undergo either radical haemorrhoidectomy (group 1) of four-pile haemorrhoidectomy (group 2) by opening sealed envelopes in the operating theatre.

In group 2, patients had diathermy excision of the three primary piles.[26] The largest remaining pile-bearing mucocutaneous bridge was then brought down by incising the proximal end of the bridge and dissecting it from the underlying circular sphincter muscle. Haemorrhoidal tissue and excess mucosa were excised. The mucocutaneous bridge was then reconstituted with 00 polyglactin-interrupted sutures.

In group 1, the anorectal mucosa was divided into thirds circumferentially and each third was dealt with in turn. Two pairs of artery forceps were used to cause further prolapse of the normal rectal mucosa above the pile-bearing area and to put this third of the anorectal circumference at a stretch. A suitable point above the dentate line was chosen and an incision made along this line for one-third of the circumference of the anal canal. The mucosal flap was then raised free from the underlying circular internal anal sphincter. Grossly evident haemorrhoidal tissue and excess mucosa were then removed. Devascularization of the flap by overenthusiastic removal of haemorrhoidal tissue was carefully avoided. The flap was then stitched to the proximal divided edge of the rectal mucosa and circular internal sphincter at that point with interrupted 00 polyglactin, thereby pulling the anal skin and mucosa upwards into the anal canal. This level was always at or above that of the previous dentate line. This procedure was repeated for the remaining two-thirds of the anal canal and haemorrhoids. Occasionally, when flap tension was excessive as a result of too much skin or mucosa, circumanal release incisions were made as required.

The results were not entirely satisfactory (Table 1). At six months, two patients with radical haemorrhoidectomy were disappointed with their outcome, ten were satisfied and two thought they had excellent surgery. In the four-pile haemorrhoidectomy group, one patient was disappointed, seven satisfied and six had excellent results. Hence we concluded that four-pile haemorrhoidectomy was significantly easier to perform and although residual tags and piles were left behind, the operation was preferred to radical haemorrhoidectomy. Currently, however, this discussion is immaterial as stapled haemorrhoidectomy adequately deals with most cases of circumferential prolapse.[28]

Table 1. Results of radical and four-pile haemorrhoidectomy.

	Group 1 ($n = 14$)	Group 2 ($n = 14$)
Age (years)*	48 (29–68)	37 (22–56)
Duration of surgery (min)*	30 (5–50)	10 (5–25)‡
Length of hospital stay (days)*	3 (2–6)	3 (2–6)
Skin-releasing incision	2†	0
Secondary or reactionary bleeding	0	0
Complete continence	14	12
Incontinence to fluid	0	1
Incontinence to flatus	0	1
Mucosal ectropion	0	0
Flap dehiscence	5	0§
Re-structuring necessary	5	0
Anal stricture	3	2
St Mark's dilators	2	2
Anoplasty	1	0
Residual skin tags or piles	2	9¶
Residual symptoms	0	2

* Values are median (range).
† Neither of these patients developed flap dehiscence.
‡ $P < 0.0001$ (Wilcoxon's rank sum test).
§ $P < 0.02$.
¶ $P < 0.01$ (Fisher's exact test).

Conventional surgical haemorrhoidectomy, moreover, is based not on a correction of pathophysiology but on ablation of symptoms. Hence, if prolapsed piles are bleeding, painful or otherwise symptomatic, these piles are excised. Piles by themselves are normal vascular cushions and are not pathological.

Prolapsed haemorrhoids are therefore not pathological unless symptomatic. Totally asymptomatic individuals can be made to engorge their anal cushions during proctoscopy by straining down or by doing the Valsalva manoeuvre. This sort of engorgement may be aggravated by straining in the squatting position. Once prolapse occurs, further engorgement of these vascular cushions occurs, leading to pain and inflammatory response. Anal spasm then prevents reduction, and pathological changes with thrombosis, oedema and inflammatory changes occur.

Chronicity is caused by repeated prolapse and congestion of these vascular cushions. The vascular cushions hence prolapse easily and allow the anal sphincters to constrict, resulting in haemorrhoidal congestion, oedema and pain.

Conventional surgical haemorrhoidectomy attacks the symptoms alone without regard to restoration of normal physiology by fixation of the congested anal cushions. Stapled haemorrhoidectomy, on the other hand, corrects the primary pathology, resulting in resolution of haemorrhoidal symptoms.[29] By an elegant reduction of prolapsed haemorrhoidal tissue, the technique then excises redundant lower rectal mucosa and fixes the prolapse back into its proper place on the wall of the anal canal.[30] Fixation of this prolapse into muscle may be important to help prevent subsequent re-dislodgment and recurrence.[29] As previously mentioned, once reduced, the engorged haemorrhoidal tissues rapidly decongest and shrink. This theory is borne out in clinical practice. Our technique of stapled haemorrhoidectomy takes into account these pathophysiological changes and attempts to carefully correct them all.[30]

However, even stapled haemorrhoidectomy on its own cannot deal adequately with very massive haemorrhoidal prolapse. Massive haemorrhoids are prolapsed haemorrhoids more than 3–4 centimetres outside the anal verge. In this situation, there is not enough space within the staple housing to contain the massive redundant tissue of the prolapsed haemorrhoids. If stapling as originally described is performed, much residual haemorrhoids will remain prolapsed and hence symptomatic relief will not be obtained. Thankfully, this situation is very rare. We have now encountered 10 cases out of more than 1600 cases of stapled haemorrhoidectomy done to date.

A modified stapled haemorrhoidectomy technique has been developed in the department to deal with massive haemorrhoidal prolapse with the use of one circular PPH stapler, and we have found it safe and efficacious. This procedure is currently being described.[31]

Stapled haemorrhoidectomy or one of its modifications is an excellent method of dealing with circumferential prolapsed haemorrhoids and indeed is our procedure of choice if surgical therapy for haemorrhoids is deemed necessary.

Conclusions

Haemorrhoidal disease is a common anorectal disease. Its aetiology is likely related to inadequate dietary fibre and straining at defecation. As a result, the supports of the submucosal anal cushions are weakened. Anal cushions are normal structures which line the anal canal. They contain arteriovenous fistulas, which increase and decrease in size according to blood flow. The variation in size has an important function in helping to seal the anal canal, and thus controlling faecal continence. When the anal cushion support is weakened, it becomes susceptible to abnormal engorgement with blood, resulting in symptomatically bleeding and prolapsing haemorrhoids.

In the treatment of haemorrhoids, other possibly life-threatening diseases, such as rectal cancer, have first to be excluded by adequate history, physical examination (including rectal digital examination) and, if necessary, endoscopy. Nonprolapsing and reducible prolapsing piles can usually be treated with preservation of the anal cushions. Fibre supplements alone are effective. However, submucosal injection, rubber band ligation or Daflon 500 may accelerate symptomatic relief. Irreducible prolapsed piles formerly treated by haemorrhoidectomy is now better tackled by stapled haemorrhoidectomy.

References

1. Thompson WHF. The nature of haemorrhoids, *Br J Surg* 1975; 62: 542–52.
2. Haas PA, Fox TA and Haas GP. The pathogenesis of haemorrhoids, *Dis Colon Rectum* 1984; 27: 442–50.

3. Thulesius O and Gjores JE. Arterio-venous anastomoses in the anal region with reference to the pathogenesis and treatment of haemorrhoids, *Acta Chir Scand* 1973; 139: 476–8.

4. Jorge JM and Wexner SD. Anorectal manometry: techniques and clinical applications, *South Med J* 1993; 86: 924–31.

5. Berstein WC. What are haemorrhoids and what is their relationship to the portal venous system? *Dis Colon Rectum* 1983; 26: 829–34.

6. Hanock BD. Internal sphincter and nature of haemorrhoids, *Gut* 1977; 62: 833–6.

7. Johanson JF and Sonnenberg A. Constipation is not a risk factor for haemorrhoids: a case-control study of potential etiological agents, *Am J Gastroenterol* 1994; 89: 1981–6.

8. Moesgaard F, Nielsen ML, Hansen JB and Knudsen JT. High fibre diet reduces bleeding and pain in patients with haemorrhoids, *Dis Colon Rectum* 1992; 25: 454–6.

9. Ho YH. Management of haemorrhoidal disease: a review. *Phlebology* 1997; 15: 3–6.

10. Ho YH and Goh HS. Current value of anorectal physiology and biofeedback in clinical practice, *Asian J Surg* 1995; 18: 244–56.

11. Nicholls J and Glass R. *Coloproctology: Diagnosis and Outpatient Management.* Berlin, Springer-Verlag, 1985.

12. Gardner E, Gray DJ and O'Rahilly R. *Anatomy: A Regional Study of Human Structure.* Philadelphia, WB Saunders, 1975.

13. Keighley MRB and Williams NS. *Surgery of the Anus, Rectum and Colon.* London, WB Saunders, 1993.

14. Jensen SL, Harling H, Tange G, Shokouh-Amiri MH and Nielsen OV. Maintenance bran therapy for prevention of symptoms after rubber band ligation of third degree haemorrhoids, *Acta Chir Scand* 1988; 154: 395–8.

15. Wadworth AN and Faulds D. Hydroxyethylrutosides: a review of its pharmacology, and therapeutic efficacy in venous insufficiency and related disorders, *Drugs* 1992; 44: 1013–32.

16. Duhault J. *Mecanism d'action de Daflon 500 mg sur le tonus veineux noradrenergique, Arteres Veines* 1992; 11: 217–18.

17. Galley P. A double-blind, placebo-controlled trial of a new venoactive flavonoid fraction (S5682) in the treatment of symptomatic fragility, *Int Angiol* 1993; 12: 69–71.

18. Damon M. Effect of chronic treatment with purified falvonoid fraction on inflammatory granuloma in the rat: study of prostaglandin E_2 and

F_2 and thromboxane B_2 release and histological changes, *Arzneimittelforschung/Drug Res* 1987; 37(11)10: 1149–53.

19. Cospite M. Double-blind versus placebo evaluation of clinical activity and safety of Daflon 500 mg in the treatment of acute haemorrhoids, *Angiology* 1994; 6: 566–73.

20. Ho YH, Foo CL, Seow-Choen F and Goh HS. Prospective randomized controlled trial of micronized flavonidic fraction to reduce bleeding after haemorrhoidectomy, *Br J Surg* 1995; 82: 1034–5.

21. Ho YH and Goh HS. Unilateral anal electrosensation—modified technique to improve quantifications of anal sensory loss, *Dis Colon Rectum* 1995; 38: 239–44.

22. Ho YH, Seow-Choen F, Tan M and Leong APFK. Randomised trial of open and closed haemorrhoidectomy, *Br J Surg* 1997; 84: 1729–30.

23. Seow-Choen F, Ho YH, Ang HG and Goh HS. Prospective, randomised trial comparing pain and clinical function after conventional scissor excision/ligation vs diathermy excision without ligation of symptomatic prolapsed haemorrhoids, *Dis Colon Rectum* 1992; 35: 1165–9.

24. Ho YH, Seow-Choen F and Goh HS. Haemorrhoidectomy and disordered rectal and anal physiology in patients with prolapsed haemorrhoids, *Br J Surg* 1995; 82: 596–8.

25. Ho YH, Seow-Choen F, Low JY, Tan M and Leong APKF. Effect of trimebutine (anal sphincter relaxant) on post-haemorrhoidectomy pain tested in a controlled prospective randomised trial, *Br J Surg* 1997; 84: 377–9.

26. Seow-Choen F and Low HC. Prospective randomized study of radical versus four piles haemorrhoidectomy for symptomatic large circumferential prolapsed piles, *Br J Surg* 82: 188–9.

27. Kraemer M and Seow-Choen F. Whitehead haemorrhoidectomy in older patients, *Tech Coloproct* 2000; 4: 79–82.

28. Seow-Choen F. Stapled haemorrhoidectomy: pain or gain, *Br J Surg* 2000; 88: 1–3.

29. Seow-Choen F. Surgery for haemorrhoids—ablation or correction, *Asian J Surg* 2002; 25: 265–6.

30. Lloyd D, Ho KS and Seow-Choen F. Modified Longo's haemorrhoidectomy, *Dis Colon Rectum* 2002; 45: 416–17.

31. Jayne D and Seow-Choen F. Modified stapled haemorrhoidectomy for treatment of massive circumferentially prolapsing piles, *Tech Coloproctol* 2002; 6: 191–3.

CHAPTER 9

Day Case and the Use of Local Anaesthesia in PPH (Stapled) Haemorrhoidectomy

KW Eu

Introduction

Stapled PPH (procedure for prolapsed haemorrhoids) haemorrhoidectomy has received tremendous enthusiasm since its first description by Longo in 1998.[1] It has the potential to be a relatively painless technique for dealing with prolapsing haemorrhoids.[2] Comparison with conventional Milligan–Morgan in randomized controlled trials reveals significant reductions in analgesic requirements and an earlier return to full activities for the stapled haemorrhoidectomy patients.[3–5] Patient satisfaction and quality-of-life assessment are certainly more favourable in the stapled haemorrhoidectomy group of patients as far as short term results are concerned.[6]

Currently, stapled haemorrhoidectomy is a more expensive procedure, although this may be partly offset by an earlier return to work and a shorter hospital stay. Conventional haemorrhoidectomy is commonly performed as a day case procedure and has no significant complications and involves minimal costs.[7,8] We therefore looked at the feasibility of doing stapled haemorrhoidectomy in an ambulatory (day case) setting in order to further decrease the final bill size for the patient.

Day Case Stapled Haemorrhoidectomy

Fifty consecutive patients who had undergone stapled haemorrhoidectomy under general anaesthesia (GA) as day cases (DCs) (mean age 41 years; 27 females) over a 12-month period were compared with 50 consecutive patients who had undergone the same procedure as in-patients (IPs) (mean age 44 years; 25 females). All cases were performed by a single consultant surgeon.

Eight DC patients (16%) were admitted from the day surgery unit for urinary retention (3), pain (3), bleeding (1) and an anaesthetic reason (1). Three of the DC patients were admitted after a mean period of 4 days with bleeding (2), one of which required surgical haemostasis; and a septic complication (1). The mean hospital stay for IP cases was 2.6 (range 1–9) days. Two IP cases were re-admitted after 4 and 11 days for bleeding and wound infection, respectively. At review 2–4 weeks after discharge, satisfaction in both groups was high. Minor staple line strictures were seen in 1 DC and 2 IP cases but all were easily dilated digitally. The mean costs incurred were significantly less for day surgery patients.

We therefore concluded that stapled haemorrhoidectomy is suitable for use in day case surgery as it is a quick and relatively painless procedure. The advantages, particularly financial, support the technique for use in an ambulatory setting, provided detailed patient advice is given.

The relatively painless nature of stapled haemorrhoidectomy perhaps makes it more suitable to be a day case procedure than conventional haemorrhoidectomy, which is already commonly performed in an ambulatory setting with satisfactory results. Recent comparisons with conventional techniques have shown a superior outcome for the stapling technique in terms of reduced pain and a shorter time to return to work. We have also shown in our institution, involving 119 in-patients (62 open diathermy, 57 stapled), that outcomes for function, satisfaction score and quality-of-life assessment between the two groups were similar. The costs incurred, however, were significantly higher in the stapled group on account of the equipment required, although this difference appeared to be partly offset by an earlier return to work. Our study on day case stapled haemorrhoidectomy demonstrated a significant reduction in cost compared with in-patient procedures, thereby allowing an additional cost recovery. The complication rates were also similar whether stapled haemorrhoidectomy was done as day-case or as in-patient. Although the initial admission rates for day case patients seem high (16%), this was so because these patients had undergone surgery in the afternoon. Thus, scheduling the ambulatory procedures for a morning operating list and providing patients with detailed advice about what to expect might prevent the need for admission.

Therefore, we concluded that stapled haemorrhoidectomy can be performed safely as a day case procedure, preferably in the morning. As the indications and techniques for stapled haemorrhoidectomy became more widely accepted and defined, the benefits of its selective use in an ambulatory setting will become increasingly apparent.

Stapled Haemorrhoidectomy Under Local Anaesthesia

The benefits of stapled haemorrhoidectomy, which include a significant reduction in pain, have already been clearly demonstrated. This also makes it possible for use in a day case setting. The prospect of performing such surgery under local anaesthesia as a day case procedure incorporates such benefits and makes the procedure feasible for patients unsuitable for day case general anaesthesia, who could otherwise require overnight stay and incur additional cost.

A prospective study was therefore embarked on to assess the suitability of stapled haemorrhoidectomy under local anaesthesia in a day case setting. Twenty patients who needed stapled haemorrhoidectomy in day surgery were recruited for the study and randomly selected to undergo either local or general anaesthesia.

For patients randomized to the local anaesthetic group, they were first given stat dose of intravenous midazolam intravenously together with Remi-Fentanyl at a dose of 1 mcg per kg body weight. Twenty units of 0.5% Marcaine with adrenaline 1 : 100,000 was injected around the perianal area and into the sphincter complex, followed by gentle digital dilatation of the anal sphincter until the plastic dilator could be easily inserted. The

Table 1. Comparison of outcomes for in-patient and day case stapled haemorrhoidectomy.

	Day cases	In-patients	p value
Total number	50	50	
Sex ratio (M/F)	23/27	25/25	NS[‡]
Mean age (range) [years]	41 (26–61)	44 (27–74)	NS
Mean stay (range) [days]	0.28 (0–6)*	2.6 (1–8)	$p < 0.05$
Number of complications (%)	14 (28)	11 (22)	NS
Number of re-admissions (%)	5 (10)[†]	2 (4)	NS
Mean additional stay for re-admission (days)	2.2	2.5	NS
Mean cost/pts ($S)	1642–72	1965–90	$p < 0.05$

* Includes eight admissions directly from the day case centre.
[†] Excludes admissions from the day case centre.
[‡] NS = not significant.

rest of the operation was as per normal stapled haemorrhoidectomy under general anaesthesia.

Overall, 18 of the 20 (10 GA and 10 LA cases) patients satisfied the criteria for discharge after recovery. One patient in each group required admission. Patient satisfaction, pain scores and post-operative complications were similar in the two groups. There was a slight increase in overall operating time in the local anaesthesic group although it was not statistically significant.

The patients' opinion on the procedure suggests that the combination of local analgesic infiltration and intravenous anxiolytic provides an acceptable combination for the duration of surgery and allows a rapid and uncomplicated recovery.[9] No patients complained of nausea, vomiting or unsteadiness. Pain was not a problem preventing discharge.

We therefore concluded that the benefits of stapled haemorrhoidectomy can be employed to facilitate the use of local anaesthesia in day case haemorrhoidectomy without compromising patient satisfaction or operative technique and valuable theatre time.

References

1. Longo A. Treatment of haemorrhoidal disease by reduction of mucosa and haemorrhoidal prolapse with a circular suturing device: a new procedure. In *Proceedings of the 6th World Congress of Endoscopic Surgery*. Bologna: Monduzzi Editore, 1998: 777–84.

2. Fazio VW. Promise of stapling technique for haemorrhoidectomy, *Lancet* 2000; 355: 768–9.
3. Seow Choen F. Stapled haemorrhoidectomy: pain or gain? *Br J Surg* 2000; 88: 1–3.
4. Mehigan BJ, Monson JR and Hartley JE. Stapling procedure for haemorrhoids versus Milligan–Morgan haemorrhoidectomy: randomised controlled trial, *Lancet* 2000; 355: 782–5.
5. Rowsell M, Bello M and Hemingway DM. Circumferential mucosectomy (stapled haemorrhoidectomy) versus conventional haemorrhoidectomy: randomised controlled trial, *Lancet* 2000; 355: 779–81.
6. Ho YH, Cheong WK, Tsang C, Ho J, Eu KW, Tang CL and Seow Choen F. Stapled haemorrhoidectomy—cost and effectiveness. Randomized controlled trial including incontinence scoring, anorectal manometry and endoanal ultrasound assessments at up to three months, *Dis Colon Rectum* 2000; 43: 1666–75.
7. Carapeti EA, Kamm MA, McDonald PJ and Phillips RK. Double-blind randomised controlled trial of effect of metronidazole on pain after day-case haemorrhoidectomy, *Br J Surg* 1998; 351: 169–72.
8. Carapeti EA, Kamm MA, McDonald PJ, Chadwick SJ and Phillips RK. Randomised trial of open versus closed day-case haemorrhoidectomy, *Br J Surg* 1999; 86: 612–13.
9. Ho KS, Eu KW, Heah SM, Seow-Choen F and Chen YW. Randomised clinical trial of haemorrhoidectomy under a mixture of local anaesthesia versus general anaesthesia, *Br J Surg* 2000; 87: 1–4.

CHAPTER 10

Anal Stenosis

CL Tang

Introduction

Anal stenosis is an abnormal fixed anatomical narrowing of the anal canal associated with a degree of functional obstruction at that level.[1] This is in contrast to the "stenosis" resulting from anal canal spasm secondary to painful lesions (commonly seen in anal fissure).

Aetiology

The aetiology may be manifold, but previous anal surgery is by far the most common cause (Table 1). Recurrent anal fissure, perianal abscess–fistula with repeated surgical procedures, and excessive excision of perianal skin in Bowen's and Paget's disease may heal with anal canal stenosis. Chronic

Table 1. Aetiology of anal stenosis.

Congenital:
imperforate anus, anal atresia

Acquired:
E.g. Lacerations
    Irradiation
    Chronic diarrhoea
    Following surgery of anal canal/low rectum

Neoplastic:
E.g. Perianal or anal cancers
    Leukaemia
    Bowen's disease
    Paget's disease

Inflammatory:
E.g. Crohn's disease
    TB
    Amoebiasis
    Lymphogranuloma venereum
    Actinomycosis

Spastic:
E.g. Chronic anal fissure
    Ischaemic

laxative abuse (especially with the use of mineral oils) over prolonged periods in inmates of nursing homes can lead to anal stenosis. Excessive removal of prolapsed haemorrhoids leaving tenuous mucosal bridges, especially in the emergency setting, often accounts for one of the commonest causes of anal stenosis.

Clinical Presentation

Patients with anal stenosis may present with a history of constipation, decreasing stool calibre, difficulty in voiding with the need to strain excessively, and tenesmus. In severe stenosis, they may only pass loose stool. They may become laxative and enema-dependent. Bleeding occurs when there is associated fissure from traumatic defecation. The diagnosis is obvious on inspection. Very often, passage of the index finger through the narrowing is impossible. The ability to pass the index finger through the narrowing is often taken to be a negative test for clinically significant stenosis. Associated surgical scars may give a clue to the aetiology of the stenosis. A biopsy is essential if a predisposing cause of the anal stenosis is suspected. The magnitude of the symptoms does not usually correspond with the anatomical findings.[2]

Treatment

The key to treatment is in the prevention of post-operative anal stenosis. Excessive removal of the anoderm is often the most common underlying cause of significant anal stenosis. Excessive excision of the perianal skin to achieve a "cosmetically" smooth and even skin contour does not always result in smooth anal function. Surgical judgement leaning towards just adequate excision of the haemorrhoidal tissue and anoderm is often prudent. Eversion of the haemorrhoidal mass and excision may often lead to excessive removal of the anoderm. In particular, the Whitehead procedure for circumferential hemorrhoids often puts the anal canal at risk of developing anal stenosis[3] and an associated mucosal ectropion as the scar contracts outwards towards the perineum. Approximately 87% of the patients with anal stenosis in one series had previous haemorrhoidectomy.[4] In a review of 704 patients[5] who had undergone excisional haemorrhoidectomy (500 elective and 204 emergency cases) over a two-year period, 3.8% developed clinical evidence of anal stenosis. No difference was seen between the elective and emergency cases.

Anal Dilatation

The treatment of anal stenosis depends on the severity and the level of the stenosis in the anal canal. Mild or moderate stenosis (tight anal canal, but permitting the passage of the index finger on pressure or forceful dilatation) may be treated with bulk laxatives, which will increase the stool calibre and provide a dilatation effect. This may be supplemented with either regular self-digital stretching or an appropriately sized anal dilator (e.g. St Mark's anal dilator). Dilatation should be demonstrated to the patient in the clinic. This may be done in a left lateral lying position or with the patient squatting and bearing down onto a well-lubricated (with 4% lignocaine jelly) finger or anal dilator. He should be encouraged to pass the finger or the dilator as far into the anal canal as he can tolerate each time, once or twice daily for two to three weeks. Good functional results

Table 2. Principles of surgical treatment for
anal stenosis.

Stool bulking
Increase anal outlet dimension
Sphincter narrowing—internal sphincterotomy
Cutaneous scarring—removal
Maintain correction
Skin advancement (in)
Mucosal advancement (out)
Colostomy

may be achieved in this manner. The additional use of topical steroids has
no documented benefits.

More severe anal stenosis (unable to pass the index finger through
the stenosis) would require some form of surgical intervention, especially
when symptomatic. The principles of surgical treatment are outlined in
Table 2.[2]

Four-finger manual dilatation performed under anaesthesia is discouraged. This may lead to excessive damage of the anal sphincters with resultant incontinence, especially in the hands of a novice. Jensen *et al.*[6] and
McDonald *et al.*[7] both reported a high rate of faecal incontinence (39% and
24% respectively) after dilatation, especially in the female patients who
already had a pre-existing anatomically short anal canal.

Sphincterotomy

Lateral internal sphincterotomy is particularly useful in dividing any
fibrotic bands. This is simple to perform, and if a single sphincterotomy
is insufficient to open up the stenosis, multiple sphincterotomies may be
done at different positions. Open sphincterotomy has the advantage of
allowing the in-growth of anoderm to maintain the increase in diameter
of the anal canal.[1] Sphincterotomy will provide immediate relief of the
pain and apprehension associated with bowel opening in these patients.
The associated complications of bleeding from inadvertently nicking the
haemorrhoidal vessels (0.3–0.8%), failed healing (2–6%) and abscess formation when the anoderm is accidentally breached in closed sphincterotomy
(0–2.3%) are infrequent and minor. However, impaired faecal continence
has been reported to vary from 11 to 25%, and late faecal incontinence of
some degree from 4 to 35%.[8,9]

Flap Procedures

Mucosal advancement flap

This procedure involves the advancement of anal mucosa into the stenotic area by way of a vertical incision made in the stenotic area perpendicular to the dentate line in the lateral position. An anal sphincterotomy and excision of scar tissue allows widening of the stenosis. The incision is then underminded about two centimetres and closed in a transverse manner with vicryl 3-0, stitching the mucosal edge down onto the skin edge of the anoderm. This creates a minor mucosal ectropion, which will keep the stenosis open. This was described by Martin and subsequently modified by Khubchandani.[2]

Y–V advancement flap

Penn described this in 1948. Essentially, a Y-incision is made with the vertical limb of the Y in the anal canal above the proximal level of the stenosis. The V of the Y is drawn on the lateral perianal skin. The skin is incised and a V-shaped flap is raised. The length-to-breadth ratio must be less than 3.0. After excision of the underlying scar tissue in the anal canal with or without an additional lateral sphincterotomy, the flap can be mobilized into the anal canal and stitched into place. This may be done bilaterally with good results[3,10,11] and relief in 85–92% of cases. Tip necrosis occurs in 10–25% of cases and stenosis may then recur.

V–Y advancement flaps

Unlike the Y–V advancement flap, the V–Y flap has the advantage of bringing a wider piece of skin into the stenosis to keep it open. The V is drawn with the wide base parallel to the dentate line about two centimetres long. A length-to-base ratio similar to that of the Y–V flap should be maintained. Scar tissue is excised. The skin the flap is incised and freed so that it may move without tension into the anal canal. Sufficient subcutaneous tissue must be mobilized with the flap, which derives its blood supply from the perforating vessels arising in the fat. The skin is then closed behind the flap to produce the limb of the Y. The treatment success rate with this flap has been reported to be as high as 96%.[3]

Island advancement flaps

Caplin and Kodner first described these.[12] The flap may be constructed in various shapes, like a diamond, a house or a U. It is mobilized from its lateral margins attached together with the subcutaneous fat after the scar tissue in the stenotic area is excised with or without a lateral sphincterotomy. This procedure has the distinct advantage of bringing a broad skin flap (up to 25% of the circumference) into the entire length of the anal canal and at the same time allowing closure of the donor site. Successful improvement of symptoms may be as high as 91%[13,14] at three years of follow-up. Eighteen to 50% had minor wound separation.[13,14]

S-anoplasty

This procedure mobilizes bilateral gluteal skin into the entire anal canal after excision of the scar tissue up to the dentate line. The incision is designed in an S shape, hence the name of the flap. The flap's breadth-to-length ratio must be more than 1.0, with a base of the limbs of the S about 7–10 cm wide. The skin is rotated to line the anal canal in a tension-free manner. This extensive procedure is rarely used. Prior full bowel preparation and peri-operative antibiotics cover are advocated.[1]

Most of the above treatment and surgical procedures will adequately deal with the post-surgical anal canal stenosis, which usually involves the lower anal canal. Occasionally, higher stenosis (above the dentate line) is encountered. In these instances, a lateral sphincterotomy or division of the fibrotic band is usually sufficient, as the anal canal is more distensible at this level. In perianal Crohn's disease-related anal stenosis, one would try to bring about symptomatic relief with anal dilatation, thereby avoiding surgical wound healing problems.

References

1. Luchtefeld MA and Mazier WP. Anal stenosis. In *Current Therapy in Colon and Rectal Surgery*, VW Fazio (ed.). Philadelphia, Pennsylvania: BC Decker, 1990; 46–59.
2. Khubchandani IT. Anal stenosis, *Surg Clin North Am* 1994; 74: 1353–60.
3. Rosen L. Anoplasty, *Surg Clin North Am* 1988; 68: 1441–6.

4. Milsom JW and Mazier WP. Classification and management of post-surgical anal stenosis, *Surg Gynaecol Obstet* 1986; 163: 60–4.
5. Eu KW, Teoh TA, Seow-Choen F and Goh HS. Anal structure following haemorrhoidectomy: early diagnosis and treatment, *Aust NZ Surg* 1995; 65: 101–3.
6. Jensen SL, Llund F, Nielsen OV and Tange G. Lateral subcutaneous sphincterotomy versus anal dilatation in the treatment of fissure in ano in outpatients: a prospective randomised study, *Br Med J* 1984; 289: 528–30.
7. MacDonald A, Smith A, McNeill AD and Finlay IG. Manual dilatation of the anus, *Br J Surg* 1992; 79: 1381–2.
8. Senagore AJ. Surgery for chronic anal fissure and stenosis. In *Complications of Colon and Rectal Surgery*, Hicks TC, Bek DE, Opelka FG and Timmcke AE (eds.). Baltimore, Maryland: Williams and Wilkins, 1996; 193–202.
9. Prager E. Common ailments of the anorectal region, anal stenosis. In *Operative Colorectal Surgery*, Block GE and Moossa AR (eds.). Philadelphia, Pennsylvania: WB Saunders, 1994; 413–14.
10. Angelchik PD, Harms BA and Stanley JR. Repair of anal stricture and mucosal ectropion with Y–V or pedicle flap anoplasty, *Am J Surg* 1993; 166: 55–9.
11. Ramanujam PS, Venkatesh KS and Cohen M. Y–V anoplasty for severe anal stenosis, *Contemp Surg* 1998; 3: 62–8.
12. Caplin DA and Kodner IJ. Repair of anal stricture and mucosal ectropion by single flap procedures, *Dis Colon Rectum* 1986; 29: 92.
13. Pidala MJ, Slezak FA and Porter JA. Island advancement anoplasty for anal canal stenosis and mucosal ectropion, *Am Surg* 1994; 60: 194–6.
14. Sentovich SM, Falk PM, Christensen MA, Thorson AG, Blatchford GJ and Pitsch RM. Operative results of house advancement anoplasty, *Br J Surg* 1996; 83: 1242–4.

CHAPTER 11

Managing Rectal Prolapse

HM Quah

Introduction

Rectal prolapse is a fairly unusual condition in which the rectum invaginates itself and descends towards the anus. "Internal intussusception", or internal prolapse, is the term used to describe the condition where the prolapse does not protrude from the anus. Overt prolapse occurs when the rectum exits the anus. Both of these conditions must be differentiated from mucosal prolapse, in which the mucous membrane of the rectum and anus protrudes; this is not a full-thickness prolapse but, rather, a manifestation of significant haemorrhoidial disease, and is treated as such.

History

The history of rectal prolapse is a long one, having been described since Egyptian times. In a detailed review of the history of this disease over time, Roberts[1] recounts the methods used by Hippocrates to treat this disease, with the application of caustics followed by reduction of the prolapse and binding of the buttocks; this is not dissimilar to the treatment of this disease in infants even today. Upside-down suspension to facilitate reduction enjoyed a long period of popularity; methods to hold the prolapse in place are a testimony to the ingenuity of the physicians treating this dramatic condition. Definitive surgical procedures to treat prolapse in the 19th century focused on perineal approaches; abdominal operations were still excessively morbid, particularly when an anastomosis of the bowel was performed. As the associated anatomical abnormalities in rectal prolapse became more understood, and as abdominal surgery became safer, anterior resection and then sigmoid resection and rectopexy became more common, beginning in the 1950s. Fixation of the rectum to the sacrum without resection became the alternative abdominal procedure at about the same time. To date, well over 100 procedures have been described to treat this condition and debate continues regarding the most appropriate approach.

Pathophysiology

Several anatomical abnormalities are present in patients with full-thickness rectal prolapse. It is still unclear whether these are primary aetiological factors or are secondary to the still unknown primary cause. These abnormalities include:

- Deep anterior cul-de-sac
- Diastasis of the levator muscles
- Loss of posterior fixation of the rectum
- Patulous anal sphincter
- Redundant sigmoid colon

All operations are designed to repair some or all of these abnormalities. The goal is to restore not only normal anatomy but, more importantly, normal function.

Early theories regarding the aetiology of prolapse centred upon the belief that the initiating factor was a sliding hernia of the cul-de-sac. This belief made the initial descriptions of the perineal rectosigmoidectomy difficult to understand. With the advent of defaecography, it became clear that the primary abnormality is intussusception of the rectum, which may be eccentric due to the presence of a deep cul-de-sac within the anterior part of the prolapse with an associated enterocele. Nevertheless, the invagination of the rectum is the inciting event.

Associated physiological abnormalities include anal incontinence in approximately 50% of patients with rectal prolapse. This is due to pudendal nerve stretch injury, with chronic denervation of the sphincters. Mechanical stretching of the sphincters by the prolapse itself is of secondary importance. Constipation is also seen in a high percentage of patients with rectal prolapse; some have evacuation abnormalities such as non-relaxing puborectalis muscle, some have perineal descent syndrome and some may have abnormal motility of the colon, as yet undefined. The presence of constipation must be taken into account when planning therapy.

Clinical Features

Rectal prolapse is a disease of the extremes of age, affecting infants up to three years old and the elderly. The disease is much more common in women in the elderly age group, by a 10–15 : 1 ratio. In children the two sexes are affected equally; and men are affected at any age, unlike women, who tend to be in the seventh to ninth decades. The majority of women are nulliparous or, at least, have not had many vaginal deliveries. Women may have other manifestations of pelvic relaxation, such as cystocele, rectocele and uterine or vaginal vault prolapse. In the past, it was believed that there were a disproportionate number of people with underlying psychiatric disturbances, particularly depression.

The clinical symptoms are primarily those of protrusion. Initially, the prolapse comes only with straining and will spontaneously reduce after defecation. As the disease progresses, anything that increases intraabdominal pressure results in prolapse, and reduction may be difficult or even impossible. Mucosal irritation results in bleeding and the passage of mucus. Incontinence and constipation are both common. Rarely, the prolapse can become incarcerated and even strangulated, requiring prompt intervention.

Rectal prolapse is generally readily appreciable on physical examination. If the patient cannot produce the prolapse, administration of a disposable enema and examination after defecation will reveal the typical intussusception with concentric folds. This must be distinguished from mucosal prolapse, in which the folds are radial in nature. Palpation of a true rectal prolapse will yield the double thickness nature of the prolapsed rectum. After reduction of the rectum, digital rectal examination should assess the function of the sphincter during rest and squeeze. Endoscopic examination, at least of the rectum, should exclude the presence of a tumour as a lead point of the intussusception. Biopsies of lesions should be performed; these include mass lesions and ulcers, which may be colitis cystica profunda or solitary rectal ulcers. Total colonic evaluation, either by air contrast barium enema or by colonoscopy, should be done in all older patients prior to planning operative treatment.

Treatment

Treatment of rectal prolapse is predominantly surgical in nature; the exception is infants, in whom reduction of the prolapse, correction of the constipation and time are most often successful in preventing operation as the fixation of the rectum to the sacrum becomes secure. Choice of operation depends on associated anatomical and functional abnormalities as well as the overall medical and functional status of the patient. In general, operations for rectal prolapse are divided into transabdominal and perineal approaches.

Abdominal approaches

Transabdominal operations are basically divided into suspension/fixation operations and resection operations. The most commonly used of these include:

- Suspension/fixation
- Ripstein: anterior suspension
- Wells: posterior suspension
- Resection
- Anterior resection
- Sigmoid resection/rectopexy

The Ripstein procedure is one of the most commonly used rectal fixation operations. It involves completely wrapping the mobilized rectum with a foreign material and suturing it to the sacrum. It gives similar results to the Wells procedure. Proponents of the suspension procedures cite the lack of an anastomosis as the significant advantage of this approach. Numerous materials and technical modifications have been tried in an effort to prevent foreign material erosion, stenosis from fibrosis and infection. Most of the suspension procedures have a recurrent prolapse rate of 0–13% when followed sufficiently long. There is also an incidence of stenosis with obstructive symptoms of 2–5%.[2]

Advocates of resection for prolapse properly point out that the problems of constipation are often relieved rather than aggravated by removing the redundant sigmoid colon. In addition, resection of the sigmoid colon results in straightening and a decrease in the motility of the left colon, and hence a reduced chance of torsion and volvulus. The other advantages of resection include the absence of foreign material and the fact that it is a relatively simple surgical procedure. Modern surgical techniques allow performance of an anastomosis with clinical leak rates of less than 3%. Proper performance of a resection for prolapse requires mobilization of the rectum, at least posteriorly. For patients with documented slow transit constipation and no pelvic outlet obstruction, subtotal colectomy has been recommended by some surgeons, with good results.[3] The combined colonic resection and rectopexy is also commonly performed. This makes use of the advantages of resection and avoids the disadvantages of rectopexy alone, especially with regard to constipation. The recurrence rates for resection rectopexy range from 2 to 8%.[3,4]

Perineal procedures

Perineal procedures in common use include:

- Encirclement (Thiersch)
- Delorme
- Perineal rectosigmoidectomy

Anal encirclement operations are designed to hold the prolapse inside the anus by tightening the anal orifice. Many technical modifications since the original silver wire have been described, all of which involve placement of a foreign body around the anus at some level. This approach is probably of historical interest only, due to the high failure rate of 20–60% and the high risk of faecal impaction.

The Delorme operation is one in which a mucosectomy is performed circumferentially to denude the muscularis of the prolapsed segment, followed by reefing of the muscle to create a barrier to prolapse. The recurrence rates in relatively small series are in the 5–21% range;[5–8] the advantage over the encirclement procedures is the lack of a foreign body and some tightening of the sphincter muscle with resultant improvement in function. This procedure, while quite commonly performed in the UK in elderly and unfit patients, is rarely used in the USA.

Perineal rectosigmoidectomy was first described by Mikulicz and re-popularized by Altemeier.[9] This operation involves transanal resection of the prolapse with repair of the lax musculature of the pelvic floor. Williams *et al.*[10] showed that inclusion of a levatoplasty procedure in patients undergoing rectosigmoidectomy significantly improves continence after operation. The recurrence rates range from 0 to 44%.[9–12]

Recurrent Rectal Prolapse[2]

Most surgical procedures described for rectal prolapse can achieve a satisfactory success rate and fairly low recurrence, with the exception of Thiersch anal encirclement. The true incidence of recurrence is, however, difficult to determine, as there is under-reporting by most authors. Also, the duration and method of follow-up are not stated in most series. It has been said that the longer the follow-up, the higher the incidence of recurrence of prolapse, which may occur up to 10 years after surgery. Mucosal prolapse, which occurs in 5–10% of patients following surgery, is not generally considered a proper recurrence; it is easily treated by rubber band ligation or simple mucosal excision.

Surgeons who strongly advise perineal procedures for rectal prolapse claim that these are less major than abdominal procedures and have the advantage of repeatability. Williams *et al.*[10] claim that a repeat perineal rectosigmoidectomy for rectal prolapse can be performed easily, with low morbidity. Proponents of abdominal surgery for rectal prolapse, however, disagree. They claim that a repeat abdominal operation can also be performed and that abdominal procedures are less likely to create a recurrence to begin with.

Not all recurrent prolapses require surgery. A trial of conservative measures should first be advised, especially if the prolapse is small and asymptomatic. However, regardless of the nature of the surgery, there is a small group of patients who have undergone multiple operations for recurrent prolapses, which have failed. There is also a group who remain severely symptomatic, for instance with continued incontinence, despite having a satisfactory correction of the anatomical rectal abnormality. These two groups of patients may benefit from the creation of a diverting colostomy, which is usually performed as a salvage procedure in less than 1% of all patients with rectal prolapse.

Recent Advances in Management

The feasibility of laparoscopic surgery in the management of rectal prolapse has been demonstrated in several recent reports, and it has attractive features.[13–15] Rectal prolapse is a benign condition and so causes no concern about resection margins. Furthermore, no resection may be needed in many instances. Mobilization of the rectum laparoscopically has been shown to be safe and effective.

Conclusion

The surgical management of rectal prolapse has evolved from the historic Thiersch anal encirclement procedure to the present laparoscopic rectopexy. Selection of the most appropriate surgical operation continues to be problematic for surgeons. At this institution we prefer a laparoscopically assisted resection rectopexy, especially in the young and fit patient with a significant history of constipation. A perineal procedure, such as Delorme or perineal rectosigmoidectomy, is usually reserved for the older, high-risk patient. One must remember that success in the management of rectal prolapse is not simply the correction of the physical and mechanical abnormality; functional aspects are also important. The ideal surgical technique should, therefore, not only be based on the elements of simplicity, recurrence and complications, but should also take into account the treatment or at least the alleviation of the functional disorder so commonly associated with rectal prolapse.

References

1. Roberts PL. History of the treatment of rectal prolapse, *Perspectives in Colon and Rectal Surgery* 1995; 8: 95–104.
2. Eu KW and Seow-Choen F. Functional problems in adult rectal prolapse and controversies in surgical treatment, *Br J Surg* 1997; 84: 904–11.

3. Madoff RD, Williams JG, Wong WD, Rothenberger DA and Goldberg SM. Long-term functional results of colon resection and rectopexy for overt rectal prolapse, *Am J Gastroenterol* 1992; 87: 101–4.

4. Watts JD, Rothenberger DA, Buls JG, Goldberg SM and Nivatvongs S. The management of procidentia. 30 years' experience, *Dis Colon Rectum* 1985; 28: 96–102.

5. Christiansen J and Kirkegaard P. Delorme's operation for complete rectal prolapse, *Br J Surg* 1981; 68: 537–8.

6. Graf W, Ejerblad S, Krog M, Pahlman L and Gerdin B. Delorme's operation for rectal prolapse in elderly or unfit patients. *Eur J Surg* 1992; 158: 555–7.

7. Gundersen AL, Cogbill TH and Landercasper J. Reappraisal of Delorme's procedure for rectal prolapse, *Dis Colon Rectum* 1985; 28: 721–4.

8. Monson JR, Jones NA, Vowden P and Brennan TG. Delorme's operation: the first choice in complete rectal prolapse? *Ann R Coll Surg Engl* 1986; 68: 143–6.

9. Altemeier WA, Culbertson WR, Schowengerdt C and Hunt J. Nineteen years' experience with the one-stage perineal repair of rectal prolapse, *Ann Surg* 1971; 173: 993–1006.

10. Williams JG, Rothenberger DA, Madoff RD and Goldberg SM. Treatment of rectal prolapse in the elderly by perineal rectosigmoidectomy, *Dis Colon Rectum* 1992; 35: 830–4.

11. Finlay IG and Aitchison M. Perineal excision of the rectum for prolapse in the elderly, *Br J Surg* 1991; 78: 687–9.

12. Johansen OB, Wexner SD, Daniel N, Nogueras JJ and Jagelman DG. Perineal rectosigmoidectomy in the elderly, *Dis Colon Rectum* 1993; 36: 767–72.

13. Solomon MJ, Young CJ, Eyers AA and Roberts RA. Randomized clinical trial of laparoscopic versus open abdominal rectopexy for rectal prolapse, *Br J Surg* 2002; 89: 35–9.

14. Heah SM, Hartley JE, Hurley J, Duthie GS and Monson JR. Laparoscopic suture rectopexy without resection is effective treatment for full-thickness rectal prolapse, *Dis Colon Rectum* 2000; 43: 638–43.

15. Kessler H, Jerby BL and Milsom JW. Successful treatment of rectal prolapse by laparoscopic suture rectopexy, *Surg Endosc* 1999; 13: 858–61.

CHAPTER 12

Solitary Rectal Ulcer Syndrome

JF Lim

Introduction

Solitary rectal ulcer syndrome (SRUS) was coined as an entity in 1969 by Madigan and Morson.[1] It is a rare condition, with a reported annual incidence of 1–3.6 persons per 100 000.[2] The majority of patients present before the age of 50 and there is a slight female preponderance.[2]

Clinical History

Patients with SRUS classically present with fresh rectal bleeding, passage of mucus, straining, tenesmus and deep rectal pain. There is almost always a history of digitation associated with dysfunctional defecation. Surprisingly, up to 25% of patients may not have any complaints.[3]

Physical examination is usually normal except for the anorectal region. The physician should actively search for rectal prolapse. Perineal descent may be present. Digital rectal examination may reveal thickening of the anterior rectal mucosa or nodular changes consistent with an ulcer.

Proctoscopy and sigmoidoscopy are crucial and may be diagnostic. On proctoscopy, one may find oedema or erythema of the anterior rectal mucosa about 4–8 cm from the anal verge. Only about half will have frank ulceration. Ulcerations may be multiple and may not be at the 12 o'clock position. If the patient is asked to strain, there might be internal intussusception present. Polypoidal lesions are seen in about 25% of cases with or without ulceration.[2,3]

Histology

The diagnosis of SRUS is confirmed on histology,[4] so biopsy is mandatory. In fact, SRUS is a misnomer as ulceration is not necessary for making the diagnosis.

The mucosa is elongated with distorted glands, especially at the base. Sometimes the glands may be displaced into the submucosa. The lamina propria is oedematous and contains a proliferation of fibroblasts. There is fibromuscular thickening, especially the inner circular layer of the muscularis propria, decussation of the two muscular layers, nodular induration of the inner layer and grouping of the outer layer into bundles. Degeneration of the upper epithelium of the crypts, surface erosion, engorgement of the superficial capillaries and a lack of inflammatory cells are classical. The differential diagnoses of these histological features are ischaemic colitis and rectal endometriosis.

Investigations

This condition is a form of pelvic floor dysfunction and is rarely isolated in presentation. As such, anal manometry and physiological testing are necessary for the work-up of the patient. A normal resting pressure, decreased squeeze pressure and hypersensitive rectum are found on anal manometry.[5,6]

Defaecography has a limited diagnostic use but is important in looking for concomitant disorders like rectocoele or rectal intussusception, which is present in up to 80% of defecograms done for SRUS.[7] A barium enema is commonly used to exclude any concomitant colonic pathology, like a cancer, but certain features might be present, like nodularity of the rectal mucosa or thickening of the rectal folds.[7] These features are not pathognomonic and I prefer to use colonoscopy. Endorectal ultrasound is also of limited use as the features of SRUS on ultrasound are not pathognomonic.

Aetiology

We are still unclear about the aetiology of this condition. The general belief is that there is repeated obstructed defecation, leading to intussusception and ischaemia of the rectal mucosa caused by pressure necrosis and fibrous obliteration of the submucosal vessels. Thomson described a different aetiology where the only abnormality is direct trauma from repeated digitation of the rectum.[8] I do not think these two theories are exclusive. It is my theory that the patient has a primary problem of obstructed defecation and excessive straining which leads to rectal mucosal prolapse or intussusception. Most of the patients have used digital manoeuvres (usually transvaginal in the female group) or enemas to aid evacuation. The direct trauma from the digit or enema introducer will cause mucosal damage, which leads to ulceration because of ischaemia and poor healing.

Treatment

Given all that I have mentioned, therapy should be aimed at restoring the pattern of normal defecation and correcting concomitant pathologies like intussusception or rectal prolapse.

The patient should be instructed in a high-fibre diet. The surgeon should explain the condition to the patient and stress the need to avoid excessive straining and digitation. If necessary, some laxatives may be required.

Biofeedback has shown promising results.[9,10] It is a form of pelvic floor retraining and an excellent opportunity for behavioural assessment.

Surgery should only be undertaken once medical treatments are exhausted or if there are anatomical abnormalities which need addressing. If there is bleeding from the ulcer, an intralesional adrenaline injection much like that for posthaemorrhoidectomy bleeding[11] can be used. In the case of occult rectal prolapse or intussusception, rectopexy should be offered. An alternative is Delorme's procedure. Of course, all patients undergoing surgery should have stool-bulking agents and laxatives in the perioperative period as well as postoperative biofeedback. There is little data that doing this will improve the results, but there is no reason why the surgery will be enough if the primary disorder is not addressed. Furthermore, results of operative treatment have not been encouraging. Sometimes surgery even aggravates the problem.

In summary, SRUS is an uncommon condition which is most challenging to manage. One must not focus on the ulcer but must remember to treat the underlying defecatory problem as well. Much of the management is medical and behavioural and operative results are less than optimal.

References

1. Madigan MR and Morson BC. Solitary rectal ulcer of the rectum, *Gut* 1969; 10: 871.
2. Haray PN, Morris-Stiff GJ and Foster ME. Solitary rectal ulcer syndrome—an underdiagnosed condition, *Int J Colorectal Dis* 1997; 12: 313.
3. Tjandra JJ, Fazio VW, Church JM *et al.* Clinical conundrum of solitary rectal ulcer, *Dis Colon Rectum* 1997; 35: 227.
4. Kang YS, Kamm MA, Engel AF *et al.* Pathology of the rectal wall in solitary rectal ulcer syndrome, *Gut* 1996; 38: 587.
5. Snooks SJ, Nicholls RJ, Henry MM *et al.* Electrophysiological and manometric assessment of the pelvic floor in the solitary rectal ulcer syndrome, *Br J Surg* 1985; 72: 131.
6. Ho YH, Ho JM, Parry BR *et al.* Solitary rectal ulcer syndrome: the clinical entity and anorectal physiological findings in Singapore, *Aust N Z J Surg* 1995; 65: 93.
7. Millward SF, Bayjoo P, Dixon MF *et al.* The barium enema appearances in solitary rectal ulcer syndrome, *Clin Radiol* 1995; 11: 187.
8. Thomson WH and Hill D. Solitary rectal ulcer: always a self-induced condition? *Br J Surg* 1980; 67: 784.
9. Binnie NR, Papachrysostomou M, Clare N *et al.* Solitary rectal ulcer: the place of biofeedback and surgery in the treatment of the syndrome, *World J Surg* 1992; 16: 836.

10. Vaizey CJ, Roy AJ and Kamm MA. Prospective evaluation of the treatment of solitary rectal ulcer syndrome with biofeedback. *Gut* 1997; 41: 817.

11. Nyam DCNK, Seow-Choen F and Ho YH. Submucosal adrenaline injection for posthaemorrhoidectomy haemorrhage, *Dis Colon Rectum* 1995; 38: 776.

CHAPTER 13

Anorectal Trauma and Foreign Bodies

KW Eu

Introduction

Anorectal trauma and perforation are uncommon in civilian practice and most surgeons are unlikely to have much experience with their management. Morbidity and mortality following rectal trauma remain considerable.[1,2] A dramatic fall in mortality following rectal perforation from 67% in World War I to 5.4% in World War II was attributed to the use of colostomy, presacral drainage, availability of antibiotics and blood transfusion.[3,4] Abcarian *et al.* in 1989 reported a mortality of 2.5% and a morbidity ranging from 2.5 to 63%, by adherence to conservative principles of "no anastomosis" in the overwhelming majority of cases.[5] However, despite this fall in mortality, controversies still remain in the management of rectal perforation.

The rectum can be injured in many ways. Gunshot wounds that traverse the pelvis, impalement injuries of the perineum, blunt trauma that causes displaced pelvic fractures and rectal foreign bodies could all cause significant rectal injury.

Full-thickness rectal wall injuries require surgical treatment regardless of the mode of injury. The location of the injury is also important, as treatment for intraperitoneal and extraperitoneal rectal injuries varies significantly. Rectal foreign bodies pose a special problem, because in addition to dealing with the rectal injury, the foreign body needs to be removed.

Diagnosis of Rectal Injuries

A rectal injury must be suspected in any patient who sustains a transpelvic wound. A rectal digital examination is essential in all such patients.

Injuries in the distal rectum may be palpable. Detection of gross blood on the glove is diagnostic of large bowel injury.

A sigmoidoscopy should also be performed in all patients at risk unless the patient is haemodynamically unstable. This is true even for patients who require a laparotomy for other injuries. Patients who are to undergo a laparotomy are best examined with the sigmoidoscope under general anaesthesia. This will allow a more complete examination.

It must be stressed that when findings are inconclusive, a rectal injury cannot be excluded. Occasionally, an acceptable alternative would be to perform a limited gastrograffin enema. A CT scan with oral, rectal and intravenous contrast may be indicated if all else fails.

Surgical Management of Full-Thickness Rectal Injuries

The most common cause of death in patients with anorectal trauma who survive the initial 48 hours is sepsis. All surgeons have stressed the role of parenteral antibiotics and this should cover both aerobic and anaerobic organisms. The antibiotics should be administered preoperatively and discontinued after two to three postoperative doses unless sepsis continues.

Intraperitoneal rectal perforations are treated like colonic perforations. When feasible, primary closures without diversion may be carried out. Proximal diversion in the form of a loop colostomy can be added if there is

Table 1. Rectal trauma result.

Author, Year	Number of patients	Morbidity	(%)
Robertson,[8] 1982	36	0	(0)
Vitale,[9] 1983	32	2	(6)
Grasberger,[10] 1983	20	2	(10)
Tuggle,[11] 1984	47	0	(0)
Magiante,[12] 1986	43	0	(0)
Brunner,[13] 1987	25	4	(16)
Shannon,[14] 1988	27	1	(4)
Burch,[1] 1989	100	4	(4)
Ivatory,[6] 1991	54	3	(5)
Total	384	16	(4)

sufficient concern about the repair. However, if the rectal perforation is not amenable to primary repair, then a Hartmann's pouch and end colostomy should be considered.

The usual treatment for full-thickness extraperitoneal rectal perforation includes:

- Proximal colostomy
- Primary repair of the injury, if possible
- Pre-sacral drainage
- Distal rectal washout

The mainstay of treatment in patients with extraperitoneal rectal perforation is faecal diversion. Both loop and end colostomy are feasible, giving similar outcomes postoperatively.[7] Whether presacral drainage, primary repair of the rectal perforation and distal rectal washout make a difference in the eventual outcome of extraperitoneal rectal perforation remains controversial. However, till a randomized trial is conducted to answer some of these controversies, these should be routinely performed.

In general, it has been reported that the mean mortality rate is 4% and the rate of intra-abdominal infection and rectal fistula formation is 12% in patients with penetrating rectal injuries (Table 1).

Rectal Foreign Bodies

Most rectal foreign bodies that require removal have been inserted transrectally. Rarely does an orally ingested object lodge in the rectum.

Most patients present with the foreign body in place and pose a special challenge to the surgeon. In addition to assessing the rectum for injury, the foreign body must be removed. Fortunately, most rectal foreign bodies can be removed transanally and do not cause significant rectal injury. However, in some cases, transabdominal surgery may be necessary.

Diagnosis and Assessment

Immediate surgery is rarely indicated unless a full-thickness perforation is identified or if the patient presents with massive haemorrhage. Rectal perforation identified should be treated as discussed earlier.

The majority of patients will present without signs or symptoms of perforation. A thorough history must be obtained, including information regarding the time of insertion and description of the object(s). The perineum should be inspected for lacerations or bruising that resulted from traumatic insertion of the foreign body. Low-lying foreign bodies may be palpable on digital examination. Plain abdominal X-rays will reveal radio-opaque objects. Sigmoidoscopy may be helpful in determining the level and orientation of high-lying foreign bodies.

Questions regarding sexual practices and the use of foreign bodies should also be asked and may be of medico-legal significance.

Retrieval of the Foreign Body

Low rectal foreign bodies can be retrieved transanally. This can be performed in either the operating theatre or the emergency room. The operating room is preferable, as it is better-equipped and conversion to a laparotomy is easy if required.

The lithotomy position is best for foreign body extraction. An effective sphincter block will allow maximal anal dilatation. If this fails, then general anaesthesia may be required.

With adequate anal sphincter relaxation, an anal retractor is inserted. Hopefully, the object can then be visualized and grasped digitally with an instrument and removed. A pair of sponge forceps is ideal in most cases for grasping foreign bodies. There are numerous other devices, including the foleys or fogarty catheters, to assist in retrieval.[15,16]

High-lying objects may need to be milked down into the low rectum via the abdomen before removing it transanally.

If transanal removal proves unsuccessful, a laparotomy will be necessary. The same is true for proximal objects that cannot be milked down into the low rectum. At laparotomy, the foreign body can then be milked down into the rectum and removed. Alternatively, a colotomy is closed primarily. The rectum and distal colon should also be carefully examined to ascertain whether other significant injuries are present which require treatment.

Conclusion

The management of anorectal trauma and foreign bodies obviously requires an individualized approach based on sound surgical principles, hence minimizing morbidity and mortality in this uncommon form of trauma.

References

1. Burch JM, Feliciano DV and Mattox KL. Colostomy and drainage for civilian rectal injuries; is that all? *Ann Surg* 1989; 209: 600–10.
2. Eu KW, Seow-Choen F and Goh HS. Unusual rectal perforation—an individualised approach to management, *Singapore Med J* 1994: 35: 79–81.
3. Wallace C. Gunshot wounds of the abdomen, *BR J Surg* 1917; 4: 679–43.
4. Taylor ER and Thompson JE. The early treatment and results there of if the injuries of the colon and rectum, *Internal Abstr Surg* 1984; 87: 209–28.
5. Orsay CP, Merlolti G, Abcarian H, Pearl RK, Nanda M and Barrett J. Colorectal trauma, *Dis Colon Rectum* 1989; 32: 188–90.
6. Ivatory RR, Licata J, Gunduz Y, Rao P and Stabil WM. Management option in penetrating rectal injuries, *Am Surg* 1991; 57: 50.
7. Lavenson GS and Cohen A. Management of rectal injuries, *Am J Surg* 1971; 122: 226.
8. Robertson HD, Ferrari BT and Ray JE. Management of rectal trauma, *Surg Gynecol Obstet* 1982; 154: 161.
9. Vitale GC, Richardson JD and Flint LM. Successful management of injuries to the extraperitoneal rectum, *Am Surg* 1983; 49: 159.

10. Grasberger RC and Hirsch EF. Rectal Trauma: a retrospective analysis and guidelines for therapy, *Am J Surg* 1983; 145: 795.
11. Tuggle D and Hwa PJ. Management of rectal trauma, *Am J Surg* 1984; 148: 806.
12. Magiante EC, Graham AD and Fabian TC. Rectal gunshot wounds: management of civilian injuries, *Am Surg* 1986; 52: 37.
13. Brunner RG and Shatney CA. Diagnostic and therapeutic aspects of rectal trauma: blunt versus penetrating, *Am Surg* 1987; 53: 215.
14. Shannon FC, Morre EE and Moore FA. Value of distal colonic washout in civilian rectal trauma: reducing gut bacterial translocation, *J Trauma* 1988; 28: 989.
15. Wigle RC. Emergency department management of retained rectal foreign bodies, *Am J Emerg Med* 1988; 6: 385.
16. Coltharst JR. How to remove a rectal foreign body, *Br J Hosp Med* 1990; 43: 329.

CHAPTER 14

Selective Versus Routine Sedation During Colonoscopy: The Surgeon Factor

F Seow-Choen, CL Tang and KW Eu

Introduction

Colonoscopy can be uncomfortable for some patients. For this reason, conscious sedation has been the prevailing practice in many centres throughout the world. All regimens for conscious sedation involve titrating for the minimal required dose and monitoring to avoid the side effects of over-sedation.[1] In frail elderly patients with concomitant cardiovascular or respiratory disorders, the risk of over-sedation with hypotension and respiratory depression may be significant.[2,3]

Some investigators have therefore questioned the need for routine sedation during colonoscopy.[4–8] Recent studies showed that given a choice, only a tenth or less of all patients will require sedation. It is well tolerated by the rest and the majority will agree to another colonoscopy procedure without sedation.[5-8] Nonetheless, some surgeons insist on routine sedation during colonoscopy as it is thought to be painful by them. In this unit routine non-sedation is preferred; conscious sedation is used only for patients who find the procedure painful. In this way we have found that most patients can be managed without sedation. Throughput as well as staff and patient satisfaction increased. We recently looked at our own experience with non-sedation during colonoscopy.

Patients and Methods

From a computerized database, all colonoscopy procedures performed in the Department of Colorectal Surgery, Singapore General Hospital, during the period from 1 April 1992 to 1 November 1998 were analyzed. Sedation in the department consists of midazolam and is normally given in 1 mg increments until the patient is comfortable during colonoscopy. Surgeons who sedated more than 70% of their patients over this period of time were classified as routine sedaters (RSs) and surgeons who did not sedate more than 70% of their patients over this period of time were classified as selective sedaters (SSs). SSs sedated patients only when pain was present during colonocopy and not as a routine before starting colonoscopy. RSs sedated all patients prior to colonoscopy. The parameters examined included age and sex of patients, diagnosis, duration of procedure, success rate of examination, complications and any mortality. A successful examination was defined as intubation of the ileum or caecum. Failure was observed due to patient intolerance, inherent difficult colonic anatomy or inadequate technique. The number of colonoscopy procedures done with sedation and without sedation was tabulated on an annual basis from 1992 till 1998.

All data were examined for symmetry of distribution using stem and leaf plots. Continuous variables were compared using a simple t-test and categorical data was analyzed using the chi-quare test. A p-value of 0.05 was deemed to be statistically significant.

Results

A total of 17 472 colonoscopy procedures were performed by seven consultant colorectal surgeons during the period of study. Prior to 1 April 1992, all patients undergoing colonoscopy were routinely sedated. There were 6460 procedures (40%) performed in the SS group by two surgeons and 11 012 procedures (60%) in the RS group by five surgeons. In our hospital, the cost of one ampoule of IV 2.5 mg Midazolam is US$1.41 and that of IV Flumazanil is US$30.58.

Patient demographics were similar between the RS group and the SS group. The mean age of the patients in the RS group was 54.3 years (s.e.m. 0.15), versus 54.6 years (s.e.m. 0.19) in the SS group ($p = 0.22$). The male-to-female ratio was 1.09 and 1.08 in the RS and SS groups, respectively ($p = 0.73$). Colonoscopic diagnosis was also similar in distribution between the two groups (Table 1). Overall the most common pathological diagnoses were haemorrhoids (12.2%), colonic polyps (9.8%), functional disorders (9.5%), cancers (6.9%) and diverticular disease (4.8%). 36.8% of colonoscopies were normal. Cancer and polyp follow-up accounted for 13.7% of all procedures done.

The mean duration of colonoscopy procedures was 7.5 min (s.e.m. 0.058) for the SS group, versus 10.2 min (s.e.m. 0.059) for the RS group ($p < 0.0001$). Successful intubation rates were similar, with success rates of 98.5% and 98.2% for SS and RS, respectively. Failure rates were similar, at 1.5% for SS and 1.8% for RS. Morbidity was low (0.1% in the SS group vs. 0.3% in the RS group; $p < 0.01$). The most common complications were respiratory depression, cardiovascular changes (e.g. bradycardia),

Table 1. Diagnosis of patients undergoing colonoscopy by selective and routine sedaters.

	Selective sedater (SS)	Routine sedater (RS)	Total (%)
Cancer	406	775	6.9
Benign neoplasm	624	1071	9.8
Imflammatory bowel disease	70	107	1.0
Ischaemic colitis	26	59	0.5
Radiation colitis	48	94	0.8
Infective colitis	2	15	0.1
Diverticular disease	331	494	4.8
Functional disorders/constipation	301	1340	9.5
Volvulus	6	12	0.1
Follow-up for cancer resection	693	1004	9.9
Polyp follow-up	149	509	3.8
Haemorrhoids	625	1479	12.2
Others, including mixed diagnoses	242	390	3.7
Normal findings	2894	3440	36.8

Table 2. Morbidity associated with patients undergoing selective and routine sedation for colonoscopy. Significant respiratory depression implies the need for reversal of Midazolam. Minor respiratory depression is not recorded.

Complication	Selective sedation	Routine sedation	p
Perforation	1	2	ns
Respiratory depression	5	26	0.02
Postpolypectomy bleeding	1	2	ns
Aspiration pneumonia	—	1	ns
Angina pectoris	—	2	ns
Total	7	33	0.01
Total Patients	6460	11 012	17 472

ECG changes and postcolonoscopic bleeding. There were only three perforations in 17 472 procedures, two of which were delayed perforation following polypectomy (Table 2). Minor respiratory depression without adverse sequelae may be common with sedation, but such data was not obtainable in this retrospective review.

Amongst the surgeons who practised selective sedation, there was a steady increase in the proportion of procedures performed without sedation, from 47% in 1993 to 90.5% (Table 3). In the group of surgeons who practised routine sedation, there was a small increase in the practice of withholding sedation, from 1.7% in 1993 to 39.6% in 1996, and then a decrease again, to 15.6% in 1998 (Table 4). RS surgeons were asked why they needed to sedate most of their patients, and the invariable answers included "because my patients need sedation as colonoscopy is painful". SS surgeons were asked the reason why most of their patients did not need sedation, and the answers always included "because most patients do not have pain during colonoscopy".

Discussion

We have shown in a small prospective randomized study at our centre that selective sedation is feasible and preferred by patients.[5] They can also better remember findings explained during colonoscopy or instructions given to them during colonoscopy if sedation is not used.

In the present larger study, patient demographics and diagnosis were similar between patients in the RS and SS groups. Since patient variables

Table 3. Percentage of sedated and non-sedated patients for selective sedating surgeons performing colonoscopy from 1992 to 1998.

Year	No sedation	Sedation
1992	0.2	99.8
1993	47	53
1994	77.7	22.3
1995	61	39
1996	84.8	15.2
1997	86.2	13.8
1998	90.5	9.5

Table 4. Percentage of sedated and non-sedated patients for routinely sedating surgeons performing colonoscopy from 1992 to 1998.

Year	No sedation	Sedation
1992	1.4	98.6
1993	1.7	98.3
1994	2.7	97.3
1995	9	91
1996	39.6	60.4
1997	26.5	73.5
1998	15.6	8.4

are similar, and as the previous colonoscopic experience of surgeons in both the RS and SS groups are similar, it would be reasonable to extrapolate that it was the individual experience and mindset of the colonoscopists that determined the use or non-use of sedation, and not patient factors. Furthermore there is no difference in caecal intubation rates or mean procedure time between routinely sedated and selectively sedated patients. Pain scores are not assessable as this is a retrospective study. It is the policy of the department to sedate patients early once pain is anything more than tolerable discomfort, and hence the proportion of the sedated patients in the SS group is about the same as the proportion of patients experiencing pain during colonoscopy. The performance of colonoscopy without sedation does call for a gentler technique with less "forceful" insertion and being constantly mindful of the need to "shorten" the loops and to keep the colonoscope "straight". Hence colonoscopists need to be aware that painless colonoscopy without routine sedation is possible and attempt such procedures until they are proficient. For routinely sedating surgeons, an increased proportion of non-sedation was implemented following our 1994 publication for one or two years. However, these surgeons are probably inherently uncomfortable with non-sedation and gradually increased their level of sedation during colonoscopy. Routinely sedating surgeons currently "do not sedate" only patients who have had an anterior resection or a left hemicolectomy. These patients normally have a very easy colonoscopy in any case.

Over the period of study, there was an increasing trend in the proportions of patients being sedated in the SS group. However, sedating surgeons continue to need to sedate their patients routinely as a rule. A simple change in mindset and increasing experience in selective sedation may therefore give the surgeon more confidence and debunk the myth that colonoscopy without sedation is painful. Ninety per cent of patients can be colonoscoped without routine sedation.[5-8] However, there will always be a minority of patients who require sedation due to a variety of factors, including some patients with a history of total hysterectomy, some patients with irritable bowel syndrome and some patients who develop severe pain even with "easy" colonoscopy.

Selective sedation improves patient–doctor interaction. The majority of patients prefer to watch the colonoscopic procedure.[5] At least some patients forget conversation and even the procedure being done following the use of midazolam.[5] A patient can choose to proceed with sedation or stop altogether if the procedure becomes uncomfortable if sedation is not given routinely before colonoscopy. For sedated patients, the wish of the patient to stop colonoscopy due to pain may not be remembered as such after reversal of sedation, often to the irritation of the dissatisfied patient, who may have to undergo another colonoscopy or a barium enema examination.[10,11]

There are also cost savings to be gained from practising selective sedation. Of the 17 472 colonoscopy procedures reviewed in this series, only 25% were performed without sedation. Within the RS group, 1548/11 012 (14%) procedures were performed without sedation. In the SS group, 4677/6460 (72%) procedures were performed without sedation. In 1998 alone, the percentage of non-sedated procedures in the SS group increased to just beyond 90%. Extrapolating from the numbers in the SS group, it is possible that 58% of the procedures (6387 colonoscopies) in the RS group could have been performed without sedation. Sedated patients also need postcolonoscopy observation for one hour on the average. Non-sedated patients, however, are discharged immediately following colonoscopy.

This would have translated to cost savings of US$204 384 and 6387 nursing hours if selective sedation had been practised universally by all during the period of study.

Conclusion

The practice of selective sedation during colonoscopy does not affect adversely the performance of colonoscopy. Besides a significant decrease in morbidity, there are cost savings to be gained for the patient and the institution if selective sedation is practised. Nonetheless, the need for routine sedation may be influenced more by the surgeon's mindset and not patient demand due to pain.

References

1. Phillips MS. Drugs and sedation for colonoscopy, *Prim Care* 1995; 22(3): 433–43.
2. Iber FL, Sutberry M, Gupta R and Kruss D. Evaluation of complications during and after conscious sedation for endoscopy using pulse oximetry, *Gastrointest Endosc* 1993; 39(5): 620–5.
3. Eckardt VF, Kanzler G, Schmitt T *et al.* Complications and adverse effects of colonoscopy with selective sedation, *Gastrointest Endosc* 1993; 49(5): 560–5.
4. Ristikankare M, Hartikainen J, Heikkinen M *et al.* Is routinely given conscious sedation of benefit during colonoscopy? *Gastrointest Endosc* 1999; 49(5): 566–72.
5. Seow-Choen F, Leong AF and Tsang C. Selective sedation for colonoscopy, *Gastrointest Endosc* 1994; 40(6): 661–4.
6. Cataldo PA. Colonoscopy without sedation, *Dis Colon Rectum* 1996; 39(3): 257–61.
7. Hoffman MS, Butler TW and Shaver T. Colonoscopy without sedation, *J Clin Gastroenterol* 1998; 26(4): 279–82.
8. Rex DK, Imperiale TF and Portish V. Patients willing to try colonoscopy without sedation: associated clinical factors and results of a randomized controlled trial, *Gastrointest Endosc* 1999; 49(5): 554–9.

9. Schutz SM, Lee JG, Schmitt CM *et al.* Clues to patient dissatisfaction with conscious sedation for colonoscopy, *Am J Gastroenterol* 1994; 89(9): 1476–9.

10. Early DS, Saifuddin T, Johnson JC *et al.* Patient attitudes toward undergoing colonscopy without sedation, *Am J Gastroenterol* 1999; 94(7): 1862–5.

11. Ward B, Shah S, Kirwan P and Mayberry JF. Issues of consent in colonosopy: if a patient says "stop" should we continue? *JR Soc Med* 1999; 92(3): 132–3.

CHAPTER 15

Sigmoid Colon Abscess: Management

CL Tang

Introduction

Sigmoid colon abscess is a common cause of colonic sepsis and is a surgical urgency requiring early attention and relevant treatment. A walled-off perforation or an abscess is the most common complication of diverticular disease. Diverticular disease is a common incidental finding at post-mortem during the evaluation of the colon. This occurs in an estimated 30% by 60 years old and 60% by 80 years old.[1] How many of these develop sigmoid colon abscess is still not clear. On the other hand, younger patients less than 50 years old who had prior symptomatic diverticular disease (67% in a series of 77 patients) tend develop more frequent future complications requiring surgery (such as abscess and fistulas).[2] In recent years, the management of sigmoid colon abscess is towards percutaneous drainage and control of the sepsis and primary resection and anastomosis. This article will review some of the treatment modalities available for sigmoid colon abscess, with particular reference to diverticular disease.

Aetiology

The various causes are shown in Table 1. Postoperative sigmoid colon abscess often results from either a minor or a delayed anastomotic leak in the early postoperative period. More often, sigmoid colon abscess is the result of a primary disease process such as a perforated colorectal cancer, diverticular disease, Crohn's disease or even suppurative appendicitis. Delayed or undiagnosed sigmoid colon injury in trauma could result in abscess formation with time. The aetiology of the abscess greatly influences the subsequent definitive treatment after control of the local sepsis and infection.

Clinical History

This may be nonlocalizing like fever, chills and rigors, malaise, anorexia, loss of weight and vomiting. Localizing left iliac fossa pain and tenderness and abdominal distension or mass are common signs. Rectal bogginess, tenesmus and urinary urgency are common. In the postoperative setting, prolonged ileus is a common presentation. Very often the abscess may progress and extend into the pelvis, the subphrenic space or the retroperitoneal space. It may also be walled off by loops of intestines, forming an interloop abscess. The differential diagnosis of acute diverticulitis includes inflammatory bowel disease, irritable bowel syndrome, ischaemic colitis, colon cancer, and gynaecologic and urologic diseases.

Table 1. Aetiology of sigmoid colon abscess.

1. Postoperative
2. Disease process
– Colorectal cancer
– Diverticular disease
– Crohn's disease
– Appendicitis
3. Trauma

Laboratory tests will reveal elevated total white counts; an abdominal X-ray may show displacement of the gas shadow of the bowel due to the abscess together with the loss of the psoas shadow. Low albumin and elevated serum alkaline phosphatase are common.

Radiological Tests

Contrast studies using barium are strongly discouraged. Barium sulphate in the presence of sepsis and bowel perforation is often difficult to remove and will lead to smouldering sepsis. Instead, a water-soluble ionic contrast is easier to handle in the presence of perforation. Such a contrast study has the advantage of ruling out any intracolonic lesions, such as a cancer and colonic perforations. Early use of water-soluble contrast enema was mooted as the most accurate and the most cost-effective means of establishing the diagnosis.[3] A barium study may be performed at least one week after the acute episode resolves.[4] Alternatively, a flexible sigmoidoscopy may be done and this is believed to be superior in detecting intraluminal lesions. Ultrasonography is less useful as it requires experience and is operator-dependent. It is often not possible in the presence of ileus and in certain habitus. Postoperative localized ascites and abscess cavities are often indistinguishable. However, in centres where the expertise is available, this may prove to be efficient and cost-effective.[5]

A CT scan of the abdomen and pelvis is perhaps the single most useful imaging. It localizes the collection, gives a clue to the possible aetiology and helps to prepare for interventional treatment. It has high sensitivity in the detection of abscess, and this is estimated to be at least three times more accurate than water-soluble enema. It is also a good predictor of the likelihood of success in medical therapy. In diverticulitis, "severe" findings indicate the likelihood of future sequelae and secondary complications. This is estimated to be about 44%, compared to the 20% in the "mild to moderate" findings in the period of 46 months[6,7] (Table 2).

Classification

Ambrosetti[6] graded the severity of diverticulitis based on CT scan findings in an attempt to prognosticate the outcome of nonoperative treatment during the initial attack (Table 3).[8] There is a higher chance of treatment failure

Table 2. CT scan and gastrografin enema grading for severity of diverticular disease.[6,7]

	Mild	Severe
CT scan	Localized wall thickening <5 mm inflammation of pericolic fat	mild findings + one of following: abscess, extraluminal air or gastrografin
Gastrografin enema	Segmental lumen narrowing tethered mucosa +/− mass effect	mild findings + one of following: extraluminal air or gastrografin

Table 3. CT scan grading and the prediction of treatment success or failure in a series of 349 patients with diverticulitis.[8]

	Treatment failure		Treatment success	
Severity	n	%	n	%
Severe	32	30	74	70
Mild	10	4	233	96

in the severe group, and even with successful treatment in this group, relapse or future complications requiring intervention are still significant. The risk of developing complications is high, at 2% per annum.

Treatment

The basic principle in conservative treatment is bowel rest, analgesia and spasmolytics for pain, antipyretics for fever and intravenous antibiotics that cover the gram-negatives and anaerobes. Abscess will need adequate drainage and this may be done either percutaneously or surgically. Percutaneous drainage has the disadvantage that interval surgery is still required, but is of much lower risk than operative drainage during acute sepsis.

Percutaneous drainage

This reduces the emergency laparotomy rate and is a particularly good option if the patient is too ill to undergo surgery. It is, however, contraindicated in multiloculation, when a source of continued infection is present, or when there is no suitable "window" for drainage and in multiple interloop abscesses. The guiding principle is to use the most dependent part and the shortest and most direct route for drainage. The tract may be dilated subsequently to promote drainage. This procedure is often done with the assistance of the intervention radiologist with either CT scan or ultrasonography guidance in consultation with the surgeon. The success rate with percutaneous drainage is high, above 80% in most series (Table 4).

It is interesting to note that the size of the drainage catheter has no impact on the response to percutaneous drainage.[15] Streptokinase may be instilled via the catheter into the abscess cavity to increase drainage and promote earlier collapse of the cavity.[16] Elective resection should be considered after one or two well-documented attacks of diverticulitis, depending on the severity of the attack and the age and medical fitness of the patient.[17] Three to four weeks after percutaneous drainage, interval colectomy is advocated, otherwise there is a tendency for recurrent discharge and drainage. Mesocolonic abscess less than 5 cm responds well to medical

Table 4. Outcome of percutaneous drainage from various studies reported.

Authors	n	Success (%)
Haaga et al. (1980)[9]	33	28 (85)
Johnson et al. (1981)[10]	27	24 (89)
Van Sonnenberg et al. (1981)[11]	55	47 (85)
Karlson et al. (1982)[12]	42	32 (76)
MacErlean et al. (1983)[13]	42	36 (86)
Schechter et al. (1994)[14]	133	103 (78)
Total	332	270 (81)

Table 5. Outcome of percutaneous drainage compared to operative drainage.[10]

	Percutaneous $n = 28$	Operation $n = 43$
Complication	4	16
Inadequate drainage	11	21
Duration drainage	17 days	29 days
Death	11	21

treatment without drainage, while other collections will require drainage. Colonoscopic or barium enema evaluation is required to exclude a sealed perforation from a colorectal cancer.

Surgical treatment

Alternatively, drainage of the abscess may be operative—transabdominal, transrectal, transvaginum, loin approach and subcostal resection. Interval colectomy may then be carried out when the sepsis is under control. Possible definitive procedures include resection without anastomosis (Hartmann's procedure), resection with immediate anastomosis, resection with immediate anastomosis and diversion as well as laparoscopic drainage and resection. Primary resections and anastomosis may be preceded by an intraoperative colonic wash-out. Other, less popular methods, which fell out of favour, were primary oversewing of the perforation, exteriorization, diverting caecostomy or colostomy with drainage and only excision of the site of perforation. The trend towards primary resection and anastomosis is mainly the result of recent improvements in anaesthesia and postoperative intensive care.

While resection without anastomosis appears to be a safer procedure, cumulative complications and mortality for a two- or three-stage procedure are ironically greater than for a primary procedure. In fact, many patients do not want to take another risk to have the stoma reversed. A review of patients who had a Hartmann's procedure and subsequently went on to closure of the colostomy puts the range between 42 and 94% (median 70%) only.[18] Cumulative mortality rates for the two- or three-stage procedure appear to be higher than for the one-stage procedure, with a median of 16% versus 5%, respectively. However, there are no randomized prospective trials comparing the treatments available in this area. Furthermore, treatment has to be individualized.

One-stage primary resection and reanastomosis is possible. In a recent prospective cohort study of 45 patients[19] who had complicated diverticular disease and had undergone primary resection and anastomosis, the incidence of anastomotic leakage, septic complication and death was correlated with the degree of peritoneal soilage based on the MPI (Mannheim Peritonitis Index). There were no significant relationships between the degree of soilage and anastomotic dehiscence. This was a significant difference from the previous recommendations of Hartmann's procedure as the first surgical choice.[20–22] Furthermore, recent studies of large bowel obstruction have shown that there is no need to perform an intraoperative colonic irrigation that will prolong operative time by at least 30 minutes.[23]

An intermediate alternative is to create a proximal diversion after primary resection to minimize sepsis should an anastomotic leak occur later. This may be an ileostomy or a colostomy and should be performed together with irrigation of the distal limb. The assumption is that closure of a loop stoma is easier than reanastomosis after a Hartmann's procedure. A recent study has shown that a defunctioning loop ileostomy has less postoperative complication after closure compared with a colostomy.[24]

In recent years, laparoscopic colectomy for diverticulitis has been successfully performed, with minimal morbidity and mortality. Benefits of laparoscopic resections were experienced in most series in which there was a shortened hospital stay, early discharge, less pain and early resumption of daily activities.[25–27] However, this technique has a significant learning phase associated with morbidity and prolonged operative time and is best left to those who do it as a daily routine.[28]

When should operation be done after successful medical treatment of the first episode of diverticulitis? Males tend to have more severe recurrent attacks and this is more significant if the individual is less than 50 years old. A younger person would naturally face a higher lifetime cumulative risk for recurrence. Severity on an initial CT scan (25% develop severe complication in 46 months in the "severe" group) would indicate the need for interval surgery as the complication rate may be unacceptably high.[6–8] This represents an estimate of greater than 60% in young men with "severe" disease compared to 30% in older patients. In contrast, less than 13% have recurrent disease in the "mild" disease group. Associated pelvic abscess requires early drainage and resection.

Conclusion

With advances in perioperative care, management of sigmoid colonic abscess may be simplified without the need for a multiple-stage procedure. Percutaneous drainage is an extremely useful adjunct and facilitates surgery by controlling sepsis.

References

1. Parks TG. Natural history of diverticular disease of the colon, *Clin Gastroenterol* 1975; 4: 53–69.
2. Anderson DN, Driver CP, Davidson AI and Keenan RA. Diverticular disease in patients under 50 years of age, *J R Coll Surg Edin* 1997; 42: 102–4.
3. Wexner SD and Dailey TH. The initial management of left lower quadrant peritonitis, *Dis Colon Rectum* 1986; 29: 635–8.
4. Veidenheimer MC. Clinical presentation and surgical treatment of complicated diverticular disease. In: Allan RN, Keighley MRB, Alexander-Williams J and Hawkins CF (eds.), *Inflammatory Bowel Diseases*, pp. 519–28. Edinburgh: Churchill Livingstone.
5. Civardi G, Di Candio G, Giorgio A, Goletti O, Ceragioli T, Filice C, Caremani M and Buscarini L. Ultrasound guided percutaneous drainage of abdominal abscesses in the hands of a clinician: a multicentre Italian study, *Eur J Ultrasound* 1998; 8: 91–9.
6. Ambrosetti P, Robert J, Witzig JA *et al.* Prognostic factors from computed tomography in acute left colonic diverticulitis, *Br J Surg* 1992; 79: 117–19.
7. Ambrosetti P, Robert J and Witzig JA. Incidence, outcome, and proposed management of isolated abscesses complicating acute left-sided colonic diverticulitis, *Dis Colon Rectum* 1992; 35: 1072–6.
8. Ambrosetti P and Morel P. Acute left-sided colonic diverticulitis: diagnosis and surgical indications after successful conservative therapy of first time acute diverticulitis, *Zentralbl Chir* 1998; 123: 1382–5.
9. Haaga JR and Weinstein AJ. CT-guided percutaneous aspiration and drainage of abscess, *Am J Radiol* 1980; 135: 1187–94.
10. Johnson WC, Gerzof SG, Robbins AH and Nasbeth DC. Treatment of abdominal abscesses, *Ann Surg* 1981; 194: 510–20.
11. Van Sonnenberg E, Willenberg J, Ferruci JT Jr, Mueller PR and Simeone JF. Triangulation method for percutaneous needle guidance: the angled approach to upper abdominal mass, *Am J Radiol* 1981; 137: 757–61.
12. Karlson KB, Martin EC, Fankunchen EI, Schultz RW and Casarella WJ. Percutaneous drainage of abdominal abscesses and fluid collections: technique, results and applications, *Diagn Radiol* 1982; 142: 1–10.
13. MacErlean DP and Gibney RG. Radiological management of abdominal abscess, *J R Soc Med* 1983; 76: 256–61.

14. Schechter S, Eisenstat TE, Oliver GC, Rubin RJ and Salvati EP. Computerized tomographic scan-guided drainage of intra-abdominal abscesses: preoperative and postoperative modalities in colon and rectal surgery, *Dis Colon Rectum* 1994; 37: 984–8. Review.

15. Rothlin MA, Schob O, Klotz H, Candinas D and Largiader F. Percutaneous drainage of abdominal abscesses: are large-bore catheters necessary? *Eur J Surg* 1998; 164: 419–24.

16. Haaga JR, Nakamoto D, Stellato T, Novak RD, Gavant ML, Silverman SG and Bellmore M. Intracavitatory urokinase for enhancement of percutaneous abscess drainage: phase II trial, *Am J Roentgenol* 2000; 174: 1681–5.

17. Wong D, Wexner S, Lowry A *et al*. The Standards Task Force. The American Society of Colon and Rectal Surgeons practice parameters for the treatment of sigmoid diverticulitis, *Dis Colon Rectum* 2000; 3.

18. Gorden P. Diverticular disease of the colon. In: Gorden P and Nivatvongs S (eds.), *Principles and Practice of Surgery for the Colon Rectum and Anus*, 2nd edition, 1999. Quality Medical Publishing, Missouri, USA, pp. 975–1043.

19. Gooszen AW, Tollenaar RA, Geelkerken RH, Smeets HJ, Bemelman WA, Van Schaardenburgh P and Gooszen HG. Prospective study of primary anastomosis following sigmoid resection for suspected acute complicated diverticular disease, *Br J Surg* 2001; 88: 693–7.

20. Tucci G, Torquati A, Grande M, Stroppa I, Sianesi M and Farinon AM. Major acute inflammatory complications of diverticular disease of the colon: planning of surgical management, *Hepatogastroenterology* 1996; 43: 839–45.

21. Belmonte C, Klas JV, Perez JJ, Wong WD, Rothenberger DA, Goldberg SM and Madoff RD. The Hartmann procedure: first choice or last resort in diverticular disease? *Arch Surg* 1996; 131: 612–15.

22. Schilling MK, Maurer CA, Kollmar O and Buchler MW. Primary vs. secondary anastomosis after sigmoid colon resection for perforated diverticulitis (Hinchey stage III and IV): a prospective outcome and cost analysis, *Dis Colon Rectum* 2001; 44: 699–703; discussion 703–5.

23. Nyam DC, Seow-Choen F, Leong AFPK and Ho YH. Colonic decompression without on-table irrigation for obstructing left-sided colorectal tumours, *Br J Surg* 1996; 83: 786–7.

24. Rullier E, Toux N Le, Laurent C, Garrelon J-L, Parneix M and Saric J. Loop ileostomy verses loop colostomy for defunctioning low

anastomoses during rectal cancer surgery, *World J Surg* 2001; 25: 274–6. Invited commentary 277–8.

25. Tuech JJ, Pessaux P, Rouge C, Regenet N, Bergamaschi R and Amaud JP. Laparoscopic vs. open colectomy for sigmoid diverticulitis: a prospective comparative study in the elderly. *Surg Endosc* 2000; 14: 1031–3.

26. Siriser F. Laparoscopic-assisted colectomy for diverticular sigmoiditis: a single-surgeon prospective study of 65 patients, *Surg Endosc* 1999; 13: 811–13.

27. Kockerling F, Schneider C, Reymond MA, Scheidbach H, Scheuerlein H, Konradt J, Bruch HP, Zornig C, Kohler L, Barlehner E, Kuthe A, Szinicz G, Richter HA and Hohenberger W. Laparoscopic resection of sigmoid diverticulitis: results of a multicenter study. Laparoscopic Colorectal Surgery Study Group. *Surg Endosc* 1999; 13: 567–71.

28. Schlachta DM, Mamazza J, Seshadri PA, Cadeddu M, Gregoire R and Poulin EC. Defining a learning curve for laparoscopic colorectal resections, *Dis Colon Rectum* 2001; 44: 21–22. Review.

CHAPTER 16

Sigmoid Diverticulitis: Current Management

PL Roberts

Introduction

Diverticular disease is a common problem in Western society and has an estimated incidence of 10 pts/100 000 per year in the United States, resulting in 200 000 admissions/year. In contrast to the East, over 95% of cases involve the sigmoid and/or descending colon.

Diverticula are saccular outpocketings of the colon. In the sigmoid colon, they are false diverticula, containing mucosa and muscularis mucosa; whereas, in the right colon, they may be false or "true diverticula" containing all layers of the bowel wall. Sigmoid diverticula have been termed acquired lesions of aging; under the age of 40, 5% of the Western population have diverticula and the incidence increases on a linear basis; thus, by age 85 over two-thirds of the population have diverticulosis. There are no long-term population-based studies looking at the risk of developing diverticulitis, given the presence of diverticulosis. It is generally accepted that 10–25% of individuals with diverticulosis will at some point develop diverticulitis.[1,2] After one attack of diverticulitis, approximately one-third of patients will develop another attack. Half of second attacks occur in the first year and 90% occur within five years. After a second attack, the majority of patients will have subsequent attacks and this has led to the recommendation for sigmoid resection after two well-documented attacks of diverticulitis.

Although diverticular disease has been called a "fiber deficiency disease of Western civilization",[3,4] this well-entrenched belief has been called into question recently, partly due to increasing reports of diverticular disease in African nations previously reporting a low incidence of the disease.[5,6] Nevertheless, a prospective cohort study of 47 888 men in the United States did find a decreased incidence of diverticular disease in patients with a low total fat and high fibre diet.[7] Other factors contributing to the development of diverticular disease include a process or segmentation described by Painter as the generation of high pressure waves in the sigmoid colon,[8] and the effect of aging which leads to decreased tensile strength of collagen and muscle fibres.[9]

Acute Diverticulitis

The signs and symptoms of acute diverticulitis include fever, leukocytosis, and left-sided abdominal tenderness with or without a mass. The differential diagnosis includes appendicitis, colon cancer, inflammatory bowel disease, gynaecologic diseases and pyelonephritis. Initial treatment consists of antibiotics and bowel rest. If the symptoms are mild, and the patient is reliable and able to tolerate a diet, outpatient therapy is considered. For patients who require in-patient hospitalization, 25–35% need surgery on initial hospitalization for diverticulitis. After resolution of an attack of diverticulitis, the colon is evaluated by a combination of flexible sigmoidoscopy and air contrast barium enema or colonoscopy at 4–6 weeks' time. Patients are counselled to remain on a high fibre diet, which has been suggested to decrease the risk of subsequent attacks of diverticulitis.[10]

Surgical Indications

The surgical indications for diverticulitis include two attacks of well-documented diverticulitis (generally of sufficient severity to require in-patient hospitalization), one attack associated with complications (such as abscess, fistula or obstruction) and the inability to exclude carcinoma.[11] One attack of diverticulitis in a patient under the age of 50 was previously considered to be an indication for elective surgery; however, recent data on the natural history of diverticulitis has suggested that young patients essentially have the same natural history as older patients[12] and therefore it is reasonable to wait for a second attack of diverticulitis before recommending resection.

Elective Resection

Mechanical and antibiotic bowel preparation is performed the day prior to surgery. All diseased and thickened bowel is removed and anastomosis is performed to the proximal rectum, as the incidence of recurrent diverticulitis is significantly lower with an anastomosis to the proximal rectum in comparison with the distal sigmoid.[13] A recent report suggested that preservation of the inferior mesenteric artery may decrease the incidence of anastomotic leakage.[14]

An open or laparoscopic resection may be performed. If a laparoscopic approach is performed, the specimen may be retried through a Pfannenstiel incision. Hand-assisted laparoscopy allows preservation of tactile sensation and may decrease the conversion rate when compared to a total laparoscopic approach.[15]

Complicated Diverticulitis and Urgent/Emergent Surgery

Fistulas

Colovesical fistulas are the most common of all diverticular fistulas and manifest with pneumaturia or polymicrobial urinary tract infections. Colovaginal, colouterine and colocutaneous fistulas may also occur. Colocutaneous fistulas rarely occur de novo and are more commonly due to a complication of prior surgery, especially if the distal sigmoid colon instead of the rectum was used for an anastomosis.[16] The majority of patients with fistulas may undergo a single-stage resection. Omentum, if available, is used to interpose between the colon and the involved organ. The fistula can generally be "pinched" off; wide resection of the involved organ (e.g. the bladder) is unnecessary.

Abscess/Perforated Diverticulitis

In an effort to categorize patients with associated abscess and perforation, the Hinchey classification was devised (Table 1).[17]

Patients with abscesses generally have ongoing pain, fever and leukocytosis. A CT scan is useful in assessing the abscess and has a therapeutic as well as diagnostic role. A small pericolic abscess (generally <2 cm) resolves with antibiotics and does not warrant percutaneous drainage. Patients with large abscesses can undergo percutaneous drainage as long as a radiographic "window" is present, thus allowing stabilization of the patients and resolution of the septic process, hopefully making possible an elective sigmoid resection as opposed to a two-stage procedure. Percutaneous drainage is contraindicated in patients with generalized peritonitis or pneumoperitoneum; these patients are best treated with resuscitation and emergent operation.

While many patients with a pericolic abscess can undergo preoperative bowel preparation and single-stage resection, this is not the case for patients who present with faecal or purulent peritonitis and require emergent operation. In such patients a two-stage procedure with an initial Hartmann resection is performed. The Hartmann procedure was first described by a French surgeon, Henri Hartmann, for treatment of rectal cancer, but is currently most commonly performed for perforated diverticulitis.[18] A 3–6-month period is generally advised prior to colostomy reversal. Adhesions and difficulties with subsequent identification of the

Table 1. Hinchey classification of perforated diverticulitis.

Stage I:	Pericolic abscess
Stage II:	Pelvic, retroperitoneal or intra-abdominal abscess
Stage III:	Purulent peritonitis
Stage IV:	Faecal peritonitis

*After Hinchey[17]

Hartmann pouch in the pelvis may make Hartmann reversal a potentially difficult undertaking.

To obviate the difficulties with identification of the Hartmann pouch, some have advocated sigmoid resection with primary anastomosis and proximal faecal diversion. A proximal loop stoma is technically easier to reverse than reversing a Hartmann pouch with the attendant potential difficulties of pelvic dissection.[19]

An additional alternative is on-table lavage and primary anastomosis. This procedure is performed in selective patients who are unable to undergo bowel preparation prior to surgery because of ileus, obstruction of the need for emergent surgery. While the traditional teaching has been to perform resection and faecal diversion in such patients, on-table lavage avoids the need for a staged procedure. We have used this technique in selected patients, who were not immunocompromised and who were haemodynamically stable intraoperatively. The technique has previously been described in detail.[20] In 33 patients with diverticular disease (Hinchey stage I–18 pts; stage II–10 pts; stage III–5 pts) who underwent on-table lavage and primary anastomosis, there was one anastomotic complication.[21] The technique may be used safely in selected patients.

On the theme of lavage, a recent report used laparoscopic peritoneal lavage as the sole modality to treat a cohort of eight patients with purulent peritonitis from diverticulitis.[22] No patient underwent sigmoid resection and at a follow-up of 12–48 months no patients required surgical resection. Although this is a small cohort of patients with a relatively short follow-up, reports such as these suggest that we should at least review some of our traditional surgical teaching regarding the treatment of complicated diverticulitis.

References

1. Parks TG. Natural history of diverticular disease of the colon: a review of 521 cases, *Br Med J* 1969; 4: 639–42.
2. Makela J, Vuolio S, Kiviniemi H *et al*. Natural history of diverticular disease: when to operate? *Dis Colon Rectum* 1998; 41: 1523–8.i.
3. Painter NS and Burkitt DP. Diverticular disease of the colon; a deficiency disease of Western civilization, *Br Med J* 1971; ii: 450–4.

4. Painter NS and Burkitt DP. Diverticular disease of the colon: a 20th century problem, *Clin Gastroenterol* 1975; 4: 3–21.

5. Ihekwaba FN. Diverticular disease of the colon in black Africa, *J R Coll Surg Edin* 1992; 37: 107–9.

6. Baako BN. Diverticular disease of the colon in Accra, Ghana, *Br J Surg* 2001; 88: 1595.

7. Aldoori WH, Giovannucci EL, Rimm EB *et al.* A prospective study of diet and the risk of symptomatic diverticular disease in men, *Am J Clin Nutr* 1994; 60: 757–64.

8. Painter NS, Truelove SC, Ardran GM *et al.* Segmentation and the localization of intraluminal pressures in the human colon, with special reference to the pathogenesis of colonic diverticula, *Gastroenterology* 1965; 49: 169–77.

9. Morson BC. Pathology of diverticular disease of the colon, *Clin Gastroenterol* 1975; 4: 37–52.

10. Larson DM, Masters SS and Spiro HM. Medical and surgical therapy in diverticular disease: a comparative study, *Gastroenterology* 1976; 71: 734–7.

11. Roberts PL, Abel M, Rosen *et al.* Practice parameters for sigmoid diverticulitis—supporting documentation, *Dis Colon Rectum* 1995; 38: 126–32.

12. Vignati PV, Welch JP and Cohen JL. Long-term management of diverticulitis in young patients, *Dis Colon Rectum* 1995; 38: 627–9.

13. Benn PL, Wolff BG and Ilstrup DM. Level of anastomosis and recurrent colonic diverticulitis, *AM J Surg* 1986; 151: 269–71.

14. Tocchi A, Mazzoni G, Fornasari V *et al.* Preservation of the inferior mesenteric artery in colorectal resection for complicated diverticular disease, *Am J Surg* 2001; 182: 162–7.

15. Targarona EM, Gracia E, Garriga J *et al.* Prospective randomized trial comparing conventional laparoscopic colectomy with hand-assisted laparoscopic colectomy: applicability, immediate clinical outcome, inflammatory response and cost, *Surg Endosc* 2002; 16: 234–9.

16. Fazio VW, Church JM, Jagelman DG *et al.* Colocutaneous fistulas complicating diverticulitis, *Dis Colon Rectum* 1987; 30: 89–94.

17. Hinchey EF, Schaal PG and Richards GK. Treatment of perforated diverticular disease, *Adv Surg* 1978; 12: 85–109.

18. Hartmann H. Cited by Corman ML. Classic articles in colonic and rectal surgery, *Dis Colon Rectum* 1984; 27: 273.

19. Veidenheimer MC and Roberts PL. *Colonic Diverticular Disease.* Blackwell Scientific, 1991.
20. Murray JJ, Schoetz DJ, Coller JA *et al.* Intraoperative colonic lavage and primary anastomosis in nonelective resection of the colon, *Dis Colon Rectum* 1991: 34: 527–31.
21. Lee EC, Murray JJ, Coller *et al.* Intraoperative colonic lavage in non-elective surgery for diverticular disease, *Dis Colon Rectum* 1997; 40: 669–74.
22. O'Sullivan GC, Murphy D and O'Brien MG. Laparoscopic manage-ment of generalized peritonitis due to perforated colonic diverticula, *Am J Surg* 1996; 171: 432, 434.

Surgical Management of Rectovaginal Fistulas

F Seow-Choen

Introduction

Rectovaginal fistulas account for about 5% of anorectal fistulas and may result in very severe and distressing symptoms for the afflicted patients. By and large, treatment is still controversial and difficult. Whereas the causes of acquired rectovaginal fistulas may be numerous, there are only a few common aetiologies (Table 1). Individualized treatment aimed at both the underlying disorder and the rectovaginal fistula itself is needed if fistula healing is to occur.

Aetiology

The commoner causes of rectovaginal fistula accounting for the vast majority of such cases include obstetrical injury, pelvic irradiation and carcinoma.

Table 1. Causes of rectovaginal fistulas.

Anal-glandular
Bartholin's abscess
Crohn's disease
Childbirth injury
Surgical injury on vaginal/rectum
Traumatic injuries
Blood disorders, including leukaemia
Pelvic irradiation
Pelvic cancers
Congenital defects

Prolonged labour as well as obstetric trauma may be responsible for 50–90% of all rectovaginal fistulas. Pelvic irradiation, especially of cervical cancer, is another leading cause of rectovaginal fistulas. Intracavitary contact radiation is more frequently implicated than external beam radiotherapy in the causation of rectovaginal fistulas. Early radiation damage includes proctitis and ulceration and one third may result in rectovaginal fistulas. The risk of fistula formation is proportional to the dose of radiation given. Inflammatory bowel disease, especially Crohn's disease, is uncommon locally but may be responsible for up to two to 22% of rectovaginal fistulas among Caucasian patients. Congenital rectovaginal fistulas may be associated with other developmental abnormalities but their management is beyond the scope of this paper. Malignant diseases of the rectum, cervix, uterus or vagina may present with rectovaginal fistulas.

Clinical Examination and Investigations

A complete pelvic examination including vaginal and rectal palpation will confirm the presence of the fistula and give important information on the size, the location, the presence of any extensions, the state of the anal sphincters as well as the occurrence of underlying diseases. Depending on the previous history and clinical examination, further investigations including transanal ultrasound, anorectal physiology, colonoscopy, small bowel enemas, fistulography or biopsies may be needed. In a fit young lady with a rectovaginal fistula of obstetric origin, the only investigations that are helpful are the anorectal physiology and the transanal ultrasonography. It is wise in the lady above 45 years of age for a colonoscopy to be performed to exclude coincidental colonic malignancy. In rectovaginal fistulas associated with pelvic irradiation for pelvic malignancy, biopsies are important to exclude residual tumours. Where a defunctioning colostomy alone is planned as the definitive or as an initial procedure for rectovaginal fistulas, the small bowel should be imaged first to exclude another, more proximal enterovaginal fistula.

Classification

Besides the aetiological classification, rectovaginal fistulas are also categorized according to their size and location. A low fistula is only slightly above the dentate line or inside the vagina fourchette. A high fistula is at least in the mid-rectum or behind the cervix. A mid fistula is in between. A fistula is small if it is less than 0.5 cm in diameter, and large if it is over 2.5 cm in diameter. Medium fistulas are 0.5–2.5 cm in diameter. Rectovaginal fistulas are simple if they are small, low and due to trauma or infection. They are complex if large, high or caused by cancer, irradiation or inflammatory bowel disease, or have had multiple failed repairs before.

Treatment

Rectovaginal fistulas caused by irradiation, neoplasms or Crohn's disease never heal spontaneously and will need surgical intervention. Spontaneous healing may occur in up to 50% of small rectovaginal fistulas due to obstetric or postsurgical causes (for example, following anterior resection).

Surgery, nonetheless, will succeed only when the patient has been optimized for the procedure. Local tissues must be as normal as possible and a period of treatment with steroids, asacol, antibiotics, hyperalimentation or a defunctioning stoma may be needed before definitive surgery is possible. If surrounding tissues are supple and healthy, no delay in surgery is needed.

A waiting period of several months to a year or more may be needed to allow inflammation and sepsis to subside before repair. In patients with failed multiple repairs, a longer waiting period may be needed.[1,2] Where a colostomy is not used, bowel preparation must be close to perfect. It is a matter of surgical preference whether constipating, diarrhoeal or normal defecatory motion is used following surgery as none has been shown to

Table 2. Surgical procedures for rectovaginal fistulas.

1.	Local repairs
	• Laying open
	• Inversion of fistula
	• Excision of fistula with layered closure and muscle interposition
2.	Anorectal advancement flaps
3.	Sphincteroplasty
4.	Sphincter-preserving transabdominal repair
	• Layer closure without resection
	• Low anterior resection/coloanal anastomosis
	• Transacral resection
	• Onlay patch anastomosis
5.	Abdominoperineal resection
6.	Defunctioning stomas
7.	Tissue transposition
	• Omentum, gracilis, etc.

be superior to any other. To date, a well-conducted trial has yet to be conducted to study this important question.

Incontinence is a major concern in patients with rectovaginal fistulas and the incidence of preoperation anal incontinence may be as high as 48%.[3] The high incidence of anal sphincter defects indicates a requirement for thorough assessment of anal sphincters before surgery for rectovaginal fistulas. The presence of an anal sphincter defect is an indication for sphincter repair, as persistent incontinence adversely affects the surgical outcome.

Surgical Approaches*

Many approaches have been described for the management of rectovaginal fistulas. The procedure of choice depends on the height of the tract from the anal verge, the quality of the local tissues, the underlying pathology as well as the experience of the surgeon. Depending on the conditions, rectal, vaginal, perineal, abdominal or transsacral approaches may be taken either alone or in combination. Local transvaginal or transanal repair may be attempted in patients following obstetrical or traumatic rectovaginal fistulas. Radiation-induced fistulas will not heal with local procedures alone and resectional procedures are preferred. No repair should be undertaken for patients with inflammatory bowel disease until the disease is well under control. Carcinomatous fistulas will require radical surgery for a cure,

---

*See Table 2.

but where palliation only is possible, resection and anastomosis may be preferred to a permanent stoma. In some patients with advanced malignancy or in poor-risk patients with radiation-induced rectovaginal fistulas, a stoma may be all that should be offered.

Local Repairs

Laying open

Laying open of rectovaginal fistulas may result in severe anal incontinence and should not be performed for any patient except those with low anovaginal fistulas. Laying open and primary suture have been used by gynaecologists for rectovaginal fistulas. The entire tract is excised and the various muscular and mucosal layers repaired with absorbable sutures. Ninety-six to one hundred per cent success has been reported with this technique.[1]

Inversion of fistulas

Inversion of small, low rectovaginal fistulas by a transvaginal approach may be used. A circular incision is initially made around the vaginal opening of the rectovaginal fistula. The vaginal mucosa is then mobilised and inverted with several purse-string sutures which obliterate and invert the fistula. The mucosa is then closed separately. Success was reported in 8 of 11 patients in one series.[4]

Local excision with layered closure

Local excision of the rectal vaginal fistula with layered closure may be accomplished by transrectal, transvaginal or transperineal routes.[5,6] The rectal and vaginal mucosa as well as the muscular layers must be mobilised sufficiently to ensure a tension-free apposition. Healing rates vary from 16% to 70%.[1,4–7]

Transphincteric Approach

The transphincteric approach described by Mason may be useful if treatment of a mid or high rectovaginal fistula is needed without having to open the abdominal cavity.[8]

Anorectal Advancement Flaps

Anorectal advancement flaps may be useful in the management of recto-vaginal fistulas. The width of the base of the flap should be at least two times the width of the apex and the flap should consist of mucosa, submucosa and circular muscle fibres. Flaps should be based distally to prevent mucosal extropion. The rectovaginal fistula is excised and the flap sutured with absorbable sutures to the anorectal wall. The vagina is normally left open for drainage. Success rates of 78–100% have been reported.[9,10] The success rate is adversely influenced by previous repairs. For those with two previous repairs the success rate was 55%, compared with 86% for those with only one previous repair.[10]

Sphincteroplasty

An overlapping sphincteroplasty through a transperineal approach corrects underlying sphincter defects and heals the rectovaginal fistula and is advantageous for patients with a sphincter defect as well. Success rates have ranged from 78 to 100%.[10,11]

Transabdominal Sphincter-Preserving Repair

Abdominal approaches will be needed for patients with multiple repairs, and carcinomatous, radiation-induced or high rectovaginal fistulas. In the simplest cases where there is no radiation damage, carcinoma or residual inflammatory changes, mobilization of the rectum and division of the rectovaginal fistula, and repair of the defects in the rectum and vagina together with omentum interposition, may be all that is required. Where local pathology dictates, resection may be necessary and gastrointestinal continuity may then be achieved by an ultralow anterior resection using staplers or by endoanal suturing where necessary. Once again, where it is possible, omental interposition is helpful in preventing recurrence as the bowel and vaginal suture line should not be in direct contact. Low anterior resection with the double stapling technique is familiar to all colorectal surgeons and is easily performed. The proximal colon must be from outside the irradiated area and must be well vascularized to prevent recurrence. Coloanal anastomosis with endoanal hard suturing or a coloanal sleeve anastomosis may also be employed where needed.

Onlay Patch Anastomosis

The onlay patch repair was described by Bricker[12] and Johnson. They mobilized the rectosigmoid and excised the rectovaginal fistula. The sigmoid colon is then divided and the distal end anastomosed to the edge of the excised rectal opening of the rectovaginal fistula. An end colostomy is then constructed. A second operation re-establishes gastrointestinal continuity. There are few advantages, in practice, over resectional surgery and this procedure is not widely practised although Bricker *et al.* reported excellent or satisfactory results in 19 of 20 patients. The advantages cited include technical ease and lesser risk of presacral bleeding and nerve damage due to incomplete rectal mobilization.

Abdominoperineal Resection

Major ablative surgery may be necessary for selected patients with extensive carcinoma or inflammatory bowel disease where the anal sphincter complex cannot be salvaged; in such cases, absominoperineal resection will cure the rectovaginal fistulas.

Defunctioning Stomas

In patients in whom major surgery may not be indicated due to poor surgical or anaesthetic risks, a defunctioning colostomy may improve considerably their quality of life. Before a trephine sigmoid colostomy is undertaken, the small bowel should be imaged to exclude concurrent proximal fistulas as the irradiated pelvis may have more than one fistula present.

Tissue Transposition

The purpose of tissue transposition is to prevent direct apposition of two suture lines and to introduce well-vascularized tissue into the area of pathology. Omentum, bulbocavernosus, gracilis, sartorius and gluteus maximum have been used.

Other Nonsurgical Approaches

Fibrin glue injected into the fistulous tract forms a coagulum which has been reported to have a success rate of up to 74%.[13] Others, including ourselves, have not been impressed by its use.

References

1. Hibbard LT. Surgical management of rectovaginal fistulas and complete perineal tears, *Am J Obstet Gynecol* 1978; 130: 139–47.
2. Graham JB. Vaginal fistulas following radiotherapy, *Surg Gynecol Obstet* 1965; 120: 1019–30.
3. Tsang CBS and Rothenberger DA. Rectovaginal fistulas: therapeutic options, *Surgical Clinic of North America* 1997; 77: 95–114.
4. Given FT. Rectovaginal fistula: a review of 20 years' experience in a community hospital, *Am J Obstet Gynecol* 1970; 108: 41–6.
5. Greenwald JC and Hoexter B. Repair of rectovaginal fistula. *Surg Gynecol Obstet* 1978; 146: 443–5.
6. Goligher JC. Rectovaginal fistula and irradiation proctitis and enteritis. In: Goligher JC (ed.), *Surgery of the Anus, Rectum and Colon*. Thomas, Springfield, 1975.
7. Lescher TC and Pratt JH. Vaginal repair of the simple rectovaginal fistula, *Surg Gynecol Obstet* 1967; 124: 137–21.
8. Mason AY. Transphincteric surgery of the rectum. *Prog Surg* 1974; 13: 66–97.
9. Hoexter B, Labow SB and Moseson MD. Transanal rectovaginal fistula repair, *Dis Colon Rectum* 1985; 28: 572–5.
10. Lowry AC, Thorson AG, Rothenberger DA and Goldberg SM. Repair of simple rectovaginal fistulas: influence of previous repairs, *Dis Colon Rectum* 1988; 31: 676–8.
11. Khandaja KS, Yamashita HJ, Wise WE Jr *et al*. Delayed repair of obstetric injuries of the anorectum and vagina: a stratified surgical approach, *Dis Colon Rectum* 1994; 37: 344–9.
12. Bricker EM and Johnston WD. Repair of post irradiation rectovaginal fistula and stricture, *Surg Gynecol Obstet* 1979; 148: 499–506.
13. Hjortrup A, Moesguard F and Kjaegard J. Fibrin adhesive in the treatment of perineal fistulas, *Dis Colon Rectum* 1991; 34: 752–4.

CHAPTER 18

Surgery for Abdominal Crohn's Disease

KW Eu

Introduction

Most patients affected by abdominal Crohn's disease ultimately undergo an operation for this condition. Patients will normally feel significantly better, with obstructive and septic symptoms relieved, an earlier return to work, lessened dietary restriction and, most importantly, the stoppage of steroid administration.

Crohn's disease is a chronic inflammatory disorder of unknown aetiology that affects the entire intestinal tract. The sites of disease involvement are typically classified into five separate locations—gastroduodenal site, small bowel, ileocolic site, colon and anorectum. Regardless of the disease location, the operative principles and surgical options are similar. In general, operative therapy is recommended for those who have developed one or more disease complications, and when the patient's quality of life is significantly impaired despite appropriate medical therapy.

Operative Indications

The indications for surgery in abdominal Crohn's disease include:

- Failure of medical therapy
- Obstruction
- Fistula or abscess
- Haemorrhage
- Growth retardation
- Perforation
- Carcinoma

The incidence of each of these indications depends upon the site of disease involvement. Symptomatic gastroduodenal disease occurs in 2–4% of patients with Crohn's disease. While bleeding and anaemia may occur, the most common presenting complaints are upper abdominal pain and symptoms of duodenal obstruction. At the Lahey Clinic, 22 out of 70 patients with gastroduodenal Crohn's disease required operative treatment, with obstruction being the principal indication in 75% of the patients.[1]

Crohn's disease of the jejunum and proximal ileum occurs in 10–20% of patients. At the Cleveland Clinic, the two commonest reasons to conduct an operation for Crohn's disease of the jejenum and proximal ileum are obstruction (55%) and fistula or abscess (32%). Failure of medical treatment (8%), bleeding (1%) and carcinoma occur much less frequently.[2]

Ileocolic Crohn's disease is the most commonest disease pattern, as it occurs in 40–50% of patients. As in small bowel disease, fistula or abscess (4%) and obstruction (35%) are the commonest operative indications, followed by failure of medical therapy (7%) and perforation (1.6%).[2]

Colonic Crohn's disease affects 20–30% of all patients with Crohn's. Fistula and abscess (35%), and obstruction (34%), once again, are common operative indications, followed by failure of medical therapy (12%) and malignancy.[2]

Patient Preparation

All patients considered for surgery should undergo similar preoperative preparation. Unless contraindicated, a thorough endoscopic and radiographic evaluation of the patient is performed. In addition, possible stoma sites are marked.

Patients with Crohn's disease often present with a wide-ranging degree of malnutrition. Except in patients who require re-operation for enterocutaneous fistulas, opinion is divided as to whether malnutrition increases morbidity.[3] Unless sepsis is present, nutritional additives do little to reverse protein malnutrition.[4] In practice, hyperalimentation is omitted if an urgent or emergent indication for surgery exists. If surgery is elective, total parenteral nutrition is used preoperatively for 5–7 days. If significant hypo-albuminaemia exists ($<2.5\,g/dL$), serious consideration is given to avoiding bowel anastomosis in favour of a temporary stoma after resectional surgery.

Preoperative mechanical bowel preparation is routinely used except in patients with obstruction. Broad-spectrum antibiotics are delivered parenterally at induction. Patients on steroids will require a stress dosing of hydrocortisone around the time of surgery, tapering at 48–72 hours postoperation.

Operative Principles

There are several types of operations that are used in the surgery of Crohn's disease. They may be classified as follows:

- Intestinal resection with or without anastomosis
- Bypass procedure: internal (e.g. gastroduodenostomy); external (e.g. ileostomy).
- Strictureplasty

Farmer *et al.* reviewed 500 cases of Crohn's disease with surgery performed.[11] Surgical resection was the commonest procedure performed for patients with ileocolic or small bowel disease, while resection with ileostomy was more frequently done for Crohn's colitis. Bypass procedures were used in 5% of cases.

Resection

Resection is the procedure of choice for Crohn's disease of the small bowel, especially when it is the patient's first operation. The majority of authors strongly favour resectional techniques over bypass procedures for most clinical situations.[12] Resectional surgery is also the procedure of choice for Crohn's colitis. Despite the high recurrence rates, segmental resection with colocolic or colorectal or anastomosis provides many Crohn's colitis patients with many years of stoma-free life.

Bypass

Bypass operations are considered reasonable options in specific circumstances. For instance, in complicated ileocaecal phlegmon densely attached to iliac vessels or retroperitoneum, exclusion bypass is reasonable with plans for future resection.

Incontinuity bypass is the preferred method of managing symptomatic gastroduodenal Crohn's disease that is refractory to medical treatment. A highly selective vagotomy may be added to prevent marginal ulceration and minimize diarrhoea.

The blowhole colostomy with ileostomy for toxic colitis and toxic megacolon is a bypass procedure that was popularized by Turnbull of the Cleveland Clinic in the 1960s. Fortunately, this procedure is infrequently used these days, due to a decline in the incidence of toxic colitis. The main reason is that toxic colitis rarely worsens to that of toxic megacolon, for which the blowhole procedure is most valuable.

Strictureplasty

For patients with multiple strictures of the small bowel, intestinal conservation may be best achieved by surgically widening the stricture—a procedure called strictureplasty. This procedure was initially used by Katariya for the treatment of tuberculous strictures involving the small bowel.[13] It was Lee and Papaioannou who pioneered this procedure for use in stricture secondary to Crohn's disease.[14] This procedure has been proven effective in relieving obstructive symptoms, with weight gain that accompanies improved food tolerance. In addition, steroid medications can often be withdrawn or reduced despite leaving disease segments behind.

The situations where strictureplasty is considered include:

- Diffuse involvement of the small bowel with multiple strictures
- Strictures in a patient who has undergone previous major resection of the small bowel
- Rapid recurrence of Crohn's disease manifesting as obstruction
- Stricture in a patient with short bowel syndrome
- Nonphlegmonous fibrotic stricture

The contraindications to structureplasty are:

- Free or contained perforation of the small bowel
- Phlegmonous inflammation, internal fistula or external fistula involving the affected site
- Multiple strictures within a short segment
- Stricture in close proximity to a site chosen for resection (one should include this in the resected specimen)
- Colonic strictures
- Hypo-albuminaemia (<2 g/dl).

At the Cleveland Clinic, complication following strictureplasties occurred in 15% of patients; most were associated with serum albumin values of less than 3.0 gm/dl.

In addition to low operative morbidity, the long-term results of strictureplasties are quite promising. Of the 116 patients followed up for a mean of 36 months at the Cleveland Clinic, 99% were relieved of obstructive symptoms and 70% had ceased taking steroids.[15] Furthermore, the median weight gain six months postoperation was 4 kg. Most importantly, symptomatic recurrence affected only 24% of the patients, and all had new strictures or perforative disease remote from the original site of the strictureplasty. Asymptomatic re-stricturing occurred in only 2.8% of the 452 strictureplasties.

Recurrence

At ten years' follow-up, small bowel and ileocolic diseases have re-operation rates of 29%, respectively.[16] Segmental colonic disease treated by limited resection with colocolic or colorectal anastomosis has been described by several institutions.[17,18] While the majority will experience symptomatic recurrence, over 75% will maintain intestinal continuity for more than a decade, thus delaying the need for permanent ileostomy.

Crohn's colitis with relative rectal sparing can be adequately treated by colectomy and ileorectal anastomosis. The success of this operation depends on the patient's age, the duration of symptoms and concomitant small bowel disease. It has been found that up to 61% of patients maintained intestinal continuity after ten years following an ileorectal anastomosis.[19]

One of the commonest problems following proctocolectomy for Crohn's colitis is the recurrence of the disease in the ileostomy or remaining small bowel. Scammell *et al.* reported a 24% and a 35% cumulative re-operative rate for recurrence at five and ten years respectively.[20] The majority (89%) of recurrence occurred within 25 cm of the stoma.

Conclusion

Crohn's disease is a perplexing pan-intestinal disease whose aetiology is unknown. Symptoms and complications vary greatly from patient to patient. Despite the fact that no cure exists, a thoughtful, well-planned therapy and appropriate timely surgical intervention, where needed, can result in maintenance of a high quality of life for affected individuals.

References

1. Murray JJ, Schoetz DJ and Nugent FW. Surgical management of Crohn's disease involving duodenum, *Am J Surg* 1984; 147: 58.
2. Farmer RG, Hawk WA and Turnbull RB. Clinical patterns in Crohn's disease: a statistical study of 615 cases, *Gastroenterology* 1975; 68: 627.
3. Higgens CS, Keighley MRB and Allan RN. Impact of preoperative weight loss on postoperative morbidity, *J Roy Soc Med* 1981; 74: 571.
4. Irving MH. The management of surgical complications in Crohn's disease: abscess and fistula. In: Allan RN, Keighley MRB, Alexander-Williams J and Hawkins C (eds.), *Inflammatory Bowel Disease*, 2nd edition, Edinburgh, UK, Churchill-Livingstone, 1990, p. 458.
5. de Dombal FT, Burtib I and Goligher JC. Recurrence of Crohn's disease after primary excisional surgery, *Gut* 1971; 12: 519.

6. Sales DJ and Kirsner JB. The prognosis of inflammatoy bowel disease, *Arch Intern Med* 1983; 143: 294.

7. Papaioannau N, Piris J, Lee ECG and Kettlewell MGW. The relationship between histological inflammation in the cut ends after resection of Crohn's disease and recurrence, *Gut* 1979; 20: A916.

8. Chardavayne R, Flint GW, Pollack S and Wise L. Factors affecting recurrence following resection for Crohn's disease, *Dis Colon Rectum* 1986; 29: 495.

9. Speranza V, Zimi M, Leardi S and Del Pap M. Recurrence of Crohn's disease: are there any risk factors? *J Clin Gastroenterol* 1986; 8: 640.

10. Adolff M, Armaud JP and Ollier JC. Does the histological appearance at the margin of resection affect the postoperative recurrence rate in Crohn's disease? *Am Surg* 1987; 53: 543.

11. Farmer RG, Hawk WA and Turnbull RB Jr. Indications for surgery in Crohn's disease: analysis of 500 cases. *Gastroenterology* 1976; 71: 245.

12. Alexander-Williams J, Felding JF and Cooke WT. A comparison of results of excision and bypass for ileal Crohn's disease, *Gut* 1972; 13: 973.

13. Katariya RN, Sood S, Rao PG *et al.* Strictureplasty for tubercular strictures of the gastro-intestinal tract, *Br J Surg* 1977; 64: 496.

14. Lee ECG and Papaioannou N. Minimal surgery for chronic obstruction in patients with extensive or universal Crohn's disease, *Ann R Coll Surg Engl* 1982; 64: 229.

15. Fazio VW, Tjandra JJ, Lavery IC, Church JM *et al.* Long term follow-up of strictureplasty in Crohn's disease, *Dis Colon Rectum* 1993; 36: 353.

16. Scammell BE, Ambrose NS, Alexander-Williams J, Allan RN and Keighley MRB. Recurrent small bowel Crohn's disease is more frequent after subtotal colectomy and ileorectal anastomosis than pan-proctocolectomy, *Dis Colon Rectum* 1985; 28: 770.

17. Sanfey H, Bayles TM and Corman JL. Crohn's disease of the colon: Is there a role for limited resection? *Am J Surg* 1984; 147: 38.

18. Longe WE, Ballantyne GH and Cahow E. Treatment of Crohn's colitis segmental or total colectomy? *Arch Surg* 1988; 123: 588.

19. Longo WE, Oakley JR, Lavery IC, Church JM and Fazio VW. Outcome of ileorectal anastomosis for Crohn's colitis, *Dis Colon Rectum* 1992; 35: 1066.

20. Scammell BE, Andrews H, Allan RN, Alexander-Williams J and Keighley MRB. Results of proctocolectomy for Crohn's disease, *Br J Surg* 1987; 74: 671.

CHAPTER 19

Surgery for Ulcerative Colitis

F Seow-Choen

Introduction

Ulcerative colitis is an ulcerating mucosal disorder of unknown aetiology, affecting mainly the large bowel. It is often chronic, with acute relapses and periods of remission. However, in many patients, the first presentation may be that of severe acute fulminating colitis. There are also associated extraintestinal symptoms which may need treatment. In addition, there is an increased risk of malignant change, especially in patients with pancolonic disease of long duration. While most patients with ulcerative colitis will be treated medically, some may need surgery.

Acute Fulminating Colitis

Acute fulminating colitis often occurs as the first presentation of ulcerative colitis. Relapse of acute colitis is rarely as severe or has the same incidence of toxic megacolon or perforation.[1] The prognosis of an acute attack of colitis depends on the extent of the disease, the depth of bowel wall penetration and the severity of the attack. The depth of ulceration correlates closely with toxic dilatation and perforation.[2] It is the occurrence of free perforation which ultimately brings about death. Toxic dilatation without perforation was associated with only a 3% death rate, compared to 41% in those that perforated.[3] Toxic dilatation is defined as a transverse colon diameter of more than 5.5 cm, although the caecum and sigmoid colon may be involved as well.

Although 30% of patients with toxic megacolon respond to conservative treatment, the ultimate prospect of retaining such a colon is very low.[4]

Early surgical intervention is probably the single most important factor in decreasing mortality in acute fulminating colitis.[5]

Patients with acute fulminating colitis in whom there is no positive improvement after 72 hours on appropriate medical therapy should be considered for emergency colectomy, without waiting for toxic megacolon to supervene.

Choice of Surgical Methods

The choice of surgical procedures used in the past has varied from blowhole colectomy, total colectomy and ileorectal anastomosis, total colectomy and ileostomy with or without a mucus fistula, to proctocolectomy.

The Turnbull blowhole procedure has no place in modern surgery, as the incidence of sepsis is very high and all patients eventually require completion colectomies anyway.

Total colectomy and ileorectal anastomosis do not seem a sensible option in a septic, sick patient with hypo-albuminaemia who is on large doses of steroids, and should not be performed.

Proctocolectomy is practised by few surgeons as the mortality rate is higher (14%), compared with total colectomy and ileostomy (6%).[6] There is no medical reason to excise the rectum in an emergency when operating on a severely ill patient. Even in patients operated on for massive colorectal haemorrhage due to ulcerative colitis, rectal packing after total colectomy is usually successful in arresting bleeding. However, in fitter patients, a two-stage restorative proctocolectomy with defunctioning ileostomy is an excellent procedure.

The safest option for severe, acute fulminating colitis is total colectomy and ileostomy. The rectal stump may be oversewn or be brought out as a mucus fistula and, therefore, the rectum should be divided at or above the pelvic brim. This procedure leaves all options open for the future. Rectal excision is necessary in up to 80% of the patients after total colectomy for ulcerative colitis, and restorative proctocolectomy will still be possible.[7] On the other hand, where rectal sparing is optimal, an ileorectal anastomosis may then be achieved.

Chronic Ulcerative Colitis

Elective surgery may also be needed for patients with persistent acute colitis, recurrent or frequent relapsing colitis, chronic disease with debilitating side effects, or side effects of drug or steroid therapy. Other situations where elective colectomy may be indicated are in patients with otherwise uncontrollable pyoderma gangrenosum, exfoliative dermatitis, persistent or recurrent monoarthropathy, and severe uveitis. Colectomy has no influence on sacroileitis or anklylosing spondylosis or hepatobiliary complications.

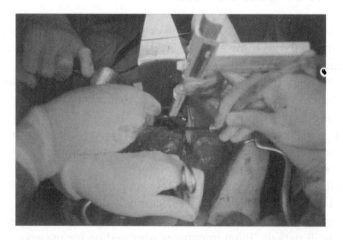

Figure 1. Transection of the anorectal junction with the help of a 30 mm linear stapler.

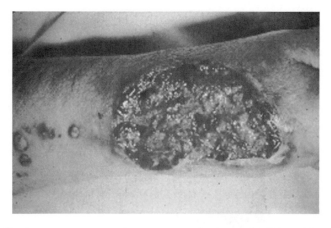

Figure 2. Pyoderma gangrenosum in a patient with ulcerative colitis, with response to colectomy.

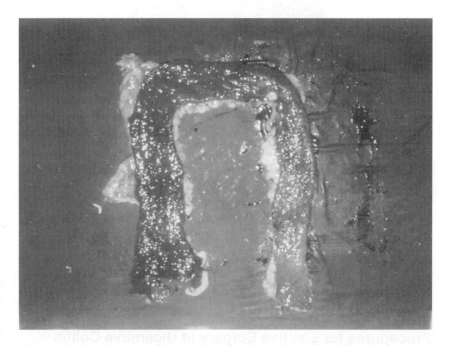

Figure 3. A resected specimen showing severe ulcerative colitis with pseudo-polyp formation.

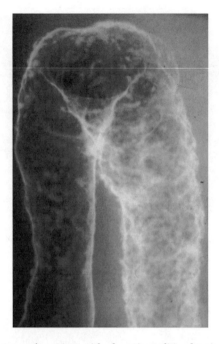

Figure 4. A barium enema of a patient with ulcerative colitis, showing loss of haustrations, pseudo-polyps and a ground-glass appearance.

The development of dysplasia or carcinoma in patients with ulcerative colitis is an indication for colectomy. The risk of malignant change is especially high, with acute-onset colitis, pancolitis, colonic dysplasia, long-standing colitis and a younger age at disease onset.[8] The risk of cancer in ulcerative colitis has been calculated to be about 0, 5 and 13% respectively after 10, 20 and 25 years of disease.[8] Furthermore, patients with previous colectomy and a retained rectum are not spared the risk of malignancy. The lack of Butyrate, a potent differentiating agent for colonic mucosa in the defunctioned rectum, may increase malignant change in such rectums. Furthermore, rectal cancer developing in the retained rectum appears to have a poor prognosis, being more frequently undifferentiated and more frequently associated with widespread dissemination.[8]

Procedures for Elective Surgery in Ulcerative Colitis

Total abdominal proctocolectomy and ileoanal anastomosis with an ileal reservoir or restorative proctocolectomy removes all large-bowel epithelium and yet preserves anal function, and is the procedure of choice in most patients with ulcerative colitis needing an elective operation.[9] The procedure, however, is normally performed only by colorectal surgeons, and few general surgeons will have any experience with it. There are variations in pouch designs, including S, W, J and H designs, although most surgeons would use about 40–45 cm of ileum to form the pouch. A well-trained and skilled surgeon should be able to perform a stapled anastomosis at or even below the dental line without actually performing a transanal mucosectomy by close anorectal dissection transabdominally below the levator ani. Mucosectomy has been blamed for increasing the incidence of postoperative incontinence and leakage. The retention of a few millimetres of colitic mucosa is not of very great consequence, fortunately. The conventional proctocolectomy and terminal ileostomy is still regarded by some general surgeons as the first-choice procedure for ulcerative colitis. In this procedure, all diseased tissues are removed and, therefore, the cancer risk is completely eliminated. The operative morbidity and mortality are also low. The disadvantages are the presence of permanent ileostomy, and that the perineal wound remains unhealed in 17–85% of patients after one year as well as by proctocolectomy itself. Proctocolectomy may result in impotence and urinary dysfunction. This may be reduced by close rectal dissection where cancer clearance is not a consideration, as well as by intersphincteric anal resection instead of wide mesorectal and perineal resections. Perineal scarring may also cause dyspareunia in females especially.

Total colectomy and ileorectal anastomosis is not often indicated in ulcerative colitis, although some surgeons recommend it for younger children. However, parents must be told that this is not a definitive procedure and there are still cancer risks.

The ileorectal anastomosis may also be used for patients who do not wish to spend time in hospital with a two-stage pouch procedure and run the risk of pelvic nerve damage. Patients, however, must have minimal rectal disease with a reasonable anal sphincter function. The ileorectal anastomosis may also be indicated as a palliative procedure for patients with colonic carcinoma and ulcerative colitis as it avoids a stoma.

Reservoir ileostomy is rarely used as a primary treatment for ulcerative colitis as the nipple valve is inherently unstable and the procedure has a high morbidity rate. The continent ileostomy has largely been superseded by the pelvic pouch procedure for patients with ulcerative colitis.

Although pouchitis or inflammation in the J pouch has been reported in up to 15% of patients following restorative proctocolectomy with an ileal J pouch, we have not seen this particular complication in any patient who did not have extra gastrointestinal manifestations before pouch construction. We feel that patients with ulcerative colitis restricted to the large bowel do very well therefore after surgery with the ileal pouch and pouchitis must be very rare or nonexistent in these patients.

References

1. Dalton HR and Jewell DP. The management of acute severe ulcerative colitis, *Ann Med* 1991; 23: 389–91.
2. Buckell NA, William GT, Bartram CP and Lennard-Jones JE. Depth of ulceration in colitis: correlation with outcome and clinical and radiological features, *Gastroenterolgy* 1980; 79: 19–25.
3. Greenstein AJ and Aufses AH. Differences in pathogenesis, incidence and outcome of perforation in inflammatory bowel disease, *Surg Gynecol Obstet* 1985; 160: 63–9.
4. Norland CC and Kirsner JB. Toxic dilation of the colon: aetiology treatment and prognosis in 42 patients, 1969; 48: 229–50.
5. Morrell P, Hawker PC, Allan RN, Dykes PW and Alexander-Williams J. Management of acute colitis in inflammatory bowel disease, *World J Surg* 1986; 10: 814–19.
6. Block GE, Moosa AR, Simonowitz D and Hassan SZ. Emergency colectomy for inflammatory bowel disease, *Surgery* 1977; 82: 531–6.
7. Binder SC, Miller HH and Deterling RA Jr. Emergency and urgent operations for ulcerative colitis, *Arch Surg* 1975; 110: 284–9.
8. O'Riordain DS and O'Lonnell PR. Completion proctectomy in ulcerative colitis, *Br J Surg* 1997; 84: 436–7.
9. Eu KW and Seow-Choen F. The role of mucosectomy and the ileoanal pouch, *Seminars Colon Rectal Surg* 1196; 7: 72–6.

CHAPTER 20

Toxic Megacolon in Ulcerative Colitis: Current Management

PL Roberts

Introduction

Ulcerative colitis is a mucosal disease which begins in the rectum and extends proximally, potentially affecting the entire colon. In Western countries it has a reported incidence of 5/100 000, with a slight female predominance. There is a bimodal distribution of disease, with peaks in the third and eighth decades. First degree relatives of affected individuals have a 15-fold increase in incidence of the disease.

The natural history of the disease is determined by the extent of the disease (patients with pancolitis have more severe disease and are more likely to require surgery) and the severity of the disease on initial presentation.[1] Ultimately, 30–40% of patients with ulcerative colitis require surgery, with

Table 1. Criteria for toxic megacolon.

Radiographic evidence of colonic dilatation:
At least three of the following:
• Fever >38°C (101.5°F)
• Tachycardia >100/min
• Leukocytosis (>10.5 × 10 9/l)
• Anaemia
In addition to the above, at least one of the following:
• Dehydration
• Altered consciousness
• Electrolyte disturbances
• Hypotension

Adapted from: Sheth SG and LaMont JT, Toxic megacolon, *Lancet* 1998; 351; 509–13.[3]

the most common indications including intractability to medical management, toxic or acute resolving colitis, growth retardation, cancer or dysplasia, complications of medical therapy and extra-intestinal manifestations of the disease.

Toxic megacolon was first described by Marshak in 1950 and was defined as total or segmental nonobstructive colonic dilatation of at least 6 cm associated with systemic toxicity.[2] The original definition has been refined to reflect the toxicity of the patients and not the X-ray findings, and generally includes those features outlined in Table 1.[3] Toxic megacolon is not specific to ulcerative colitis and may also occur with Crohn's disease, infectious colitides such as clostridium difficile colitis, salmonella, shigella, campylobacter, amebiasis and cytomegalovirus. Patients with ulcerative colitis and Crohn's disease have about a 1–5% lifetime risk for the development of toxic colitis.[4,5] With earlier recognition and prompt treatment of colitis, the incidence of toxic megacolon in inflammatory bowel disease is decreasing.

Pathophysiology

The role of nitric oxide in the pathogenesis of toxic megacolon has been examined. Mourelle and colleagues studied nitric oxide synthase in patients who underwent surgery for toxic colitis, patients with active ulcerative colitis (pancolitis) without megacolon and patients who underwent resection for colorectal cancer (controls).[6] The amount of nitric oxide and the inducible form of the enzyme were significantly increased in the muscle layer in toxic megacolon patients, especially in the more dilated segments. The activity of the enzyme decreased with steroid administration and with the use of oral nonabsorbable antibiotics.[6] The amount of nitric oxide and the inducible form of the enzyme were significantly increased in the muscle layer in toxic megacolon patients, especially in the more dilated segments. The activity of the enzyme decreased with steroid administration and with the use of oral nonabsorbable antibiotics.

Toxic megacolon produces pronounced dilatation and thinning of the bowel wall. In addition, acute inflammation is seen in all layers of the bowel wall, with myocyte degeneration, necrosis and replacement by granulation tissue with shortening of muscle fibres.

Clinical Features

Toxic megacolon is a complication of pan-colitis and affects males and females equally. The highest risk for the development of toxic megacolon is early in the course of the disease and up to 30% of patients present within three months of diagnosis and 60% present within the first three years of diagnosis.[7,8] A variety of factors may trigger ulcerative colitis, including medications such as anticholingerics, antidiarrhoeals, narcotics and rapid wean and/or discontinuation of 5-ASA products or steroids. Other factors include recent barium enema examination or endoscopic examination, superimposed infection such as clostridium difficile, amebiasis, cytomegalovirus or HIV, and smoking cessation. An interesting question is whether toxic megacolon could potentially be prevented by the identification of those individuals with severe colitis who will most likely require a colectomy. Carbonnel examined 46 patients with severe colitis (which was defined by the endoscopic presence of extensive deep ulcerations) and 39 patients with moderate colitis.[9] Colonoscopy was performed by an expert endoscopist. Only 3 of 46 patients with severe colitis avoided surgery, compared with 30 of 39 patients with moderate colitis, suggesting that surgery should be performed sooner in such patients instead of persisting with a long course of medical management.

The role of cyclosporine has also been examined in patients with severe colitis as it is the only drug which has been shown to control severe colitis unresponsive to steroids. The major side effects of cyclosporine include seizures, renal insufficiency and the development of opportunistic infections. It has been reported to induce remission in 50–80% of patients with severe ulcerative colitis who have failed intravenous steroids.[10,11] The long term response rate is 40–60%, and thus of the entire cohort the long term remission rate is between 20 and 50%.

Treatment

The initial management of toxic megacolon includes bowel rest, fluid resuscitation, correction of electrolyte imbalances and administration of intravenous steroids. Specific infectious agents such as clostridium difficile are treated. Broad spectrum parenteral antibiotics are considered. Serial abdominal X-rays and examinations are performed. Surgical and enterostomal consultations are obtained early in the course of the patient's hospitalization. Medical therapy is successful in up to 50% of patients.[1] Persistent fever suggests the presence of a localized abscess or perforation. If a patient does not improve within 48 hours, expeditious colectomy is strongly recommended. Preoperative marking of the intended stoma site is performed ideally by a trained enterostomal therapist. The operation of choice is total abdominal colectomy and ileostomy. The rectal stump may be dealt with in a variety of ways, including simple staple or suture closure of the stump, bringing the stump out as a buried mucous fistula and performing tube drainage of the rectum. Preservation of the omentum or use of a bioresorbable membrane may ease re-entry into the abdomen at the time of the subsequent ileoanal pouch procedure. Although toxic megacolon was previously associated with a mortality rate of 19–29%,[12] the current mortality rates are 0–2% and are probably due to early recognition, better intensive medical management, earlier surgical intervention and better postoperative care. The mortality rates are determined by the incidence of associated perforation of the colon. The presence of perforation is associated with a fivefold increase in surgical mortality.[13]

Miscellaneous

Cytomegalovirus (CMV) is associated with ulcerative colitis and has been increasingly recognized as a triggering factor. CMV is a highly specific herpes virus that is spread by person-to-person contact, blood transfusion and tissue transplantation. The symptoms of CMV colitis include diarrhoea, vomiting and abdominal pain and are virtually indistinguishable from ulcerative colitis. Detection and subsequent treatment of CMV may help to avoid the need for colectomy.

In 19 patients with severe steroid-resistant ulcerative colitis, proctoscopy without air insufflation and rectal biopsy revealed CMV in seven rectal biopsies and one in the buffy coat.[14] Five patients were subsequently treated successfully with gancyclovir and foscarnet and only one required colectomy.

Toxic megacolon is increasingly recognized as a manifestation of severe clostridium difficile colitis, and at our institution we are seeing increasing numbers of patients with severe c diff colitis. These patients are frequently hospitalized for other reasons and have multiple other medical comorbidities. A uniform finding in such patients has been impressive thickening of the colonic wall and sequestration of large amounts of fluid. While patients with clostridium difficile colitis are often adequately treated with oral metronidazole, patients with severe disease often have an ileus and, accordingly, consideration should be given to administration of intravenous metronidazole and irrigation of the colon with vancomycin with a rectal tube or through the colonoscope. Colonoscopy can be considered for decompression and has been shown to be safe in selected patients.[15] Patients who fail to respond to medical treatment may require colectomy; however, mortality rates are quite high.[16,17]

References

1. Farmer RG, Easley KA and Rankin GB. Clinical patterns, natural history and progression of ulcerative colitis: a long-term follow-up of 1116 patients, *Dig Dis Sci* 1993; 38: 1137–46.
2. Marshak RH, Lester LJ and Friedman AI. Megacolon: a complication of ulcerative colitis, *Gastroenterology* 1950: 16: 768–82.
3. Sheth SG and Lamont JT. Toxic megacolon, *Lancet* 1998; 351: 509–13.
4. Grieco MB, Bordan DL and Geiss DL. Toxic megacolon complicating Crohn's disease, *Ann Surg* 1980; 191: 75–80.
5. Fazio VW. Toxic megacolon in ulcerative colitis and Crohn's colitis, *Clin Gastroenterol* 1980; 9: 389–407.
6. Mourelle M, Casellas F, Guarner F *et al.* Induction of nitric oxide synthase in colonic smooth muscle from patients with toxic megacolon, *Gastroenterology* 1995; 109: 1497–502.

7. Jalan KN, Circus W, Cord WI *et al*. An experience with ulcerative colitis: toxic dilatation in 55 cases, *Gastroenterology* 1969; 57: 68–82.

8. Langholz E, Munkholm P, Davidsen M *et al*. Course of ulcerative colitis: analysis of changes in disease activity over years, *Gastroenterology* 1994; 107: 3–11.

9. Carbonnel F, Lavergne A, Lemann M *et al*. Colonoscopy of acute colitis: a safe and reliable tool for assessment of severity, *Dig Dis Sci* 1994; 39: 1550–7.

10. Sandborn WJ. A critical review of cyclosporine therapy in inflammatory bowel disease, *Inflammatory Bowel Diseases* 1995; 1: 48–63.

11. Lichtiger S, Present DH, Kornbluth A *et al*. Cyclosporine in severe ulcerative colitis refractory to steroid therapy, *N Engl J Med* 1994; 330: 1841–5.

12. Strauss RJ, Flint GW, Platt N *et al*. The surgical management of toxic dilatation of the colon: a report of 28 cases and review of the literature, *Ann Surg* 1976; 184: 682–8.

13. Roy MA. Inflammatory bowel disease, *Surg Clin North Am* 1997; 77: 1419–31.

14. Cottone M, Pietrosi G, Martorana G *et al*. Prevalence of cytomegalovirus infection in severe refractory ulcerative and Crohn's colitis, *Am J Gastroenterol* 2001; 96: 773–5.

15. Triadafilopoulos G and Hallstone AE. Acute abdomen as the first presentation of pseudomembranous colitis, *Gastroenterology* 1991; 101: 685–91.

16. Rubin MS, Bodenstein LE and Kent KC. Severe clostridium difficile colitis, *Dis Colon Rectum* 1995; 38: 350–4.

17. Trudel JL, Deschenes M, Mayrand S *et al*. Toxic megacolon complicating pseudomembranous enterocolitis, *Dis Colon Rectum* 1995; 38: 1033–8.

CHAPTER 21

Massive Haemorrhage in Inflammatory Bowel Disease

D Lloyd

Introduction

Massive gastrointestinal haemorrhage is rare in IBD. It is more often seen in Crohn's than UC and recurrence is common when it is treated conservatively. An endoscopically treatable lesion when there is massive bleeding in IBD is uncommon.[1]

A good history and examination are mandatory in all cases of GI bleeding, as 1.5% of all surgical emergencies in the general population are due to lower GI bleeding[2] and there are many reports in the literature on massive gastrointestinal haemorrhage in IBD that is not directly due to colitis.[3,4]

Crohn's Disease

Crohn's disease is a transmural inflammatory process that can effect the gastrointestinal tract anywhere from the mouth to the anus. Commonly there are intervening segments of normal mucosa and because of this it is generally referred to as regional enteritis. Massive haemorrhage in Crohn's disease creates a diagnostic dilemma, as the disease can effect both the small and the large intestine.

Upper GI Tract

More commonly, massive GI bleeding occurring in Crohn's is from an unrelated entity. Peptic ulcer disease is known to accompany Crohn's in up to 15% of patients.[5] The high use of aspirin-containing compounds, nonsteroidal anti-inflammatory drugs and steroid therapy in this population increases the risk of peptic ulceration or bleeding from GI irritation. So gastroscopy +/− gastric aspiration is mandatory in these patients.

Small Intestine

In patients with small bowel Crohn's disease, there may be multiple diseased segments. Isolating the bleeding source from specific sites can be extremely difficult, as blood can back-wash proximally as well as being present down-stream.

Crohn's disease is a chronic relapsing condition, and during the course of the patients' active disease they may be subjected to multiple laparotomies and small bowel resections. The aim is to be as conservative as possible when resecting the small bowel in Crohn's, as there is a great risk of ending up with too little remaining small bowel to adequately keep up with their nutritional needs—a condition called "short gut syndrome".

If the small bowel is full of blood, it desirable to have the bleeding segment accurately isolated to enable as limited a resection as possible. The advent of mesenteric angiography in the 1960s[6] has greatly enhanced the ability to isolate the bleeding site preoperatively. Recently, mesenteric angiography has also become a therapeutic tool.[7–9] Once the bleeding site has been isolated, selective angiographic infusion of vasopressin into the feeding artery will control the haemorrhage in up to 71% of patients.[10]

Therapeutic angiography is not without risk. Vasopressin infusions may cause hypertension, bradycardia, coronary vasoconstriction, bowel wall ischaemia, peripheral vascular ischaemia or catheter-related thrombosis.[11]

Mesenteric angiography can also be used to allow the selective embolization of the feeding vessel.[8,11–13] The main associated complications are infarction of the bowel wall (a greater risk in the large bowel), ischaemia and stricture formation.[14,15]

If these measures fail, the mesenteric catheter may be left in place so that intraoperative angiography can be performed.[16] At surgery, metallic clips are placed along the mesenteric margin of the bowel to more accurately localize the site of bleeding at angiography, thus enabling a limited bowel resection and preserving the maximal amount of small bowel.

Occasionally the bleeding site is still unable to be isolated. Passing a paediatric colonoscope orally may help find the bleeding site.[17] Once past the ligament of Treitz, the abdominal operator is able to thread the scope along the small bowel looking for the source of bleeding both by direct vision and by transillumination of the small bowel wall. This technique may negate the need to perform an enteroscopy via a mid-small-bowel enterotomy—avoiding the potential complications of a small bowel incision and subsequent closure, which in active Crohn's has an increased risk of complications.

Colon

Massive bleeding in Crohn's colitis is as rare as bleeding from Crohn's small bowel lesions. Mesenteric angiography is currently the procedure of choice, being both diagnostic and therapeutic. But colonoscopy is increasingly becoming the first line investigative method for what looks to be bleeding from a colonic source.[5]

Segmental colonic disease occurs in less than 10% of patients with Crohn's disease.[18–20] Bleeding may occur from an isolated segment, and segmental colectomy in this situation is feasible. More commonly, bleeding occurs with fulminent colitis or toxic megacolon. Treatment should consist of subtotal colectomy, end ileostomy and mucous fistula.[5] At laparotomy, the rectum must be examined for ongoing rectal bleeding.

Emergent surgery is undertaken if there is increasing colonic dilatation, continual bleeding or haemodynamic instability after 4–6 units of blood have been transfused, perforation, peritonitis, no clinical improvement within 24 hours of initiation of medical therapy, or if any worsening of the patient's condition occurs.[5]

Ulcerative Colitis

Massive haemorrhage in ulcerative colitis is occasionally the principal reason for emergency colectomy. The frequency of severe haemorrhage in ulcerative colitis ranges from 0 to 4.5%, with a mean of 2.2%. However, this rare complication accounts for approximately 10% of all urgent colectomies for ulcerative colitis.[21] It is usually associated with fulminant colitis or toxic megacolon, but not in every case. Massive bleeding has occurred from bleeding pseudopolyyps or unrelated causes such as angiodysplasia or diverticular disease.[3,9]

In the elective setting for ulcerative colitis, total proctocolectomy with J pouch ileo-anal anastomosis is the operation of choice. Most centres perform a subtotal colectomy and end ileostomy when the patient has fulminant colitis or toxic megacolon, with a restorative procedure planned in the future.

In cases of massive haemorrhage in ulcerative colitis, when a subtotal colectomy is performed, there is a 12% reoperative rate for rebleeding from the rectal stump.[21] There is a case for performing a restorative procedure initially if there is active bleeding from the rectal stump at the time of surgery and the patient is not toxic. When the patient is toxic and has massive bleeding from the rectal stump, an option is to pack the rectal stump for 24–48 hours after performing a subtotal colectomy. The bleeding usually settles, and a proctectomy and restorative procedure can be preformed at a later date when the patient is stable.

If the patient is immunocompromised (suffering from AIDS, immunosuppressed or undergoing chemotherapy) CMV colitis/enteritis can be a cause of massive GI haemorrhage from both the large and the small bowel. The patient's symptoms and signs can mimic fulminant ulcerative colitis and it is only on biopsy, when cytomegalovirus inclusions are seen, that the diagnosis is made.[4,22]

In summary, massive haemorrhage in IBD is rare and requires a multidisciplinary approach involving surgeons, physicians and radiologists. More common causes of GI bleeding must not be overlooked.

References

1. Pardi DS *et al*. Acute major gastrointestinal hemorrhage in inflammatory bowel disease, *Gastrointest Endosc* 1999; 49(2): 153–7.
2. Stower MJ *et al*. Surgical emergencies and manpower, *Ann R Coll Surg Engl* 1984; 66: 117–19.
3. Martinez-Caballero A *et al*. Ulcerative colitis and colonic angiodysplasia associated with a lower digestive hemorrhage: their diagnosis by 99-technetium-labelled red blood cells, *Rev Esp Enferm Dig* 1997; 89(1): 51–4.
4. Roskell DE *et al*. HIV-associated cytomegalovirus colitis as a mimic of inflammatory bowel disease, *GUT* 1995; 37: 148–50.
5. Strong SA. Crohn's disease, In *Surgery of the Colon & Rectum* (eds. Nicholls RJ and Dozois RR), pp. 636–8. Churchill Livingstone, New York.
6. Baum S *et al*. The operative radiography demonstration of intra-abdominal bleeding from undetermined sites by percutaneous selective celiac and superior mesenteric angiography, *Surgery* 1965; 58: 797–805.
7. Browder W *et al*. Impact of emergency angiography in massive lower gastrointestinal bleeding, *Ann Surg* 1986; 204: 530–6.
8. Rosch J *et al*. Selective arterial infusions of vasoconstrictors in acute gastrointestinal bleeding, *Radiology* 1971; 99: 27–36.
9. Cavaluzzi JA *et al*. Vasopressin control of massive hemorrhage in chronic ulcerative colitis, *Am J Roentgenol* 1976; 127(4): 672–5.
10. Clark RA *et al*. (1981) Acute arterial gastrointestinal hemorrhage: efficacy of transcatheter control, *AJR* 136: 1185–9.
11. Gomes AS *et al*. Angiographic treatment of gastrointestinal hemorrhage: comparison of vasopressin infusions and embolization, *AJR* 1986; 146: 1031–7.
12. Uflacker R. Transcatheter embolization for treatment of acute lower gastrointestinal bleeding, *Acta Radiol* 1987; 28: 425–30.
13. Palmaz JC *et al*. Therapeutic embolization of small bowel arteries, *Radiology* 1984; 152: 377–82.
14. Mitty HA *et al*. Colonic stricture after transcatheter embolization for diverticular bleeding, *AJR* 1979; 133: 519–21.
15. Rosenkrartz H *et al*. Post-embolic colonic infarction, *Radiology* 1982; 142: 47–51.

16. Fazio VW *et al*. (1980) Intraoperative angiography and the localization of bleeding from the small intestine, *Surg Gynecol Obstet* 1980; 151: 637–40.
17. Leong AFP-K and Seow-Choen F. Lower gastrointestinal bleeding. In *Surgery of the Colon & Rectum* (eds. Nicholls RJ and Dozois RR), p. 772. Churchill Livingstone, New York.
18. Farmer RG *et al*. Long-term follow-up of patients with Crohn's disease: relationship between the clinical pattern and prognosis, *Gastroenterology* 1985; 88: 1818–25.
19. Shivananda S *et al*. Crohn's disease: risk of recurrence and reoperation in a defined population, *Gut* 1989; 30: 990–5.
20. Goligher JC. Surgical treatment of Crohn's disease affecting mainly or entirely the large bowel, *World J Surg* 1988; 12: 186–90.
21. Robert JH *et al*. Management of severe hemorrhage in ulcerative colitis, *Am J Surg* 1990; 159: 550–5.
22. Cheung AN *et al*. Cytomegalovirus infection of the gastrointestinal tract in non-AIDS patients, *Am J Gastroenterol* 1993; 88(11): 1882–6.

CHAPTER 22

Perianal Crohn's Disease

JF Lim

Introduction

Crohn's disease is a chronic inflammatory condition that can affect any part of the gastrointestinal tract. The presence of perianal Crohn's disease is usually evident on clinical examination. Anal manifestation is rarely seen in isolation. As such, evaluation of the entire gastrointestinal tract is an important part of management.

Clinical Presentation

Patients with colonic disease are more likely to manifest anal symptoms. As Crohn's disease has a bimodal age distribution, with the elderly group having a predilection for distal disease, it is more common to see perianal disease in this group. Patients can present with asymptomatic skin tags, fissures, abscesses, simple and complex fistulas or incontinence as a sequela from previous overzealous surgery.

Patients with asymptomatic skin tags should be advised against surgery, as this is often complicated by nonhealing ulcers. Patients with haemorrhoids or symptomatic skin tags should be treated by local measures such as increasing dietary fibre, oral micronized purified flavonidic fraction (e.g. Daflon®) or sclerotherapy/rubber-band ligation. Definitive haemorrhoidectomy should be reserved for those with severe complications like haemorrhage, as surgery is fraught with complications. Jeffrey *et al.* showed that in 21 patients treated for haemorrhoids, 10 developed complications and 6 of these eventually required proctectomy.[1] Since their paper, most surgeons have found surgery in this group of patients equally frustrating.

Anal Fissure

While the majority of cases of anal fissures in patients with Crohn's disease are located in the "usual" 6 or 12 o'clock location, a significant number of patients suffer from multiple, cavitating or eccentrically located fissures. If uncomplicated, the patient should be treated nonoperatively with topical agents, antidiarrhoeal medication and medication for coexisting proximal disease. The majority have a self-limiting course and surgery should be reserved for the complex or persistent cases.

Lateral sphincterotomy is the procedure of choice, as the rate of healing is excellent (up to 88% in one group[2]). Advancement flaps are rarely indicated, as most of these patients have coexistent proximal disease, which contributes significantly to the occurrence of fissures. If the fissure is persistent despite sphincterotomy, proctectomy (if the rectum is involved macroscopically or microscopically[3]) or defunctioning colostomy may be required. One important thing to note is that if a previously painless fissure becomes painful, the surgeon should be wary of underlying anal abscess, which needs urgent drainage.

Perianal Abscess

Perianal abscesses should be treated in the same way regardless of whether the patient has a history of Crohn's disease or not. An aggressive search for a fistula tract or the addition of postoperative antibiotics has not been clearly shown to be of benefit.

For recurrent disease, the surgeon should try to locate the fistula tract and insert a draining seton. In our experience using Prolene sutures or silastic vascular loops, the patients tolerated long-term loose seton drainage well. However, if sepsis is recurrent despite this, a defunctioning colostomy is necessary to aid healing.

Fistula-in-Ano

This problem remains the most challenging one facing surgeons today. In the past, due to the fear of nonhealing wounds, definitive fistula surgery was frowned upon. The problem has not been so much one of a nonhealing wound as of new fistulas forming. Hence the preservation of a functional anus remains the main objective.

For low fistulas, a simple fistulotomy will suffice. The results have been encouraging, with success of over 80% in most series. However, there are occasions when the wound fails to heal and becomes a chronic ulcer. Such cases should be treated symptomatically and medical management instituted.

For high fistulas, the management would depend on the location and complexity of the fistula, the presence of concomitant proctitis or anal canal disease, and previous surgery.

In the case of a high transphincteric fistula without evidence of proctitis (macroscopic or microscopic), a loose seton or fistulectomy with a rectal mucosal advancement flap is acceptable. The loose seton controls sepsis and, provided the patient has no hang-ups, can be a good long-term option. If there is concomitant proximal disease, medical treatment would be necessary. While activity of intestinal and of anal disease appear to be parallel, there is little definitive evidence that resection of diseased intestine will heal the anal disease.

When proctitis is present with a high fistula, a loose seton with concomitant medical therapy should be the first line of treatment. If anal sepsis is difficult to control, proximal diversion with an ileostomy or colostomy may help improve symptom control, but reversal of the stoma has rarely led to long-term control of the fistula. If these measures fail, then an abdominoperineal resection might be needed. Caution must be taken in view of a raised incidence of delayed perineal wound healing.

Occasionally, long-course antibiotics have been tried for treating simple anal fistulas, with metronidazole having a reported success rate of 50%, but I am skeptical about this as this success rate has not been reproduced for fistulas-in-ano of patients without Crohn's disease.

Recently, Infliximab (an anti-TNF α antibody) has been tried, with a response rate of 71% and a healing rate of 39% within eight weeks. However, there was a relapse rate of 64% at one year for respondents.[4]

For patients with faecal incontinence from prior surgery, an attempt of sphincteroplasty would not be unreasonable but, if done, it should be covered with proximal diverting stoma.

One rarely seen but important thing is the possibility of development of carcinomatous change in a persistent Crohn's ulcer or fistula, and one must be wary of it.

In summary, managing a problem of perianal Crohn's disease is challenging but a surgeon should be unfazed by this, as the results are usually satisfying. Remember that the aim is to restore function and not anatomy.

References

1. Jeffery PJ, Ritchie JK and Parks AG. Treatment of haemorrhoids in patients with inflammatory bowel disease, *Lancet* 1977; 1: 1084–5.
2. Fleshner PR, Schoetz DJ, Roberts PLand *et al*. Anal fissure in Crohn's disease: a plea for aggressive management, *Dis Colon Rectum* 1995; 38: 1137–43.
3. Chrysos E *et al*. Rectoanal motility in Crohn's disease, *Dis Colon Rectum* 2001; 44(10): 1509–13.
4. Ouraghi A *et al*. Infliximab therapy for Crohn's disease anoperineal lesions, *Gastroenterologie Clinique et Biologique* 2001; 25(11): 949–56.

CHAPTER 23

Clinical Manifestations of Familial Adenomatous Polyposis

F Seow-Choen

Introduction

Familial adenomatous polyposis (FAP) is an autosomal dominant condition originally known as familial polyposis coli. Gardner's triad initially described an FAP syndrome of multiple epidermoid cysts, multiple osteomas and familial polyposis.[1] The number of known associated conditions, both malignant and benign, has now increased significantly. Some of these lesions cause morbidity and mortality whilst others are clinical markers for the genotype only. Abnormal structures can be found in tissues from all three primary embryonic layers.[2]

Abnormalities Arising in Tissues of Endodermal Germ Layer Origin

Colorectal polyps

The main pathology in FAP is the presence of multiple adenomatous polyps in the large intestine, most of which arise in the second decade of life. Colorectal adenomas, however, have been detected in an 18-month-old child. Rarely polyps arise in older adult life in what is called attenuated FAP.

Affected individuals may have as many as 10 000 or, rarely, less than 200. There is a 100% risk of malignant transformation in at least one adenoma by middle age. Timely surgery is necessary to prevent the development of colorectal carcinoma. This is normally performed at the end of the second decade of life.

Gastric polyps

Several types of gastric polyps are associated with FAP. The most common are fundic glandular cysts, which are usually harmatomatous and have no malignant potential.[2] However, about 10% of patients have gastric adenomas and sometimes gastric carcinomas can occur. Hyperplastic polyps have also been reported.

Duodenal/periampullary polyps

Duodenal polyps may be found in the majority of patients with FAP.[2,3] These polyps are most numerous in the second and third parts of the duodenum, especially around the periampullary region. Duodenal and periampullary carcinomas are common and are the second-most-common cause of cancer mortality in patients with FAP, after colorectal resection. Bile in FAP has a co-carcinogenic effect.[4] Sulindac NSAID's and COX-2 inhibitors may prove to be useful adjunct drugs for the prevention of duodenal polyps.[5]

Small bowel polyps

Adenomas are not infrequently found in the terminal ileum and may also occur in the jejunum. These small intestinal polyps may result in ileal or jejunal carcinoma although risks are small.[6]

Gall bladder, bile duct, pancreas and pancreatic duct tumours

Hepatobiliary and pancreatic ductal adenomas and their malignant counterparts, together with pancreatic carcinoma, have been reported with increasing frequency in patients with FAP.[7]

Thyroid carcinoma

Young females under 35 years of age have a 160×-greater-than-expected risk of developing thyroid papillary carcinoma if they have FAP.[8]

Other endocrine tumours

Other endocrine tumours, including adrenal carcinomas,[9] multiple endocrine neoplasia type 2b, pituitary adenomas and pancreatic islet cell tumours, have also been reported.[10]

Abnormalities Arising from Tissues of Mesodermal Germ Layer Origin

Skeletal abnormalities

Osteomas of the skull, jaw and, less commonly, other parts of the skeletal system are commonly found.[11] Occult osteomas may occur in more than 90% of patients with FAP. These lesions are of no clinical significance except in identifying affected individuals before the development of colorectal polyposis.

Dental abnormalities

Dental pathology was described as part of the original Gardner's syndrome. These abnormalities include early caries with tooth loss, supernumerary teeth, odontomas, dentigerous cysts and impacted permanent teeth.[11]

Hepatoblastoma

There is a higher-than-expected incidence of hepatoblastoma in the off-spring of patients with FAP, some of which will present as stillbirths.[12]

Desmoids

Desmoids (or fibromatosis) are found in about 10% of patients in FAP.[13] Two types of desmoid tumours are recognized: the intra-abdominal type and the musculo-aponeurotic type. Intra-abdominal desmoids are very vascular tumours. They may be well-encapsulated or diffuse, and may occur within the mesentery or in the retroperitoneal region. Musculo-aponeurotic desmoids are usually more fibrous and may occur in the abdominal wall, within scar tissues or even within aponeurotic sites away from the abdomen. These tumours have varying growth rates in individual patients: in some, growth is rapid, others show a very slow growth rate, and in a few, actual regression may be seen. Growth is said to be stimulated by pregnancy and surgery although the relationship may be related to the time lapsed and not to the actual events. Intra-abdominal desmoids are very difficult to remove totally, have a high recurrence rate, and may bleed uncontrollably during surgery. Patients may also present with ureteric obstruction due to retroperitoneal desmoids. Patients with FAP have been noted also to have a high incidence of postoperative intestinal obstruction which may be related to a disorder of fibrous tissue formation.

Abnormalities Arising from Tissues of Ectodermal Germ Layer Origin

Cutaneous lesions

Epidermoid and sebaceous cysts are rare in the normal prepubertal patient. The presence of these cysts is therefore an indicator that a particular individual has inherited the gene.[14] Absence of cysts, however, does not mean that the gene has not been inherited. Unusual skin pigmentation and discoloration have also been described in relation to FAP.[14]

Central nervous system tumours

Turcot and his colleagues described two siblings in a family with colonic polyposis in whom astrocytoma and medulloblastoma had occurred. The relationship of Turcot's to FAP has given rise to considerable debate recently and the matter is still in doubt, partly because these tumours present at an early age and often prior to the development of colonic polyps.[15]

Congenital Hypertrophy of the Retinal Pigment Epithelium

Congenital hypertrophy of the retinal pigment epithelium (CHRPE) does not have any malignant potential, but it has some significance clinically as a diagnostic marker of the presence or absence of the gene for FAP. These lesions in patients carrying the gene for FAP may be multiple and appear at birth or shortly thereafter. Multiple or bilateral lesions have a very high specificity and sensitivity as a clinical marker but patients with FAP have been known to have none. These ocular lesions are discrete, usually darkly pigmented and may be round, oval or bean-shaped, with a surrounding depigmented halo. The lesion size may range from 0.1 to 1.0 or more times the diameter of the optic disc.[16] Small solitary or unilateral lesions are sometimes found in the normal population. Angoid streaks in the retina suggestive of connective tissue disorders have also been reported.

Conclusion

FAP is a multiple-system disorder. Awareness of the plethora of clinical manifestations of FAP is helpful in planning an appropriate treatment strategy for the affected patient. More recent genetic studies have shown the relation between APC gene variation[17–20] and the phenotypic spectrum.

References

1. Gardner EJ. Follow-up of a family group exhibiting dominant inheritance of a syndrome including intestinal polyps, osteomas, fibromas and epidermal cysts, *Am J Hum Genet* 1962; 14: 376–90.

2. Seow-Choen F, Neale KF, Landgrebe JC, Bussey HJR and Thomson JPS. A review of physical abnormalities in familial adenomatous polyposis, *Sing Med J* 1991; 32: 139–42.

3. Seow-Choen F, Neale K, Landgrebe JC, Bussey HJR and Thomson JPS. A review of physical abnormalities in familial adenomatous polyposis, *Sing Med J* 1991; 32: 139–42.

4. Spigelman AD, Thomson JPS and Philips RKS. Cholecystectomy, duodenogastric reflux and polyposis, *J R Soc Med* 1989; 82: 436–7.

5. Seow-Choen F, Vijayan V and Keng V. Prospective randomised study of sulindac versus calcium and calciferol for upper gastrointestinal polyps in familial adenomatous polyposis, *Br J Surg* 1996; 83: 1763–6.

6. Ross JE and Mara JE. Small bowel polyps and carcinoma in multiple intestinal polyposis, *Arch Surg* 1974; 108: 736–8.

7. Komorowski RA, Tresp MG and Wilson SD. Pancreaticobiliary involvement in familial polyposis coli/Gardner's syndrome, *Dis Colon Rectum* 1986; 29: 55–8.

8. Plail RO, Bussey HJR, Glazer G *et al.* Adenomatous polyposis: an association with carcinoma of the thyroid, *Br J Surg* 1987; 74: 377–80.

9. Painter TA and Jagelman DG. Adrenal adenomas and adrenal carcinoma in association with hereditary adenomatosis of the colon and rectum, *Cancer* 1985; 55: 2001.

10. Perkins JT, Blackstone MO and Riddell RH. Adenomatous polyposis coli and multiple endocrine neoplasia type 2b: a pathogenetic relationship, *Cancer* 1985; 55: 375–81.

11. Carl W and Sullivan WA. Dental abnormalities and bone lesions associated with familial adenomatous polyposis: report of cases, *J Am Dent Assoc* 1989; 119: 137–9.

12. Li FP, Thurber WA, Seddon J *et al.* Hepatoblastoma in families with polyposis coli, *JAMA* 1987; 257: 2475–7.

13. Lotfi AM, Dozois RR, Gordon H *et al.* Mesenteric fibromatosis complicating familial adenomatous polyposis: predisposing factors and results of treatment, *Int J Colorect Dis* 1989; 4: 30–6.

14. Leppard B and Bussey HJR. Epidermoid cysts, polyposis coli and Gardner's syndrome, *Br J Surg* 1975; 62: 387–93.

15. Kropilak M, Jagelman DG, Fazio VW *et al.* Brain tumours in familial adenomatous polyposis, *Dis Colon Rectum* 1989; 32: 778–82.

16. Burn J, Chapman PD, Wood CM *et al.* Eye examination in the assessment of carrier risk for familial adenomatous polyposis (FAP), *Int J Colorect Dis* 1990; 5: 59.

17. Cao X, Eu KW, Seow-Choen F, Zhao Y and Cheah PY. Topoisomerase-I- and Alu-mediated genomic deletions of the APC gene adenomatous polyposis, *Hum Genet* 2001; 108: 436–42.

18. Cao X, Eu KW, Seow-Choen F, Zao Yi and Cheah PY. APC mutation and phenotype spectrum of Singapore familial polyposis patients, *European J Human Genome Genetics* 2000; 8: 42–8.

19. Cao X, Eu KW, Seow Choen F and Cheah PY. Germline mutations are frequent in the APC gene but absent in the β-latenin gene in familial adenomatous polyposis patients, *Genes, Chromosomes & Cancer* 1999; 25: 396–8.

20. Cao X, Eu KW, Seow-Choen F and Cheah PY. Molecular and clinical profiles of familial adenomatous polyposis patients, *Frontiers in Human Genetics* 2001; 245–59.

CHAPTER 24

Singapore Polyposis Registry

C Loi

Introduction

The Singapore Polyposis Registry was founded in 1989 by the Department of Colorectal Surgery and is based at the Singapore General Hospital. It was recognized by the Ministry of Health in February 1990 as a national registry to promote nationwide registration of FAP and has a significant cancer prevention and screening programme.

The main objective of establishing a National Polyposis Registry is cancer prevention. A basic contention of primary health care (PHC) is that individuals and communities must be educated to take more control over their health and to learn to work with health personnel. This calls for appropriate education for the health of both individuals and communities, in accordance with the ancient proverb "Prevention is better than cure". Hence the importance of family surveillance and examination. This must be constantly emphasized to prevent death from colorectal cancer. Therefore, it is important that FAP families, doctors and registries work together as partners and are collaborators in care. Thus, the importance of a polyposis registry becomes apparent. The Singapore Polyposis Registry is intended to be a comprehensive source of information for patients and doctors. It also manages other inherited syndromes, such as hereditary nonpolyposis colorectal cancer (HNPCC) and other cancer family syndromes.

Currently, we have 69 FAP families with 160 affected members; 328 members are at-risk individuals. So far, the youngest of the patients in the Singapore Polyposis Registry who have had proctocolectomy was 13 years old and the youngest patient found to have colorectal cancer was 17 years old.

Significance of FAP

FAP is a hereditary autosomal dominant condition. Screening plays an important role since there is a 100% risk of developing colorectal cancer and it can reduce the cancer mortality rate for FAP patients. FAP is a genetic condition caused by a faulty gene. The FAP gene is one of the many thousands of genes carried in our chromosomes which determine our physical characteristics. Any child of a person with FAP has a 50:50 chance of inheriting the faulty gene.

The true incidence of FAP is unknown, but approximates 1:8000 to 1:10000 in epidemiological studies. Polyposis registries have been established in many parts of the world. There is a need for a registry for FAP families in every nation, in order to collect and maintain such information and records. Currently, there are more than 50 registries which have been established worldwide. Registries are established to help clinicians to identify, treat, support and follow up people with or at risk of developing colon cancer. They aim to maintain a cancer prevention focus through efficient information management, and to improve the prognosis and prevent cancer. Thus, the key features of a successful registry are to be able to save lives by early detection and prevention of cancer.

Aims of the Singapore Polyposis Registry

1. To identify and register all FAP families in Singapore so that the high risk individuals may be offered the most up-to-date screening procedures and treatment so as to prevent cancer.
2. To ensure efficient care of patients and their families, and to promote and carry out research that will advance our knowledge of polyposis.
3. To work in collaboration with other colleagues and departments, such as general practitioners, histopathology, endoscopy, surgery, etc.
4. To study genetic markers of disease and identify phenotypic manifestations.
5. Affiliation to the Leeds Castle Polyposis Group, an international body which co-ordinates the exchange of clinical data and research, in order to tap world experience in this condition and to keep up with the latest advances in this field.

How the Polyposis Registry Works

General practition-　→　Notify Registry　→　Singapore Polypo-
ers / medical cen-　　　　　　　　　　　　　sis Registry
tres with polyposis　　　　　　　　　　　　Department of
patients　　　　　　　　　　　　　　　　　Colorectal Surgery
　　　　　　　　　　　　　　　　　　　　　Singapore General
　　　　　　　　　　　　　　　　　　　　　Hospital
　　　　　　　　　　　　　　　　　　　　　Outram Road
　　　　　　　　　　　　↓　　　　　　　　Singapore 169608
　　　　　　　　　　　　　　　　　　　　　Tel.: 6321-3615
　　　　　　　　　　　　　　　　　　　　　Fax: 6326-5432
Coordinator fills up forms and builds up family tree.

Services Provided by the Polyposis Registry

To doctors:

- Verifying patient pedigree information for compilation of an accurate family history.
- Assisting in identifying, tracing and alerting at-risk family members.
- Facilitating the regular screening of at-risk and affected patients by contacting them either by calling or by sending reminders.
- Providing information to doctors and patients, including genetic testing.
- Making a preclinical diagnosis of FAP through the detection of the FAP gene at the Molecular Biology Laboratory of the Department of Colorectal Surgery.

To patients and at-risk family members:

- Providing information about the FAP condition.
- Helping them and their doctor complete the family tree, and offering screening.
- Disseminating information.
- Organizing support groups.
- Providing support.
- Offering counselling.

Workflow of the Polyposis Registry

The function of the Registry is to co-ordinate patient care, the construction of a pedigree and family trees, and the collection of medical information. The Registry is also involved with clinic co-ordination, administration and research studies involving individuals with undiagnosed genetic colorectal cancers. Staff act as liaison between families and their physician and offer counselling to individuals and families with FAP.

Advice is also given to patients on appropriate surveillance for FAP, and the patient is referred back to his or her own doctor for management, including any decision on surgery. The workflow (Fig. 1) of the Singapore Polyposis Registry is important to ensure that the aims of the Registry are

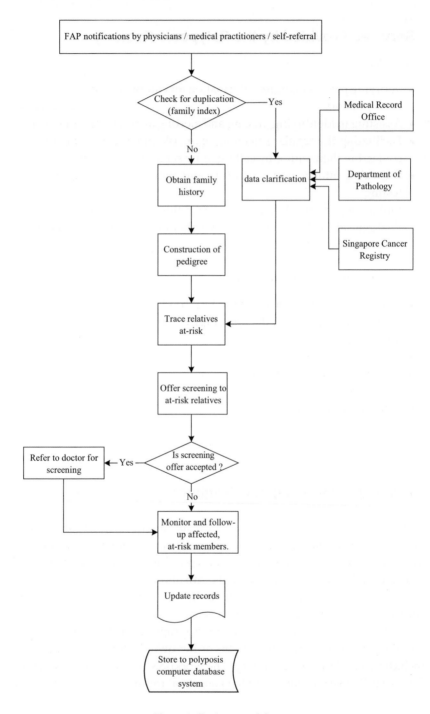

Figure 1. Registry workflow.

met. The Registry also assists doctors in the screening of all at-risk people and the follow-up of all FAP patients.[1]

Methods of Screening

CHRPE screening (optional)

CHRPE (congenital hypertrophy of retinal pigment epithelium) means pigmented ocular lesions. CHRPE screening is done with the ophthalmologist, with no fee charged at all. Appointments with the ophthalmologist are arranged by the Registry staff.

Endoscopic screening

Sigmoidoscopic or colonoscopic screening is commenced (where appropriate) at about the age of 12 years. However, in some instances, it is better to wait until 14 or 15 years of age, when the emotional immaturity of puberty is stabilized, but before later adolescent years.

Genetic screening

The Registry provides access to genetic blood testing and co-ordination of the diagnostic tests. A genetic blood test will only be offered as a form of screening to the relatives at risk if mutations are found for the proband. Genetic blood tests for the proband are done without charge, whereas a fee will be charged for the relatives at-risk. All affected patients and relatives at-risk will then be followed up with counselling in respect of the genetic results and any necessary referrals to the physician for endoscopy are made. Once a particular gene mutation has been documented in a family, at-risk family members have the choice of being tested for the presence of that particular mutation. Those who do have the gene are required to continue sigmoidoscopic surveillance regularly.

Patient Scheduling

Following screening, a comprehensive treatment plan including recommended procedures will be made by individual doctors. Several guidelines have been published but there is no definitive version at the moment.

Monitoring and Following up Affected/At-Risk Members

Registry staff facilitate appointments for surveillance, investigation, treatment and follow-up of FAP patients and all at-risk relatives who have yet to accept screening for FAP. Further screening, such as upper gastrointestinal endoscopy and a careful examination, may be considered for extracolonic features for a recently diagnosed FAP patient. Family surveillance examinations and results with copies of histology reports, surgery and biopsy results will be traced from patients or family members, hospital records, clinics or pathology laboratory etc. and updated in the computer database. All at-risk relatives, including those in refusal or denial, are recalled regularly to ensure that the most affected relatives and at-risk members of a family are offered screening and treatment.

Ensuring That All Affected Relatives Are Offered Treatment

Treatment

Registry staff will co-ordinate and facilitate appointments for surveillance, investigation and follow-up of FAP patients and the at-risk relatives. If screening is confirmed positive, appointments will be arranged by the Registry staff for the affected relatives to further discuss with the surgeon the appropriate prophylactic surgery for them.

Support

Providing support is about improving the care of those diagnosed with FAP or cancer and giving counselling either in person or over the phone, before or after treatment is necessary. It is essential that the Registry demonstrates responsiveness to calls, letters or e-mail and promotes good communication skills with patients and family members, again before or after surgery. In addition, support groups may be organized to help families support each other annually. Visits are made to affected patients and relatives before and after surgery in the hospital ward or clinic as necessary to give support.

Counselling

Genetic counselling with FAP patients and their family members occurs during or after the diagnosis of FAP, i.e. before and after treatment. A typical counselling session will include dissemination of information by educating the family about the hereditary nature of FAP, the clinical and management aspects of FAP, the risks of developing cancer and the consequences of genetic blood test results if these are positive. Counselling is required as an empathetic approach to the patient and their family is paramount.[5]

Polyposis Computer Database System

The clinical functions of a FAP registry involves maintaining an accurate and up-to-date database apart from co-ordinating surveillance, facilitating treatment, assisting in organizing diagnostic tests, offering counselling and providing support. Therefore, the database is essential, as it is a resource for both patients and their families and for the primary care giver. The Polyposis Registry therefore serves as a data collection centre. Here again, confidentiality of the data will be ensured to protect the privacy of all family members in the Registry.

Collaborative Groups

The Polyposis Registry provides vital data for epidemiological, patho-genetic and therapeutic research trials on patients with rare inherited disorders of hereditary colonic cancer. Also, the intention of the Polyposis Registry is to collect information on FAP and allied diseases throughout the nation, and to preserve this information for generic epidemiology and surveillance to help understand the natural history of hereditary colorectal cancer. Collaborative Groups have been formed in an endeavour to understand, share and plan co-operative studies so as to achieve the aim of cancer prevention. Registries can help improve research capabilities by sharing data and ideas.

A polyposis registry is required to form liaisons between leading regional cancer experts, primary care providers, consumers and public health personnel. It supports numerous projects where regional activities or perspectives will enhance progress in our understanding of hereditary colorectal cancer. Active participation in the Leeds Castle Polyposis Group plays a valuable role by bringing together people from many disciplines.[5]

Leeds Castle Polyposis Group

The Leeds Castle Polyposis Group was established in 1985 at Leeds Castle in Kent, England, by Sir Ian Todd, KBE, with the aim of understanding the aetiology, clinical features, prevention and treatment of FAP. This group holds an international research forum with meetings every second year. In fact, the term "familial adenomatous polyposis" (FAP) was named by the Leeds Castle Polyposis Group for the nature of the most common intestinal abnormality without implying restriction to the colon. National and regional registers worldwide are represented in the Leeds Castle Polyposis Group since its establishment in 1985. Various groups have now combined to form the HNPCC (hereditary non-polyposis colorectal cancer) group as well, which started in 1997 to accommodate, discuss and plan co-operative studies in nonpolyposis families.

Conclusion

The success of society greatly depends on the overall level of health of its people, because good health enables individuals to have productive and fulfilling lives, which contribute to overall economic and social stability. The participation and collaboration of general practitioners, physicians, specialists, patients, family members or even the public motivates the Registry to further realize its goals.

All FAP patients and their families, even foreigners who are working in Singapore, deserve to be registered with the Singapore Polyposis Registry. The Registry welcomes contact with persons or groups who share its interests or who feel they can contribute to the realization of its objectives.

References

1. Bulow S, Burn J and Neale K. The establishment of a polyposis register, *Int J Colorectal Dis* 1993; 8: 34–8.
2. Herrera Lemuel. *The Leed's Castle Polyposis Group: Familial Adenomatosis Polyposis*. Alan R Liss, Inc, 1990, pp. 155–8.

3. Goh HS. Singapore Polyposis Registry, *Annals of the Academy of Medicine* 1992; 21, No. 2 (Mar.).

4. Peterson Gloria M. Genetic counseling and predictive genetic testing in familial adenomatous polyposis, *Seminars in Colon & Rectal Surgery* 1995; 6, No. 1 (Mar.), pp. 55–60.

5. Spigelman Allan D, Hodgson Shirley V and Thomson James PS. Management of familial adenomatous polypsis, *Bailliere's Gastroenterology* 1992; 6, No. 1, pp. 75–93.

6. Stern Hartley S and Smith A. Recognition, screening, and medical management of familial adenomatous polyposis, *Seminars in Colon & Rectal Surgery* 1995; 6, No. 1 (Mar.), pp. 19–24.

CHAPTER 25

Physical Manifestations of HNPCC

F Seow-Choen

Introduction

Hereditary non-polyposis colorectal cancer (HNPCC) is a much-talked-about but still relatively little-understood disease. Most patients come from one of two types of families described as Lynch Type I and Lynch Type II. Multiple members of the Lynch Type I families present with colonic cancers. Members of the Lynch Type II families may also develop extracolonic cancers, particularly of the female reproductive tract and of the urothelium. Both syndromes, however, lack the extensive colonic polyposis seen with familial adenomatous polyposis, although small numbers of polyps may still be seen. Colorectal cancer is the most common cancer seen in HNPCC, whilst HNPCC accounts for up to 5% of all colonic cancers.[1,2]

Cancer cells in patients with HNPCC and in some sporadically occurring disease have a unique type of genetic abnormality, represented by

Table 1. Amsterdam II criteria.

1. At least 3 relatives with an HNPCC-associated cancer
2. One should be a first degree relative of the other two.
3. At least 2 successive generations should be affected.
4. At least 1 CRC should be diagnosed before the age of 50.

variations in the length of microsatellite DNA repeat regions.[3] Microsatellites are short segments of repeating DNA bases. Microsatellite instablity (MSI) is a change of any length due to either insertions or deletions of repeating units in a microsatellite.[4]

Cancers showing MSI are due to a failure to repair errors by DNA polymerase during DNA replication. Mutations in the mismatch repair genes (MMR) lead to MSI. At least seven genes are involved in mismatch repair in humans. The proteins derived from these genes act in a complex manner. Cells that have lost some of this mismatch repair function are therefore unable to identify mismatch defects and develop extensive microsatellite instability. The genetic hallmark of HNPCC is MSI and over 90% of such patients demonstrate MSI.

Diagnostic Criteria for HNPCC

In 1990 the International Collaborative Group on HNPCC published the Amsterdam criteria to help identify those likely to have HNPCC.[5] These criteria had a low sensitivity and many families were not identified. The Amsterdam criteria II were issued in 1999 and included cancers of the endometrium, ureter, renal pelvis and small bowel.[6] However, family history is often not well known, especially in adopted or illegitimate children or those from separated families. In addition, patients from "small" families may not have enough data to fulfil the criteria adequately.

Guidelines were therefore introduced to identify cancer families likely to demonstrate MSI.[7] However, about 15% of sporadically occurring colorectal cancers demonstrate MSI as well. Hence not all MSI positive tumours are associated with HNPCC.

If a genetic mutation is identified, clinical screening of the other family members becomes possible. Those who have not inherited the mutation have a colorectal cancer risk no higher than that of the general public.

Table 2. The Bethesda criteria.

Tumours should be tested for MSI in the following situations:
1. Individuals with cancer in families meeting the Amsterdam criteria.
2. Individuals with 2 HNPCC-related cancers, including synchronous and metachronous colorectal cancer or endometrial, ovarian, hepatobiliary, gastric carcinoma, small bowel adenocarcinoma, transitional carcinoma of the renal pelvis or ureter.
3. Individuals with colorectal cancer and a first degree relative with colorectal cancer and/or HNPCC-related cancer and/or a colorectal adenoma in which one of the cancers was diagnosed at age <45 years and the adenoma was diagnosed at age <40 years.
4. Individuals with colorectal cancer or endometrial cancer at age <45 years.
5. Individuals with right-sided colonic cancer with an undifferentiated pattern on histopathology diagnosed at age < 45 years.
6. Individuals with singnet ring cell type cancer diagnosed at age <45 years.
7. Individuals with adenomas diagnosed at age <40 years.

Genetic testing for HNPCC is particularly important in the younger colorectal cancer patient. The most commonly mutated genes in patients with HNPCC are MLH1, MSH2 and, less commonly, PMS2, PMS1 or MSH6.

Colorectal cancer is the most common malignancy in HNPCC and colonoscopy screening must be carried out in all members of affected families at the appropriate age. The optimal colonoscopic screening interval may need to be shorter than that for sporadic cancers.[9]

Annual transvaginal ultrasound and endometrial aspiration should begin between the ages of 25 and 35 years. Screening for gastric, hepatobiliary and urothelial cancer by regular gastroscopy, transabdominal ultrasound of the biliary tree, cystoscopy and urine cytology should be carried out for families known to have a tendency to develop these malignancies.

Clinical Characteristics of Patients with HNPCC

The mean age of onset of cancers in patients with HNPCC is about 20 years younger than the general population. Patients with Lynch II are at risk of developing multiple cancers in other organs, principally of the urothelium and the female genital tract.

Cancers in patients with HNPCC predominantly occur on the right side of the colon compared to cancers in non-HNPCC patients. Histologically carcinomas tend to be poorly differentiated or mucinous and are more likely to demonstrate signet ring cells.[10]

The Role of Prophylactic Surgery

Prophylactic colorectal surgery is controversial, as about 15% of patients with HNPCC may not develop malignancy. Colonoscopic screening, however, reduces the incidence of colorectal cancer. Prophylactic colectomy is therefore not absolute in all cases. Surgery however, should be considered for those who are unwilling to comply with a strict screening programme or those for whom colonoscopy is technically difficult.

However, patients with HNPCC who already have colorectal cancer should have a total colectomy since metachronous cancers are common.[11] The other option is a proctocolectomy and ileal pouch anal anastomosis. Patients with an MSH2 mutation may be at higher risk of developing rectal cancer and the presence of this genetic mutation may indicate the need for rectal resection at the same time. There is no evidence at present to offer prophylactic hysterectomy and bilateral salpingo-oophorectomy for patients with HNPCC undergoing colectomy.

References

1. Dunlop MG. Colorectal cancer, *BMJ* 1997; 314: 1882–5.
2. Aarnio M, Mecklin JP, Aaltonen LA, Nystrom-Lahti M and Jarvinen HJ. Life-time risk of different cancers in hereditary nonpolyposis colorectal cancer (HNPCC) syndrome, *Int J Cancer* 1995; 64: 430–3.
3. Ionov Y, Peinado MA, Malkhosyan S, Shibata D and Perucho M. Ubiquitous somatic mutations in simple repeated sequences reveal a new mechanism for colonic carcinogenesis, *Nature* 1993; 363: 558–61.
4. Forrington SM, McKinley AJ, Carothers AD, Cunningham C *et al*. Evidence for an age-related influence of microsatellite instability on colorectal cancer survival, *Int J Cancer* 2002; 98: 844–50.
5. Vasen HFA, Mecklin J-P, Meera Khan PM and Lynch HT. The International Collaborative Group on Hereditary Non-Polyposis Colorectal Cancer, *Dis Colon Rectum* 1991; 34: 424–5.
6. Vasen HF, Watson P, Mecklin JP and Lynch HT. New clinical criteria for hereditary nonpolyposis colorectal cancer (HNPCC, Lynch syndrome) proposed by the International Collaborative Group on HNPCC. *Gastroenterology* 1999; 116: 1453–6.
7. Boland CR, Thibodeau SN, Hamilton SR, Sidransky D *et al*. A National Cancer Institute Workshop on microsatellite instability for cancer

detection and familial predisposition: development of international criteria for the determination of microsatellite instability in colorectal cancer, *Cancer Res* 1998; 58: 5248–57.

8. Loukola A, delaChapelle A and AaHonen LA. Strategies for screening for hereditary non-polyposis colorectal cancer, *J Med Genet* 1999; 36: 819–22.

9. Vasen HF, Nagengast FM and Khan PM. Interval cancers in hereditary non-polyposis colorectal cancer (Lynch syndrome), *Lancet* 1995; 345: 1183–4.

10. Mecklin JP, Sipponen P and Jarvinen HJ. Histopathology of colorectal carcinomas and adenomas in cancer family syndrome, *Dis Colon Rectum* 1986; 29: 849–53.

11. Box JC, Rodriguez-Bigas MA, Weber TK and Petrelli NJ. Clinical implications of multiple colorectal carcinomas in hereditary non-polyposis colorectal carcinomas, *Dis Colon Rectum* 1999; 42: 717–21.

Population Screening for Colorectal Cancer

CL Tang

Introduction

Colorectal cancer is presently the most common cancer among both males and females in Singapore. Local incidence rates are comparable to some of the highest incidence rates in the world. Individuals face a moderate-to-high risk of developing colorectal cancer in their lifetime.[1] Despite improvement in diagnosis, surgical treatment and adjuvant chemotherapy, survival from colorectal cancer has not been significantly changed. One of the major reasons is the late presentation of the disease by the time clinical symptoms occur. In 1999 alone, more than half of all the new patients treated in the Department of Colorectal Surgery presented with either loco-regional or distant disease. This compares with only 10% for Dukes' A at the time of surgical resection. Early treatment of cancer is effective, but late diagnosis in Singapore continues to occur against the background of the widespread availability of acceptable tests that can be used for initial screening. Furthermore, follow-up examinations of abnormal screening tests like colonoscopy and double-contrast barium enema are not only easily available, but may also be safely and accurately performed. In initial screening, not only cancer is detected, but because of the phenotypic appearance of polyps and the natural history of the adenoma–carcinoma progression of polyps, removal of these polyps will result in reduced colorectal cancer risk. This natural history of the disease permits subsequent surveillance through repeat screening at intervals.[2]

If an earlier stage at diagnosis improves survival, then, translated into a population setting, is screening effective? How should we go about doing it? What is the impact of screening, including costs, on the individuals and the community? This short review will highlight some of the screening tests available and recent results of randomized trials for colorectal cancer population screening, as well as discuss some of the issues, and the impact, of population screening.

Screening Tools

Most colorectal cancer screening programmes aim to select a high-risk subpopulation through the use of a simple screening test, followed by detailed screening of those individuals tested positive by the initial test. Such two-tiered screening is believed to reduce costs and morbidity, since definitive tests like colonoscopy are expensive and manpower-intensive as well as invasive to perform in many parts of the world. Each screening test has its own characteristic effectiveness (true predictive value) and accuracy (false predictive value). Effectiveness and accuracy often vary inversely, according to the complexity and the inconvenience and risks involved for the individual. While the method or test used for screening is critical to the success of a screening programme, as we will discuss later, it is certainly not the sole determinant.

Screening tools available in current practice include (1) recent-onset symptoms, (2) digital rectal examination (DRE), (3) faecal testing for occult blood (FOBT), (4) imaging, either with contrast X-rays or endoscopically, a part or all of the large intestines.

Recent-Onset Symptoms

This is widely practised clinically and is based on the reporting of classical or suspicious symptoms of colorectal cancer. Commonly, the symptoms include a history of bleeding per rectum, change in bowel habits, reduction in stool calibre, tenesmus, abdominal pain and anaemia. None of these symptoms are specific and often, by the time symptoms appear, as evidenced by the stage of cancer at diagnosis in our department database, the disease is advanced, making cure difficult. Interestingly, in a small study[2] involving patients presenting with bleeding per rectum of new onset after the age of 40 years who were undergoing colonoscopy, two-thirds of the colorectal cancers detected were confined to the bowel wall (i.e. Dukes' A and B). In reality, most of the early symptoms experienced are dismissed by the individual as "probably not significant" or as something minor like "haemorrhoids". It would thus appear that a policy of health education alone is not sufficiently compelling for voluntary screening and early detection.

Digital Rectal Examination

Digital rectal examination (DRE) as part of a physical examination in those over 50 years of age is prudent clinical practice and certainly essential in the evaluation of bleeding per rectum. However, due to its obvious insensitivity and as it has, at best, been estimated to detect only 10% of the colorectal cancer, DRE is usually done in conjunction with other screening tests, such as the faecal occult blood test or sigmoidoscopy.

Faecal Occult Blood Tests

In the last 20 years, this modality of screening has been rigorously tested, and the process of evaluating its use is often complex. Three principal groups of faecal occult blood tests (FOBTs) are available, with different features in each (Table 1). The earliest stool guaiac test works on the principle of the pseudo-peroxidase activity of heme either in its free form or bound to its apoprotein (as haemoglobin, myoglobin and certain cytochromes). This produces a bluish colour on the test paper when the developing solution is applied. They do not react with degradation products of heme which lack

Table 1. Major features of principal FOBTs.

	Guaiac	Immunochemical	Heme-porphyrin
Test basis	Peroxidase	Immunoreactive Hb	Porphyrins
Compounds detected	Hb (all), Mb (all), All hemes, Nonhemeperoxidases	Hb (human) Globin (human)	Hb (all), Mb (all), All hemes, heme porphyrins
Method	Chromogen	HA, ELISA, latex, particle-based immunodetection	Solvent extraction & fluorimetry
Dietary restrictions	Yes	No	Yes
Effect of medication	Yes (vitamin C, NSAIDS, aspirin)	Yes (aspirin, NSAIDS may produce positive results)	Yes
Effect of diet	Yes (red meat, peroxidases)	No	Yes (red meat)
Equipment	None	Method-dependent	Fluorimeter
Processing	A few minutes	Method-dependent	4–8 hours

peroxidase activity. As the reaction is not specific for blood, dietary peroxidase of plant or animal origin will produce a positive test result. Similarly, drugs with reducing properties such as vitamin C will produce a false negative result. Thus dietary restrictions are necessary to reduce false positive results. The nature of the test does not permit localization of the bleeding and may also test positive in the presence of lower-gastrointestinal-ulcer-inducing drugs like aspirin and NSAIDS.

In contrast, the immunochemical tests are the most chemically selective and specific for human globin and some of the early degradation forms. Herein lies the advantage, as no dietary restrictions are necessary. Nonhuman haemoglobin is also not known to produce a false positive test. However, drugs related to gastrointestinal bleeding may test positive. Technologies used in these tests include enzyme-linked immunosorbent assays (ELISA), double immunodiffusion, qualitative haemagglutination and latex haemagglutination. They are now available in easy-to-use office test kits, just like the stool guaiac tests. Used in early population trials in Japan since 1992, this test has a major drawback—the instability of haemoglobin in the stool sample (in the region of hours only) if stored and transported at room temperature from the time of collection in the home to arrival in the laboratory. The quality of the monoclonal antibody in different batches of the test kit may also vary at the stage of production and subsequent storage. In order to reduce the degradation of haemoglobin in the stool and hence maintain the sensitivity of the test, a stabilizing solution is often used to put the stool specimen for transport back to the laboratory. This is often stable for up to three days in the buffer media. In mass screening, modification of the principle using spectrographic techniques in the analysis allows quantification and improves the sensitivity of detection, but usually at the expense of specificity.

The heme-porphyrin tests are specific for di-carboxylic porphyrins and detect intact heme in any form and its porphyrin degradation products. Fluorescent spectrometry is required and permits rather accurate quantification. This method is not often used in the population setting.

The choice of test has impact on the type of cases detected. Haemoglobin and its derivatives found in the stool are dependent on the site of the bleeding. Gastric and proximal small bowel bleeding would result in greater heme degradation products as opposed to distal colonic bleeding, as blood in the colon has less time for degradation[5] (Table 2). Furthermore, there is a degree of overlap between blood loss in the normal gastrointestinal tract (estimated to be up to 1.5 ml per day, mean 0.5 ml/day + 0.4 (SD)) and patients with colorectal neoplasia. Thus a test that depends on detection of haemoglobin and its degradation products will necessarily discriminate incompletely between normal and cancer patients[3] (Table 3).

The amount of bleeding from the tumour is dependent not on the stage but on the site and even size.[4] Proximal cancers bleed the most, while adenomas bleed less than cancers. Small adenomas of less than 1 cm are unlikely to be outside the normal range[5] (Table 4). The amount of bleeding varies from day to day. Multiple stool guaiac tests over different days will improve sensitivity, but testing of greater than three gives little added benefit and will worsen specificity.[7]

Table 2. Predicted balance of haemoglobin derivatives in faeces according to the site of blood loss.[4]

Derivative	Site of Bleeding		
	Gastric	Proximal colon	Distal colon
Intact haemoglobin	−	+	++
Intact heme	+	+	++
Porphyrins	+++	++	+

Table 3. Estimated sensitivity of different FOBTs to the source and amount of gastrointestinal blood loss.

Test type	Blood Loss (ml/day)	
	Colonic	Gastric
Heme-porphyrin	>2	>2
Guaiac	>0.5	10–20
Immunochemical	>0.25	>100

Table 4. Comparison of sensitivities for colorectal cancer and adenoma of three types of FOBTs.[6]

Lesion	No patients	Hemoccult	HemeSelect	HemoQuant*
Cancer	107	95 (89%)	104 (97%)	76 (71%)
Adenomas				
≥ 1 cm	45	19 (42%)	34 (76%)	19 (42%)
< 1 cm	36	6 (17%)	13 (36%)	11 (31%)

*Positive if HemoQuant value is greater than 2 mg/g.

The method of sampling and handling of the sample has significant impact on the stool guaiac test results. Stool coming into contact with toilet bowl water before sampling may lead to leaching of the haemoglobin. In fact, a paper saddle placed across the toilet bowl has been proposed. A thick film on the card can lead to errors in reading and a false positive result. Different areas of sampling is encouraged while straining at defecation or obtaining the specimen through a digital exam should be avoided as trauma to the anorectal region may lead to blood in the stool. Hard stool returns fewer positive results than loose stool. Delay in transport may lead to excessive degradation of the haemoglobin. Subject acceptance of sampling and handling of faecal material plays an important role in accurate sampling.

The crude sensitivity in individuals screened with the guaiac FOBT (Hemoccult II) is estimated to be in the region of 50–75% and as high as 90% for hydrated Hemoccult II (Table 5). These are based on individuals who are known to have colorectal cancers and are probably symptomatic. However, in reality, if the test is applied to a population setting, compliance and multiple factors influence the outcome. The predictive values

Table 5. Relationship between sensitivity and compliance.

Test	Proportion of cancers detected (%)	Compliance (%)	Comment
Digital examination	<10	95–100	Gives no information on the large bowel.
FOBT	40–80	50–80	Cheap, low sensitivity, needs follow-up colonoscopy.
Rigid sigmoidoscopy	20–30	Up to 35	Cheap, convenient, needs colonoscopy follow-up.
Flexible sigmoidoscopy	50–65	Not known	Simple, requiring no sedation. Needs colonoscopy if positive.
DCBE	85–95	Not known	Less expensive than colonoscopy.
Colonoscopy	95–99	Not known	Very high sensitivity and specificity. Permits biopsy, expensive, requires bowel preparation, and risk of perforation/bleeding.

are thus lower for cancers and adenomas in the Nottingham,[8] Funen[9] and Goteborg[10] trials (53, 59 and 27% respectively). These are based on the two-year follow-up for interval or "screen-missed" cancers detected after the initial screening test.

The Hemoccult II stool guaiac test is perhaps the most-studied FOBT used for population screening. Five major trials[8–12] (Table 6) (four randomized controlled trials and one nonrandomized controlled trial) involving a total of about 180 000 people in each arm testing annual or biennial FOBT compared to a no-test group have all yielded colorectal cancer mortality reduction with testing. In a recent meta-analysis,[13] those allocated to screening had a reduction in colorectal cancer mortality of 16% (relative risk 0.84, CI 0.77–0.93). When adjusted for screening attendance, the reduction rises to 23% (relative risk 0.77, CI 0.57–0.89).

Population trials using immunochemical tests in the west are much fewer. In Japan, an immunochemical test by legislation was used in population screening since 1992. The Japanese Ministry of Health and Welfare targeted 2.5 million individuals aged 40 years and above for screening. Data was available for 1 083 097 in a survey.[14] 76 323 (7.0%) tested positive. This is far above those seen in all the guaiac FOBT trials (ranging from 1 to 2.1%, 5.8% with hydration). 70% underwent further evaluation and 2017 (2%) were found to have a colorectal cancer. About half of these were early cancers. These results are comparable to the guaiac FOBT trials. Compared

Table 6. Summary of trials of haemoccult (HO) screening for colorectal cancer.

	Minnesota, USA[11]	Nottingham, UK[8]	Goteborg, Sweden[10]	Funen, Denmark[9]	New York, USA[12]
Study population	Volunteers, 50–80 yrs	From GP records, 50–74 yrs	Residents of Goteborg, 60–64 yrs	Random sample, 45–74 yrs	Clients attending NY medical clinic, > 40 yrs
Total numbers Assigned to screening	46 551 Annual: 15 570 Biennial: 15 587	107 349 53 464	68 308 34 153	140 000 Annual: 61 938 Biennial: 30 970	– Annual: 21 756 Biennial: 12 974
Screening periods	Randomly assigned to annual/biennial and control groups, 1975–1982 & 1986–1992	Started 1981; offered biennially	Started 1982; rescreening offered to all screen groups 16–24 mths later	1985–1990, 3 screens done	Screen and control groups offered s'copy and screen group offered HO testing
Follow-up periods Compliance with screening	Follow-up continues Per cent of screenings completed: Annual gp: 75.2% Biennial gp: 78.4% Proportion completing all screening: Annual gp: 46.2% Biennial gp: 59.7%	Follow-up continues Rescreening to compliers only 1st round: 53% completed HO 2nd round: 77% compliance with rescreening	Follow-up continues 1st round: 63% both HO and questionnaire 12%—questionnaire only 2nd round: 60% both HO and questionnaire tests 14% questionnaire only	Follow-up continues Rescreening to compliers only 1st round: 67% completed 2nd round: 93% of those invited (prev compliers) completed tests 3rd round: approx. 92% of those invited (prev compliers twice) completed tests	Follow-up ceased 1984 1st round compliance: Regular attenders: 70% First presenters: 80% Compliance in next 2 rounds ↓ to 20% and then 16% for first presenters
Screening test positivity rate	9.8% (rehydrated) 2.4% (unhydrated) 82.5% were rehydrated slides	1st round: 2.3% 2nd round: 1.7%	4 cohorts 1st round: 1.9% (unhydrated) 5.8% (rehydrated) 6.3% (rehydrated) 8.0% (rehydrated)	1st round: 1.0% 2nd round: 0.8% 3rd round: 0.9%	Regular attenders: 1.4% First presenters: 2.6%

Positive predictive value of test for colorectal cancer	5.8% (unhydrated) 2.2% (rehydrated)	1st screen: 10.2% of HO pos 2nd screen: 8.5% of HO pos	2nd round: 8.0% (prev unhyd gp) 4.8% 5.6% 14.3% Overall, 5% Follow-up as at Oct. 92	1st screen: 17.7% of HO pos 2nd screen: 8.4% of HO pos	Overall: 10.7% of HO pos 1st presenters: 17%; no further data for regular attenders
Total colorectal cancers	At 13 yrs' follow-up Annual: 323 (50% screen detected) Biennial: 323 (39% screen detected) Control: 356	At 5 yrs' follow-up (ave 3 yrs) Screen gp: 181 (42% screen detected) Control gp: 123	At mean follow-up of 7 and 3 yrs for first 2 cohorts Screen gp:132 (61% screen detected) Control gp: 191	At 38 mths' follow-up Screen gp: 147 (34% screen detected) Control gp: 115	At 9 yrs' follow-up (rate per 1000) Regular attenders: Screen gp: 10 Control gp: 10.4 1st attenders: Screen gp: 9.8 Control gp: 7.2 Overall: 39% of HO pos
Proportion of colorectal cancers detected in the early stage (Dukes' A, B)	At 13 yrs' follow-up, staging available for 91% of cancers Annual: 64.8% Biennial: 57.8% Control: 58.6%	Staging for 98% of cancers Screen gp: 61.5% Control gp: 44.5%	All cases staged Screen gp: 61.6% Control gp: 43.1%	Staging for 93.5% of cancers Screen gp: 61.2% Control gp: 45.3%	All cases staged Screen gp: 59.2% Control gp: 51.4%
Colorectal cancer mortality	At 13 yrs' follow-up Annual: 5.9% Biennial: 8.3% Control: 8.8%	Mortality data not available Follow-up continues	Mortality data not available Follow-up continues	At 38 mths' follow-up mortality per 1000 Screen gp: 2.4 Control gp: 2.9 ($p = 0.24$)	At 9 yrs' follow-up Mortality per 1000 per year Screen gp: 0.42 Control gp: 0.58

Table 6 (continued)

	Minnesota, USA[11]	Nottingham, UK[8]	Goteborg, Sweden[10]	Funen, Denmark[9]	New York, USA[12]
Statistical significance	Statistically significant with 33% reduction in cancer mortality between annual and screen groups No difference between biennial and control groups	Significantly lower proportion of early cancers in control group than in screen-detected group	No significant difference in early cancers in control group from screen group Trend towards more favourable staging of HO-detected cancers	No significant difference in deaths from cancer between screen and control groups to date Significantly lower proportion of early cancers in control than in screen group	Borderline statistically significant ($p = 0.053$) difference in cancer mortality between screen and control groups for 1st presenters No difference in cancer mortality between regular attenders and control groups
Any adverse outcomes of screening/follow-up investigation?	12 246 colonoscopies: * 4 perforations * 11 serious bleeding * (rate 12 per 10 000)	1774 colonoscopies: * 7 complications with 6 requiring surgery * (rate 39 per 10 000)	BE and sigmoidoscopy used † 2108 flexible sigmoidoscopy * 3 perforations from polypectomy 1987 BE—no complications 190 colonoscopies for BE pos * 1 bleeding * 2 perforations	No information on complications of colonoscopy	No information given
Losses to follow-up	1% no medical records found	Follow-up continues	Follow-up continues	4 participants at 3 yrs	3% of all participants

† From: Kewenter J and Brevinge H. Endoscopic and surgical complications of work-up in screening for colorectal cancer, *Dis Colon Rectum* 1996; 39: 676–80.

HO: haemoccult test.

to the Nottingham trial, which has the highest FOBT positivity of the five randomized trials (2.7 per 1000 screened with rehydrated slides and 0.9 per 1000 with unhydrated slides), the immunochemical test gave a cancer detection rate of 1.9 per 1000 screened. The rates are similar in using the "intention-to-screen" principle, taking into account compliance. It would appear that for the immunochemical test, although more sensitive than the guaiac test in detecting occult blood, the specificity for cancer is similar or at best slightly better. This may lead to a greater number of subsequent colonoscopes or barium enema. However, the polyp detection rate is more elevated for the immunochemical tests, which may account for the lower specificity for colorectal cancer with increased sensitivity for blood detection. Data on interval cancer detection is not available in the Japanese series and this may shed more light on the precision of an immunochemical test.

Sigmoidoscopy

The rationale of using a flexible sigmoidoscope for screening lies in the fact that up to two-thirds of the colorectal cancer is within the reach of the scope. Its secondary function in screening is the detection of index polyps, which will necessitate a subsequent full colonoscopy. Approximately 30% of cancers proximal to the splenic flexure have an index lesion situated distally.[15]

Sigmoidoscopy is a lesser procedure than a full colonoscopy and in some countries, like the US and the UK, it can be performed effectively and safely by trained nurse practitioners, with minimal discomfort.[16–18] In fact, as our present population ages, the demand on medical practitioners in the hospital for screening flexible sigmoidoscopy may outstrip the supply and there will be an increasing need to train not only general practitioners but also nurse practitioners in this procedure.

This may be easily performed in the office setting 30 minutes after a Fleet enema. Although rigid sigmoidoscopy has often been said to be able to visualize to the distal sigmoid colon, in practice, passing the scope to beyond the rectosigmoid junction is achievable in 40–70% of those scoped. A finer paediatric scope may be more successful and comfortable for the individual.[19] Likewise, a flexible sigmoidoscope may theoretically be able to visualize to the descending colon and splenic flexure region; in effect, the numbers that achieve this end-point may be small.

Early trials of sigmoidoscopy involved the rigid scope and were nonrandomized case-controlled trials susceptible to selection bias. In a large trial within the Kaiser Permanente Medical Care Programme comparing 261 fatal cases of colorectal cancer within the reach of the sigmoidoscope and 868 matched controls, the adjusted odds ratio for having had at least one sigmoidoscopy was 0.41. In some of the remaining descriptive trials,[20,21] there was a trend towards detection of early disease translating into better survival for individuals having tumours within the reach of the sigmoidoscope. In a pooled analysis of 14 studies using the flexible sigmoidoscope for screening about 11 000 individuals, 30 cancers were detected and 24 of these were localized disease.[22]

While, empirically, flexible sigmoidoscopy screening should reduce mortality from colorectal cancer, its true effectiveness will still not be clear until the results of an MRC-sponsored trial and an NCI trial involving 148 000 over 50 years of age mature by 2006 and 2008 respectively. In a small trial,[23] 3744 individuals between 50 and 75 years old undergoing screening in a general practice were randomized into one of the three groups comparing flexible sigmoidoscopy, FOBT (Hemoccult) and sigmoidoscopy with FOBT. FOBT missed one cancer and 30 adenomas seen in the combined group.

Colonoscopy

While colonoscopy is the "gold standard" in screening for colorectal cancer and has a widely accepted role and proven track record in screening for high-risk individuals, its use in population screening in a moderate risk setting is still largely unknown. It requires full bowel preparation and inconvenience—which will reduce compliance—if used as a screening tool. However, its major concern is costs and associated complication rates, including death. A significant amount of resources is required for a colonoscopy, not to mention the extra effort on the part of the individual, who could be no less than highly motivated.

Perforation and bleeding after polypectomy is a concern. In the Minnesota trial,[11] 12 246 colonoscopies were done, with 4 perforations and 11 haemorrhage cases (rate 12 per 10 000). In the Goteborg trial,[10] 2298 endoscopies (mainly flexible sigmoidoscopy) and DCBE were performed, with a complication rate reported as 30 per 10 000. In the Nottingham trial,[8] 1774 colonoscopies were done, with 7 complications, 6 requiring surgery giving a rate of 39 per 10 000. In the Japan series[14] of 53 536 examinations, 248 complications were reported (rate 46 per 10 000). Twelve deaths were reported. Thus, whilst colonoscopy is a relatively safe procedure with low rates of complications, it is not devoid of complications and is particularly a concern as the number scoped is very large in a population screening setting.

Double Contrast Barium Enema

The double contrast barium enema (DCBE) requires a proper bowel preparation for accurate diagnosis of small lesions like polyps. As it is less invasive than colonoscopy, the risk of perforation is lower, but still exists. The American Society of Radiologists standards stipulate that the enema should be of a quality sufficient to detect 90% of the colorectal cancer and 80% of the polyps greater than 1 cm in diameter. However, it is known to miss small polyps, which is less likely in colonoscopy. There is also involved cost and exposure to radiation. What is perhaps more significant is the need to perform a colonoscopy if the DCBE is positive for confirmation and biopsy. As a tool in population screening, unlike the barium meal in Japan for gastric cancer, its role is still unknown. However, in some trials, this modality is used in combination with other tests.

Other Screening Tools on the Horizon

Technology is advancing rapidly. Novel screening methods that will improve not only sensitivity but also specificity and compliance are being developed. Virtual colonography using existing CT scan technology and computer software for reconstruction is available in Singapore. At the moment, such techniques are still in the evaluation phase, and may be time-consuming and expensive, and further tests are required.[24] Reconstruction of the images is automated and easy but interpretation may take between 15 and 60 or even more minutes per patient. The latest technology has made it possible to use computerized algorithms to screen the colonographs, thereby cutting down on the time required for interpretation. Robotics is being developed for use in colonoscopy and is aimed at reducing complications of the procedure. It will take the technicality of "scoping" off the operator so that relatively untrained individuals may operate the procedure. This will allow wider and safer practice.

A more exciting area of development is telemetry colonoscopy (or capsule colonoscopy), in which a capsule is swallowed and is allowed to pass into the lower gastrointestinal tract. This capsule is slightly bigger than a tablet and comprises in the prototypes (e.g. the Given M2A capsule video endoscope) a system of lenses with usually four microcameras that allow two pictures to be taken every second. The digital information is transmitted to a recording receiver worn around the waist and the information may be played back in a video. The capsule is powered by its own battery and it is possible to obtain relatively good images of the small intestines without a need to fast for the examination. Novel markers for colorectal cancer in stool are also tried. These commonly include tumour markers like *k-ras*, TP-53 and APC shed in the stool by the tumour but recovered for analysis by recombinant DNA microanalysis techniques. This is made easier with the development of microarray analysis. Such techniques may be so sensitive and specific that screening for faecal occult blood may be a thing of the past.

Finally, with the unravelling of the human genome, excitement awaits with the possibility of a genetic test for a "predisposition" to future colorectal cancer risks.

Strategies in Population Colorectal Cancer Screening

Dividing the population into risk profiles (i.e. high, moderate and low) according to a family history of colorectal cancer or medical conditions that predispose to colorectal cancer (e.g. ulcerative colitis, familial adenomatous polyposis coli, FAP, and hereditary nonpolyposis colorectal cancer (HNPCC)) can help to focus scarce screening resources on a group that is at greatest risk. However, this does not address the bulk of the local population, who are probably in the moderate risk group, and it is here that a screening programme has to be decided.

The obvious would be to limit the age at which screening should be done. The incidence of colorectal cancer in the general population of Singapore, where there is no significant family history, like in Western countries, rises steeply from the age of 50 years, peaking in the late 50s and 60s, and plateaus somewhat by 80 years old. A screening programme targeted at those above 50 years of age would be prudent.

The choice of an initial screening test is very much a subject of debate. As alluded to earlier, it is population screening trials studying the end

Table 7. Stage distribution in FOBT trials.

Stage	Nottingham, UK		Funen, Denmark		Goteborg, Sweden	
	Scn %	Ctrl %	Scn %	Ctrl %	Scn %	Ctrl %
A	22.8	11.8	28.8	9.6	30	12
B	32	34.7	29.4	36.3	23	24
C	24.3	32.9	19.0	29.3	31	38
D	20.9	20.6	22.7	24.8	16	26
Adenomas	1338	400	232	109	440	50
Adenomas (≥1 cm)	835	244	167	62	234	21

points of survival after diagnosis and treatment that give the most conclusive evidence of benefit. Secondary indicators such as a stage migration from advanced disease to earlier disease at diagnosis are an important consideration (Table 7). A stage migration without corresponding survival benefits may be the result of lead-time bias when in fact the clinical course of the disease is not altered with early detection and treatment. In the large prospective trials listed, there is a migration towards a corresponding earlier stage accompanied with survival benefits.

The diagnosis of polyps that are tested positive to the screening test and the amount of polypectomies, especially of high risk polyps (greater than three in number, size of greater than 1 cm, and severe dysplasia), all contribute to "increased survival" which is not directly measured in cancer survival figures. Such a policy of aggressive removal of polyps through screening has been shown in the National Polyp Study in the US to reduce cancer incidence and has been cited as one of the possible reasons for the less rapid increase in the incidence of colorectal cancer in the US in recent years.

In practice, compliance and sensitivity of the screening tool are closely related. A tool that is very sensitive but has a low compliance works poorly towards prevention of colorectal cancer death. Compliance is also dependent on the sociocultural environment. This would certainly be greater if there is active legislative participation when mandatory FOBT is enacted (e.g. Japan since 1992) or when the means is provided as part of an insurance health screening programme in many countries, like the US and Germany. Perhaps in the local context, when the costs may be entirely borne through Medisave or similar insurance policies is attractive. Endorsement by regulatory bodies is useful. These include the US Preventive Services Task Force, the American Cancer Society and the American Gastroenterological

Association. Through the Balanced Budget Act of 1997 in the US, it is standard for periodic sigmoidoscopy and FOBT for all Medicare beneficiaries above 50 years of age. Despite this, ironically, less than 30% of persons for whom screening is recommended have been screened.[25] Aversion to the nature of the problem and the procedures used for screening have presented major barriers to compliance in screening.

The interval of screening is a major consideration when cost-effectiveness is considered. In the Minnesota trial, the annual FOBT group performs better than the biennial group in detecting colorectal cancer. Three consecutive samples is better than one sample but, beyond this, specificity declines in stool guaiac tests. Immunochemical tests, being more specific for human haemoglobin, requires one test to two consecutive tests annually or biennially. A complete colonoscopy is believed to reduce the risk of cancer incidence to below that of the population over the next five years and, based on polyp and tumour incidence and progression rates, a 10-year colonoscopy may suffice to produce significant reduction in mortality (Table 8). The index colonoscopy in fact effectively risks re-stratifying individuals into those who form polyps and those who do not, in addition to the early detection of colorectal cancer. Those who have polyps detected will undergo annual surveillance till they are clear of polyps and then at 3–5-year intervals, under current prevailing practice. Thus a strategy of a 10-yearly colonoscopy (assuming a 10-year polyp recurrence after an index colonoscopy) is presumably more cost-effective than a strategy involving an annual FOBT screen. This will save on the manpower and resources for monitoring and repeated testing of the cohort. The overall cost in the prevention of a single death needs to be known in order to assess cost-effectiveness. This must be a necessary factor in not only the visible outward costs of the test, but also the manpower costs in delivering and developing the test kits. The costs of treating complications as a result of screening such as colonoscopic perforation or bleeding after polypectomy have to be considered as part of the cost-effectiveness equation. There is therefore an urgent need for prospective randomized controlled trials in the general population for the evaluation of different modalities in reducing mortality and cost-effectiveness, especially in the local context as this varies widely from place to place depending on cost and resources.

Any screening programme will prove to be a burden on the current health care delivery and infrastructure. Facilities and manpower are

Table 8. Cost-effectiveness using base-case assumptions.[26]

Strategy	Years of life gained per 100 000 screened	Added cost per 100 000 screened	Cost per added year of life
Assuming a 5-year polyp dwell:			
Annual FOBT	5150	$70 000 000	$13 581
Flexible sigmoidoscopy × 3 yrs	3910	$53 000 000	$13 554
Flexible sigmoidoscopy × 5 yrs	3370	$40 200 000	$11 947
Flexible sigmoidoscopy × 10 yrs	1900	$38 300 000	$20 122
Colonoscopy × 3 yrs	6690	$120 900 000	$18 076
Colonoscopy × 5 yrs	6100	$87 700 000	$14 383
Colonoscopy × 10 yrs	3680	$81 500 000	$22 171
Assuming a 10-year polyp dwell:			
Annual FOBT	5880	$58 200 000	$9906
Flexible Sigmoidoscopy × 3 yrs	3990	$51 900 000	$13 001
Flexible Sigmoidoscopy × 5 yrs	3580	$37 800 000	$10 541
Flexible Sigmoidoscopy × 10 yrs	3130	$24 900 000	$7966
Colonoscopy × 3 yrs	6820	$118 800 000	$17 424
Colonoscopy × 5 yrs	6500	$82 900 000	$12 750
Colonoscopy × 10 yrs	5930	$55 100 000	$9287

Calculations are based on a set of base assumptions including the cost of the screening test, the cost of subsequent evaluation, the cost of treating the complications arising from testing, and so on. The complication and incidence rates are based on the results from the Minnesota trial.

required for the conduct of the programme, test kit development, performance of the diagnostic colonoscopy, and auditing of the results. Health care costs may be increased with early diagnosis and treatment. Existing standards of health care must not be compromised.

Conclusion

In conclusion, there is compelling data to support population screening for colorectal cancer. Early detection improves cancer survival and the stage of the disease at diagnosis. Whilst this may be confounded by lead-time bias, length-time bias and screening bias, the impact of these has not been consistently and conclusively borne out in randomized prospective controlled trials. Further undocumentable risk reduction is experienced with a policy of polypectomy as, if these are left unremoved, if sufficiently large, they will lead to colorectal cancer. It is the choice of screening modality and the cost-effectiveness in any programme that are debatable. Population-based randomized controlled trials are urgently needed to identify the most effective modality.

References

1. Chia KS, Seow A, Lee HP and Shanmugatharatnam K. Cancer incidence in Singapore 1993–1997. Singapore Cancer Registry Report No. 5.
2. Watson and Junger, WHO Public Health Papers No. 34.
3. Goulston KJ, Cook I and Dent OF. How important is rectal bleeding in the diagnosis of bowel cancer and polyps? *Lancet* 1986; ii: 261–6.
4. Young GP and St John DJB. Selecting an occult blood test for use as screening tool for large bowel cancer, *Front Gastrointest Res* 1991; 18: 135–56.
5. Macrae FA and St John DJB. Relationship between patterns of bleeding and Hemoccult sensitivity in patients with colorectal cancers or adenomas, *Gastroenterology* 1982; 82: 891–8.
6. St John DJ, Young GP and Alexeyeff MA. Evaluation of new occult blood tests for detection of colorectal neoplasia, *Gastroenterology* 1993; 104: 1661–8.
7. Thomas WM, Pye G, Hardcastle JD and Mangham CM. Faecal occult blood screening for colorectal neoplasia: a randomised trial of three days or six days of tests, *Br J Surg* 1990; 77: 277–9.
8. Hardcastle JD, Chamberlain J, Sheffield J, Balfour TW, Armitage NC and Thomas WM. Randomised, controlled trial of faecal occult blood screening for colorectal cancer: results of the first 107 349 subjects, *Lancet* 1989; May 27; 1160–4.
9. Kronborg O, Fenger C, Worm J, Pederson SA, Hem J, Bertelsen K and Olsen J. Causes of death during the first 5 years of a randomised trial of mass screening for colorectal cancer with faecal occult blood test, *Scand J Gastroenterol* 1992; 27: 47–52.
10. Kewenter J, Brevinge H, Haglind E and Ahren C. Screening, rescreening and follow-up in a prospective randomised study for detection of colorectal cancer by faecal occult blood testing, *Scand J Gastroenterol* 1994; 29: 468–73.

11. Mandel JS, Bond JH and Church TR. Reducing mortality from colorectal cancer by screening for faecal occult blood, *New Engl J Med* 1993; 328: 1365–71.

12. Winawer SJ, Flehinger BJ, Schottenfeld D and Miller DG. Screening for colorectal cancer with faecal occult blood testing and sigmoidoscopy, *J Natl Cancer Inst* 1993; 85: 1311–18.

13. Towler BP, Irwig L, Glasziou P, Weller D and Kewenter J. Screening for colorectal cancer using the faecal occult blood test, hemoccult, *Cochrane Database Syst Rev* 2000; (2): CD001216.

14. Committee for a nationwide totaling of mass screening for gastrointestinal cancers: a nationwide totaling of mass screening for gastrointestinal cancers, *J Gastroenterol Mass Surv* 1995; 33: 200–18.

15. Selby JV. Targeting colonoscopy, *Gastroenterology* 1994; 106: 1702–5.

16. Schoen RE, Weissfeld JL, Bowen NJ, Switzer G and Baum A. Patient satisfaction with screening flexible sigmoidoscopy, *Arch Intern Med* 2000; 160: 1790–6.

17. Schoenfeld P, Piorkowski M, Allaire J, Ernst R and Holmes L. Flexible sigmoidoscopy by nurses: state of the art 1999, *Gastroenterol Nurs* 1999; 22: 254–61.

18. Schoenfeld PS, Cash B, Kita J, Piorkowski M, Cruess D and Ransohoff D. Effectiveness and patient satisfaction with screening flexible sigmoidoscopy performed by registered nurses, *Gastrointest Endosc* 1999; 49: 158–62.

19. Taffinder NJ, Gould SW, Wan AC, Taylor P and Darzi A. Rigid videosigmoidoscopy vs conventional sigmoidoscopy: a randomized controlled study, *Surg Endosc* 1999; 13: 814–16.

20. Hertz RE, Deddish MR and Day E. Value of periodic examination in detecting cancer of the rectum and colon, *Postgrad Med* 1960; 17: 290.

21. Gilbertsen VA. Proctosigmoidoscopy and polypectomy in reducing the incidence of colorectal cancer, *Cancer* 1974; 41: 1137–9.

22. Selby JV. Clinical trials in screening sigmoidoscopy. In *Colorectal Cancer*, Winawer SJ (eds.). Raven Press, New York, 1985, pp. 291–301.

23. Verne JE, Aubrey R, Love SB, Talbot IC and Northover JM. Population based randomized study of uptake and yield of screening by flexible sigmoidoscopy compared with screening by faecal occult blood testing, *BMJ* 1998; 317: 182–5.

24. Summers RM, Beaulieu CF, Pusanik LM, Malley JD, Jeffrey RB Jr, Glazer DI and Napel S. Automated polyp detector for CT colonography: feasibility study, *Radiology* 2000; 216: 284–90.

25. Tomeo CA, Colditz GA, Willett WC, Giovannucci E, Platz E, Rockhill B, Dart H and Hunter DJ. Harvard report on cancer prevention: volume 3: prevention of colon cancer in the United States, *Cancer Causes Control* 1999; 10: 167–80.

26. Wagner JL, Tunis S, Brown N, Ching A and Almeida R. Cost-effectiveness of colorectal cancer screening in average-risk adults. In *Prevention and Early Detection of Colorectal Cancer*, Young GP, Rozen P and Levin B (eds.). WB Saunders, New York, 1996, pp. 321–41.

CHAPTER 27

Molecular Genetics of Colorectal Cancer

PY Cheah

Abstract

How does the information explosion from molecular genetics translate into clinical practice? There are three conceivable ways such information can impact on clinical management of colorectal cancer (CRC) patients. First, the possibility of presymptomatic genetic testing for familial CRC is within reach, at least for familial adenomatous polyposis (FAP) patients. Second, various molecular markers are now being identified for better prognostication. Third, the exciting new field of drug screening and design may eventually impact on chemotherapy. This chapter describes the use of the protein truncation test (PTT) as a presymptomatic tool for screening FAP family members; the prognostic significance of p27 and β-catenin composite marker in predicting disease-free survival; and the use of an individualized, three-dimensional culture system for assessing chemosensitivity of patients to anticancer drugs.

Introduction

Cancer, specifically colorectal cancer (CRC), is caused by the complex interplay of environmental and genetic factors over time. The colon and rectum is the passage in the human body that collects all the waste the body rejects, and hence it is constantly exposed to all kinds of environmental mutagens ingested or produced by the body. Many studies link various dietary factors to the aetiology of CRC.[1] Coupled with the high turnover rate of the colonic cells (the whole intestinal epithelium replaces itself approximately every 3–4 days), it is no wonder that it is one of the most susceptible organs to cellular dysregulation leading eventually to cancer. Yet not everybody who is exposed to the same mutagens gets CRC. Those who have mutations in genes that are critical in controlling cell proliferation or apoptosis—the two rate-limiting processes in cancer growth—are more likely to succumb to the daily deluge of mutagens than others.

The model that colorectal tumorigenesis occurs via the progression of adenomatous polyps to carcinoma through the accumulation of mutations in a series of genes[2] has now been generally accepted. Nevertheless, recent development has led to various modifications of the model.[3] The majority of CRC patients are over 60 years old. These are sporadic cases attributable to spontaneous mutations in both copies of a series of genes or loci over time. However, about 20% of CRC involves young patients who are likely to have inherited a copy of the mutated gene. Individuals with such germline mutations are at a much greater risk of developing tumours than the sporadic cases since the probability of acquiring a single somatic mutation is exponentially greater than the probability of acquiring two such mutations.[4] There are three major forms of hereditary CRC—familial adenomatous polyposis (FAP), heritable nonpolyposis colorectal carcinoma (HNPCC), and early-onset CRC, whose genetic predisposition has not been clearly delineated (Fig. 1).

FAP is an autosomal dominantly inherited form of CRC in which the colon and rectum of the patient is carpeted with hundreds to thousands of adenomatous polyps by the second or third decade of his life. Patients often develop extracolonic manifestations (ECMs) such as osteomas, desmoids, retinal lesions, and brain and thyroid tumours. FAP has always been the model system for studying colorectal tumorigenesis, because polyp specimens are easily available and the penetrance of the disease is virtually 100%, i.e. the risk that one of these polyps will progress to cancer is 100% if they are not removed in time. The adenomatous polyposis coli (*APC*) gene

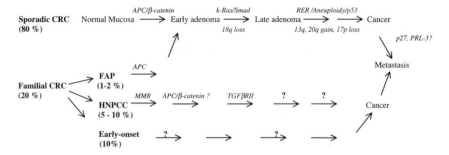

Figure 1. A modified multistage colorectal carcinogensis model. The genes/chromosomes listed are by no means exhaustive and there are many missing links, denoted by question marks. MMR—mismatched repair; TGFβRII—transforming growth factor-β receptor type II; RER—replication error. This figure is updated from Fig. 1 of Ref. 3.

at chromosome band 5q21 was first found to cosegregate with FAP. Subsequently, mutations in the *APC* gene were found in over 80% of both FAP[5] and the sporadic CRC,[6] thus strongly implicating *APC* to be the initiator or gatekeeper gene[7] in both sporadic CRC and FAP (Fig. 1).

Protein Truncation Test as a Presymptomatic Genetic Test for FAP Screening

More than 98% of the *APC* mutations reported to date are translation-terminating mutations resulting in truncated proteins.[8] A direct genetic test for FAP thus became feasible with the development of the protein truncation test (PTT). The PTT[5,9] combines polymerase chain reaction (PCR) with *in vitro* transcription and translation techniques to detect translation-terminating mutations. Unlike linkage study, no detailed family history is required to carry out the test.

Although the *APC* gene has been extensively studied in the Caucasian population, it has not been previously described in the Singapore families, who are predominantly Chinese. We used the PTT to screen the entire *APC* gene for germline mutation in 43 unrelated FAP families registered with the Singapore Polyposis Registry in the Singapore General Hospital, Singapore. About 10 ml of blood was collected from 179 members of these families.

The *APC* coding sequence is 8.5 kilobases long and contains 15 coding exons. It was amplified by 6 overlapping PCR/RT-PCR segments

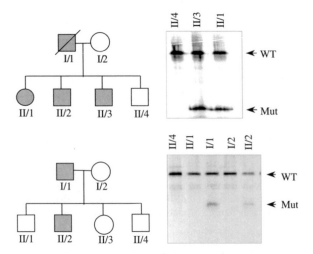

Figure 2. PTT results from representative FAP families. PTT was carried out whenever blood was available. The full-length protein (WT) is found in all members of the family. FAP patients from the same family have truncated proteins (Mut) of the same size and unaffected members have no truncated protein. In the pedigrees, FAP patients and unaffected members of the family as diagnosed by colonoscopy are represented by filled and unfilled symbols, respectively. This figure is adapted from Fig. 1 of Ref. 14.

corresponding to nucleotides 1-1800 (Segment 1.1), 1041–2514 (Segment 1.2), 2056–3831 (Segment 2), 3297–5410 (Segment 3), 4783–7011 (Segment 4) and 6364–8543 (Segment 5), as previously described.[10] The unpurified PCR product was *in vitro* transcribed and translated into protein with the TNT/T7 coupled reticulocyte lysate system (Promega) and ran on SDS-PAGE gel. The truncated protein, if any, would migrate faster on the gel than the full-length protein (Fig. 2).

We found *APC* germline mutation in 35 of the 43 families (81%). The detailed analysis of 151 members of these 35 FAP families shows that the mutated *APC* gene was found in all 82 FAP patients. In fact, truncated proteins were found in some young at-risk individuals and subsequent colonoscopy confirmed the presence of polyps. None of the 69 individuals clinically diagnosed as unaffected members have the truncated protein. There was thus no false positive or false negative case in the PTT analysis of the 151 members from these 35 families. In other words, there is a 100% correlation between clinical diagnosis by colonoscopy and molecular diagnosis by PTT. Figure 2 shows representative PTT results for two of the

FAP families. The sensitivity and specificity of the PTT test are thus 81% and 100%, respectively.

In contrast to clinical diagnosis by colonoscopy (which can only determine postsymptomatically who amongst the members of the family are FAP patients), PTT can detect FAP carriers presymptomatically, i.e. before polyps appear. Thus, patients can be better counselled and prophylactic colectomy timed to ensure compliance. More importantly, for unaffected members of the family, the relief from emotional turmoil and stress cannot be measured in monetary terms. Nevertheless, the cost saved from unnecessary repeated colonoscopy for unaffected members is highly significant.[11]

Sequencing analysis of the PCR fragments giving rise to truncation confirms the mutation at nucleotide level in all 35 families. Twenty-six different mutations were found, 13 of which (50%) are novel. These include two genomic rearrangements deleting the whole of exon 11 and exon 14 possibly mediated by the Topoisomerase I and Alu elements, respectively.[12] These large interstitial deletions would have been missed by techniques which analyse individual exons separately. Nine families have the same (AAAGA) deletion at codon 1309, indicating that like in the Caucasian families, codon 1309 is also the mutation "hotspot" for the Singapore FAP families. The detailed description of the *APC* germline mutations and the genotype–phenotype correlation have been reported elsewhere.[13,14]

In order not to miss truncating mutations at the very ends of the *APC* coding region, we sequenced the 5′ and 3′ ends (covering the first 400 and last 300 nucleotides, respectively) of the PCR fragments for the eight families without PTT-detectable mutations. No further mutation was found. The probability of finding a missense mutation amongst the 36 families is very low indeed, as less than 2% of *APC* germline mutations are missense mutations.[15] Furthermore, there are doubts as to whether missense mutations are disease-causing as observations from others and ourselves suggest that the APC protein has to be truncated in order to be inactivated.

Since the function of *APC* is to target β-catenin for degradation,[16] activating β-catenin mutations could conceivably substitute for *APC* in the initiation of sporadic colorectal cancers lacking *APC* mutation. A recent study[17] has provided evidences to substantiate this claim. The role of β-catenin mutation in FAP, however, remains unclear. We therefore screened for β-catenin germline mutations in the eight families lacking detectable

APC mutation. We focused on exon 3, as all the β-catenin mutations reported to date[17,18] involve either the GSK-3β phosphorylation sites (codons 33, 37, 41 and 45), the codons next to these sites (e.g. codons 32 and 34) or the interstitial deletion of exon 3. No β-catenin germline mutation was found in these eight families, indicating that β-catenin mutation cannot substitute for *APC* mutation in the initiation of the FAP syndrome.[10] The molecular data thus suggest that these families may have germline mutation in other genes.

Phenotypic analysis indicates that these patients have different clinical features from FAP patients with *APC* mutations and can be further classified into two groups by the characteristics of the polyps, atypical ECM and age of diagnosis. Genotypic and phenotypic heterogeneity suggests therefore that FAP patients without detectable *APC* germline mutation constitute distinct variants that could possibly aid in the identification of new candidate genes for CRC.[19]

For heritable nonpolyposis colorectal cancer (HNPCC), another dominantly inherited form of CRC in which the patients have few polyps in the colon but, nevertheless, have an accelerated rate of CRC (Fig. 1), the benefit of genetic testing is less clear. This is because, unlike FAP, the penetrance of HNPCC is not 100%. Furthermore, there are at least six mismatch repair (MMR) genes (*MLH1*, *MSH2*, *MSH6*, *MSH3*, *PMS1*, *PMS2*) that can be mutated (although the first two are the most frequent), thus rendering the screen for germline mutation very laborious and nonexhaustive. Moreover, in contrast to a Caucasian series,[20] the rate of microsatellite instability (MI), the hallmark of HNPCC, in Singapore's young CRC patients is not significantly different from that for older, sporadic patients, suggesting that population screening for germline MMR mutations is unlikely to be cost-effective.[21] Nevertheless, MI can conceivably be an additional criterion other than clinical diagnosis based on the expanded Bethesda criteria[22,23] to aid in identifying HNPCC families for targeted surveillance.

Other than FAP and HNPCC, there is another 10% or so familial or early onset CRC whose genetic predisposition remains unclear (Fig. 1) but is more likely to be of lower penetrance and multigenic in nature. Recent studies of Caucasian populations have implicated the cyclin D1 gene, an important cell cycle regulator, in the early onset and survival of several cancers, including CRC.[24,25] The cyclin D1 G870A single nucleotide polymorphism (SNP), resulting in more stable protein,[26] is one promising candidate that is currently being investigated in the local context.

Prognostic Significance of the p27[kip1] Cyclin-Dependent Kinase Inhibitor and β-Catenin Oncogene

Currently, the best prognostic marker for survival from CRC is the histological stage at presentation of the disease, which is dependent on the depth and breadth of invasion. Patients with tumours confined to the colonic wall (Stage I/II) generally have a 90% chance of surviving more than five years. In contrast, patients with lymph-node metastasis (Stage III) have a 50–75% chance of surviving five years while patients with distant metastasis (Stage IV) have a 0–10% chance to survive beyond five years. Up to 10% of the Dukes A/B patients, however, succumbed to local recurrence of the disease or metachronous metastasis. Moreover, similarly staged patients, e.g. Stage III patients, can have vastly different survival rates. It is thus important that independent markers other than tumor staging be found to better categorize patients for management and adjuvant therapy after surgery.

There is increasing evidence to suggest that the pathogenesis of many tumours is characterized by the deregulation of the cell cycle, leading to uncontrolled cell proliferation and/or inhibition of apoptosis or programmed cell death. p27, a cyclin-dependent kinase inhibitor (CDKI) of the cip/kip family, regulates progression from late G1 into the S-(DNA synthesis) phase by binding to and inhibiting the cyclin E/CDK 2 complex, which is required for entry into the S-phase. p27 is thus an important negative regulator of proliferation. A current model proposed p27 to be the central signal coordinating the varying signals from the external environment and serving as a threshold for progression into the S-phase or an exit from the cell cycle.[27] A recent study[28] has also indicated that p27 can inhibit the function of the cyclin E/cdk 2 complex in centrosome duplication. The precise duplication and segregation of centrosome is necessary for normal cell cycle progression.

Several recent studies of various tumours have found a significant correlation of p27 expression with patient survival ranging from breast,[29–31] gastric,[32,33] pituitary,[34] prostate,[35] non-small-cell lung carcinomas,[36,37] oral tongue squamous cell carcinomas[38] to CRC. Nevertheless, there has been at least one study that reported conflicting results.[39] The authors reported a positive correlation between p27 expression and the progression of human esophageal squamous cell carcinomas. p27 expression was found to be independently associated with poor prognosis. The consequence of p27 overexpression in human cancers thus remains unclear.

In one CRC study,[40] the authors found that the five-year overall survival rate of patients with strong p27 expression is 20% higher than for patients with no/weak p27 expression. In a second CRC study,[41] p27 expression was shown to be inversely correlated to the degree of tumour malignancy by Dukes' staging. However, there was no survival data. Thomas *et al.*[42] reported in a small series of primary and metachronous metastases pairs that p27 expression in the latter was significantly lower than in the former. The authors suggested that down-regulation of p27 may play a role in the development of metastases in these tumours. In contrast to these studies, Ciaparonne *et al.*[43] reported that in their series of mucosa, adenomatous polyps, hyperplastic polyps and colorectal tumours, there was no consistent up- or down-regulation of p27 expression, suggesting that p27 expression was not altered during colorectal carcinogenesis. No survival data was reported in the study.

We evaluated the expression of p27 in 136 paraffin-embedded archival tumor specimens of Singapore CRC patients in association with five-year overall survival[44] by immunohistochemistry. Kaplan–Meier survival curves show that the down-regulation of p27 was significantly related to higher mortality ($p = 0.04$; log-rank test). Nevertheless, there are individuals whose tumours exhibit high p27 expression but who survive for only a short period. This observation supports the hypothesis that a panel of tumour markers should better predict overall survival for an individual than any single marker alone in accordance with the multistage model of tumorigenesis.[2] We have previously shown that another potential prognostic marker in breast cancers, NM23, is not a good indicator in CRC as its expression is not significantly correlated to five-year overall survival of the patients.[45]

The majority of sporadic CRC has inactivating mutations in the adenomatous polyposis coli (*APC*) or activating mutations in the β-catenin gene (Fig. 1). These mutations disrupt the multiprotein complex which targets β-catenin for degradation, resulting in the accumulation and subsequent nuclear translocation of β-catenin. Once in the nucleus, β-catenin binds to the T-cell transcription factor (Tcf) to coactivate downstream target genes. Two of the target genes identified are c-Myc[46] and cyclin D1.[47–49] Biochemical studies have also shown that ectopic expression of c-Myc induces the synthesis of cyclin D1 and D2 proteins, which antagonize the association of p27^{kip1} with Cdk 2, thus allowing the cell to progress through the G1/S checkpoint.[50,51]

We assessed the expressions of β-catenin, c-Myc and cyclin D1 in association with the patients' disease-specific survival and other clinical features on the same series of tumour specimens with p27 data (but excluding Stage IV specimens) by immunostaining with the respective monoclonal antibodies. Intense nuclear overexpression of β-catenin (but not lack of cell membrane or cytoplasmic expression) is a significant predictor of poor survival by both univariate ($p = 0.0029$; Fig. 3A) and multivariate analyses ($p = 0.004$; risk ratio = 3.8). This suggests that β-catenin has to be retained in the nucleus to function as an oncogene. More importantly, none of the patients with high nuclear β-catenin and low p27 expressions survived five years or more while 65% of those with all other combinations of the two markers did ($p < 0.0001$; Fig. 3B). This composite of p27 and β-catenin, p27b12, is also a significant and independent prognostic factor ($p = 0.001$; risk ratio = 9.7). Overexpression of c-Myc tends to be associated with higher mortality but the expression of cyclin D1 has no prognostic significance. Thus the data suggests that the composite p27 and β-catenin (but not c-Myc and cyclin D1) marker can stratify CRC patients into markedly different survival groups, especially for the Stage III patients, whose survival seems the most variable.[52] p27 and β-catenin are therefore potentially useful biomarkers for clinical management and targets for therapeutic intervention.

Assessing Chemosensitivity with the Individualized and Three-Dimensional Histoculture System

Numerous attempts have been made to develop reliable, cost-effective and rapid assays for assessing the chemosensitivity of cancers to antineoplastic drugs. Traditionally, cell lines have been used for *in vitro* drug efficacy assays. However, monolayer cultures have been shown to be much more sensitive to drugs than the *in vivo* situation, partly because they do not have a three-dimensional configuration and drug response is often a function of tissue architecture.[53] It has also been shown that some tumour-specific antigens, such as TAG-72, are expressed in three-dimensional cultures but not in monolayer cultures.[54] Tumour-specific antigens are important for tumour diagnosis, prognosis and possibly therapy. On the other hand, xenografts involving the transplant of human tumors to nude mice take too long (30–50 weeks) to yield results and are therefore of limited use to most

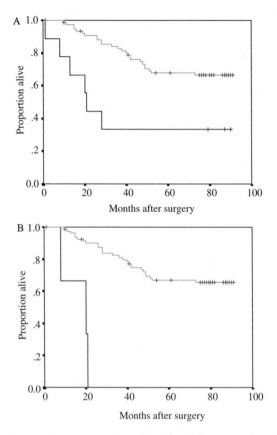

Figure 3. Kaplan–Meier survival analysis for β-catenin (A) and p27b12 (B) expressions for the entire series ($n = 87$). (A) β-catenin nuclear expression as low (gray) or high (black) (log-rank test; $p = 0.0029$) and (B) p27b12 expression as 1.00 (gray) or 2.00 (black) (log-rank test; $p < 0.0001$). p27b12 has a score of 2 when p27 expression is low and β-catenin nuclear expression is high and a score of 1 for all other combinations of the two markers. This figure is adapted from Fig. 2 of Ref. 52.

cancer patients. Moreover, results obtained in xenografts may not be representative of human response. In some instances, the xenograft tumours behave more like mouse tumors than human tumours. Thus, effective human drugs may be missed if a xenograft is used.[55] The cost of animal maintenance for xenografts may also be prohibitive. Furthermore, human cancers that have been identically classified using standard histopathological criteria have been shown to respond differently to chemotherapy.[56] Different individuals may have different sensitivity or resistance to the same drug. There is thus a need to develop an individualized, three-dimensional system to screen for the best drug for postoperative therapy.

We have successfully established a relatively rapid, three-dimensional and individualized histoculture system, based on an adaptation of the method pioneered by Hoffman and coworkers,[57,58] for chemosensitivity studies in primary CRC. Freshly resected cancers from individual patients were microdissected and cultured on floating pig-skin collagen up to a month at 37°C. We are able to achieve a high success rate of viable culture (84%) as well as keep the contamination rate low (10%). The *in vitro* histo-culture system is able to mimic the *in vivo* situation and maintain the tissue architecture of tumours before culture (Fig. 4). The histocultured tumours were also able to maintain tissue antigenicity, such as the expression of the CEA antigen.

Proliferation of the tissues was measured by the bromodeoxyuridine (BrdU) immunostaining technique.[59] The mean BrdU labelling index (LI) was about 40%. In one study,[60] we used the BrdU immunostaining tech-niques to measure the proliferation index of histocultured tumours treated with 1–10 mM sodium salicylate, an aspirin metabolite. The majority of the histoculture tumours showed a dose response to sodium salicylate, i.e. a decrease in BrdU labelling with increased dose. The dose–effect relation-ship is analysed by curve-fitting the experimental data to the modified E max model, as described below:[61]

$$E = E_0 \cdot [1 - C^n/(K^n + C^n)].$$

E is the LI as a percentage of control, C is the drug concentration, E_0 is the baseline effect in the absence of drug, K is the drug concentration at one-half E_0 and n is the curve shape parameter. K is equivalent to IC_{50}, the concentration needed to produce 50% inhibition.

We found that the chemosensitivity of individual tumours to sodium salicylate varied and can be divided into four groups, ranging from the most sensitive (group A), the typical sigmoidal response (groups B and C) and the nonsensitive (group D). Specimens in group C have an IC_{50} value that exceeds the physiologically relevant concentrations (1–3 mM)[62,63] and therefore cannot be considered to be sensitive to sodium salicylate for clinical purposes. In other words, only specimens in groups A and B show chemosensitivity to sodium salicylate within the physiological concentrations. The varying chemosensitivity of tumours to sodium sali-cylate highlighted further the need for a clinically relevant system to tailor chemotherapy to the individual patient. Preliminary data also indicates

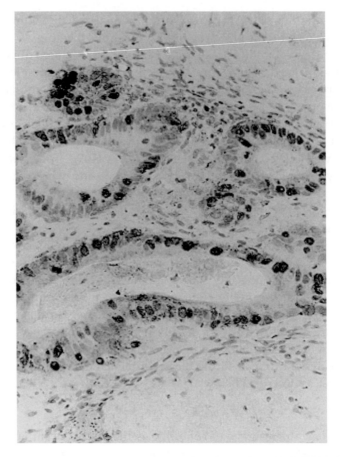

Figure 4. A representative histocultured colorectal cancer section with BrdU labelling. The tissue architecture was similar to the fresh cancer, with no observable change in cell type or differentiation.

the possibility of achieving the same inhibitory effect with a lower dose if exposure time is extended.

Furthermore, the chemosensitivity of individually cultured tumours can be correlated to the patients' clinicopathological parameters, which could provide some insight into the behaviour of the tumours. Our data, for example, has revealed that right-sided tumours (tumours to the right of the splenic flexture) were apparently not sensitive to sodium salicylate within the physiologically relevant concentrations.[60]

Conclusion

Much ground has been gained in understanding the molecular basis of CRC since the model of multistage colorectal tumorigenesis was first proposed in 1990.[2] In the postgenomics era, the challenge would be to apply this knowledge for better health care management. To this end, the laboratory has established the PTT for the screening of FAP family members. We have also made inroads into establishing a molecular profile for individual patients for better prognostication and management. Further, we have established the three-dimensional and individualized histoculture system, which offers high potential for individualized treatment, new anticancer drug screening and tumour biology study.

Acknowledgements

The contributions from various members of the laboratory, Xia Cao, Yanqun Liu, Jocelyn Yao, Poh Heok Choo and Yi Hong, are gratefully acknowledged. Thanks are also due to the surgeons in the department and Dr Ivy Sng from the Department of Pathology, SGH, who provided the fresh and paraffin-embedded tumour specimens, and the Singapore Polyposis Registry for pedigree and clinicopathological data retrieval. The studies described in this chapter are partially funded by the National Medical Research Council of Singapore, the Singapore Cancer Society and the Department of Clinical Research, SGH.

References

1. Cheah PY. Hypotheses for the etiology of colorectal cancer—an overview, *Nutr Cancer* 1990; 14: 5–13.
2. Fearon ER and Vogelstein B. A genetic model for colorectal tumorigenesis, *Cell* 1990; 61: 759–67.
3. Cheah PY, Eu KW and Seow-Choen F. Update of genetics in colorectal carcinomas: genetic instability and somatic evolution, *Ann Acad Med Singapore* 2000; 29: 331–6.
4. Knudson AG. Hereditary cancer: two hits revisited, *J Cancer Res Clin Oncol* 1996; 122: 135–40.

5. Powel SM, Peterson GM, Krush AJ *et al*. Molecular diagnosis of familial adenomatous polyposis, *N Engl J Med* 1993; 329: 1982–7.

6. Miyoshi Y, Nagase H, Ando H *et al*. Somatic mutations of the APC gene in colorectal tumors: mutation cluster region in the APC gene, *Hum Mol Genet* 1992; 1: 229–33.

7. Kinzler KW and Vogelstein B. A genetic model for colorectal tumorigenesis, *Cell* 1996; 87: 159–70.

8. Beroud C and Soussi T. APC gene: database of germline and somatic mutations in human tumors and cell lines, *Nucl Acids Res* 1996; 24: 121–4.

9. Roest PAM, Roberts RG, Sugino S, van Ommen GB and den Dunnen JT. Protein truncation test (PTT) for rapid detection of translation-terminating mutations, *Hum Mol Genet* 1993; 2: 1719–21.

10. Cao X, Eu KW, Seow-Choen F and Cheah PY. Germline mutations are frequent in the APC gene but absent in β-catenin gene in familial adenomatous polyposis patients, *Genes Chromosomes & Cancer* 1999; 25: 396-8.

11. Cromwell DM, Moore RD, Brensinger JD, Petersen GM, Bass EB and Giardiello FM. Cost analysis of alternative approaches to colorectal screening in familial adenomatous polyposis, *Gastroentrology* 1998; 114: 893–901.

12. Cao X, Eu WK, Seow-Choen F, Zhao Y and Cheah PY. Topoisomerase-1- and Alu-mediated genomic deletions of the APC gene in familial adenomatous polyposis, *Hum Genet* 2001; 108: 436–42.

13. Cao X, Eu WK, Seow-Choen F, Zhao Y and Cheah PY. APC mutation and phenotypic spectrum of Singapore familial adenomatous polyposis patients, *Eur J Hum Genet* 2000; 8: 42–8.

14. Cao X, Eu WK, Seow-Choen F and Cheah PY. Molecular and clinical profiles of Singapore familial adenomatous polyposis patients. In *Frontiers in Human Genetics*, World Scientific, Singapore, 2001, pp. 245–59.

15. Laurent-Puig, Beroud C and Soussi T. APC gene: database of germline and somatic mutations in human tumors and cell lines, *Nucl Acids Res* 1998; 26: 270–3.

16. Korinek V, Barker N, Morin PJ *et al*. Constitutive transcriptional activation by a β-catenin-Tdf complex in APC$^{-/-}$ colon carcinoma, *Science* 1997; 275: 1784–6.

17. Sparks AB, Morin PJ, Vogelstein B and Kinzler KW. Mutational analysis of the APC/β-catenin/Tcf pathway in colorectal cancer, *Cancer Res* 1998; 58: 1130–4.

18. Iwao K, Nakamori S, Kameyama M *et al*. Activation of the β-catenin gene by interstitial deletions involving exon 3 in primary colorectal carcinomas without Adenomatous Polyposis coli mutations, *Cancer Res* 1998; 58: 1021–6.

19. Cao X, Hong Y, Eu WK, Seow-Choen F and Cheah PY. Two phenotypically distinct familial adenomatous polyposis variants with no detectable APC/CTNNB1/AXIN germline mutations. Submitted to *J Med Genet*.

20. Liu B, Farrington SM, Petersen GM *et al*. Genetic instability occurs in the majority of young patients with colorectal cancer, *Nature Med* 1995; 1: 348–52.

21. Yao J, Eu KW, Seow-Choen F, Vijayan V and Cheah PY. Microsatellite instability and aneuploidy rate in young colorectal-cancer patients do not differ significantly from those in older patients, *Int J Cancer* 1999; 80: 667–70.

22. Syngal S, Fox EA, Eng C, Kolodner RD and Garber JE. Sensitivity and specificity of clinical criteria for hereditary non-polyposis colorectal cancer associated mutations in MSH2 and MLH1, *J Med Genet* 2000; 37: 641–5.

23. Terdiman JP, Gum JR Jr, Conrad PG *et al*. Efficient detection of hereditary nonpolyposis colorectal cancer gene carriers by screening for tumour microsatellite instability before germline genetic testing, *Gastroenterology* 2001; 120: 21–30.

24. Kong S, Amos CI, Luthra R, Lynch PM, Levin B and Frazier ML. Effects of cyclin D1 polymorphism on age of onset of hereditary nonpolyposis colorectal cancer, *Cancer Res* 2000; 60: 249–52.

25. Kong S, Wei Q, Amos CI *et al*. Cyclin D1 polymorphism and increased risk of colorectal cancer at young age, *J Nat Cancer Inst* 2001; 93: 1106–8.

26. Betticher DC, Thatcher N, Altermatt HJ, Hoban P, Ryder WDJ and Heighway J. Alternate splicing produces a novel cyclin D1 transcript, *Oncogene* 1995; 11: 1005–11.

27. Steeg P and Abrams JS. Cancer prognostics: past, present and p27, *Nature Med* 1997; 3: 152–4.

28. Lacey KR, Jackson PK and Sterns T. Cyclin-depencent kinase control of centrosome duplication, *Proc Natl Acad Sci USA* 1999; 96: 2817–22.

29. Catzarelos C, Bhattacharya N, Ung YC *et al*. Decreased levels of the cell-cycle inhibitor p27[kip1] protein: prognostic implications in primary breast cancer, *Nature Med* 1997; 3: 227–30.

30. Porter PL, Malone KE, Heagerty PJ *et al.* Expression of cell-cycle regulators p27^{kip1} and cyclin E, alone and in combination, correlate with survival in young breast cancer patients, *Nature Med* 1997; 3: 222–5.

31. Tan P, Cady B, Wanner M *et al.* The cell cycle inhibitor p27 is an independent prognostic marker in small (T$_{1a,b}$) invasive breast carcinomas, *Cancer Res* 1997; 57: 1259–63.

32. Mori M, Mimori K, Shiraishi T *et al.* p27 expression and gastric carcinoma, *Nature Med* 1997; 3: 593.

33. Yasui W, Kudo Y, Semba S, Yokozaki H and Tahara E. Reduced expression of cyclin-dependent kinase inhibitor p27^{kip1} is associated with advanced stage and invasiveness of gastric carcinomas, *Jpn J Cancer Res* 1997; 88: 625–9.

34. Dahia PLM, Aguiar RC, Honeggar J *et al.* Mutation and expression analysis of the p27/kip1 gene in corticotrophin-secreting tumors, *Oncogene* 1998; 16: 69–76.

35. Yang RM, Naitoh J, Murphy M *et al.* Low p27 expression predicts poor disease-free survival in patients with prostate cancer, *J Urol* 1998; 159: 941–5.

36. Esposito V, Baldi A, De Luca A *et al.* Prognostic role of the cyclin-dependent kinase inhibitor p27 in non-small cell lung cancer, *Cancer Res* 1997; 57: 3381–5.

37. Yatabe Y, Masuda A, Koshikawa T *et al.* p27^{kip1} in human lung cancers: differential changes in small cell and non-small cell lung carcinomas, *Cancer Res* 1998; 58: 1042–7.

38. Mineta H, Miura K, Suzuki I *et al.* Low p27 expression correlates with poor prognosis for patients with oral tongue squamous cell carcinoma, *Cancer* 1999; 85: 1011–17.

39. Anayama T, Furhita M, Ishikawa T, Ohtsuki Y and Ogoshi S. Positive correlation between p27^{kip1} expression and progression of human esophageal squamous cell carcinoma, *Int J Cancer* 1998; 79: 439–43.

40. Loda M, Cakor B, Tam SW *et al.* Increased proteasome-dependent degradation of the cyclin-dependent kinase inhibitor p27 in aggressive colorectal carcinomas, *Nature Med* 1997; 3: 231–4.

41. Fredersdorf S, Burns J, Milne AM *et al.* High level expression of p27^{kip1} and Cyclin D1 in some human breast cancer cells: inverse correlation between the expression of p27^{kip1} and degree of malignancy in human breast and colorectal cancers, *Proc Nat Acad Sci USA* 1997; 94: 6380–5.

42. Thomas GV, Szigeti K, Murphy M, Draetta G, Pagano M and Loda M. Down-regulation of p27 is associated with development

of colorectal adenocarcinoma metastases, *Am J Pathol* 1998; 153: 681–6.

43. Ciaparrone M, Yamamoto H, Yao Y *et al.* Localization and expression of p27 kip1 in multistage colorectal carcinogenesis, *Cancer Res* 1998; 58: 114–22.

44. Yao J, Eu KW, Seow-Choen F and Cheah PY. Down-regulation of p27 is a significant predictor of poor overall survival and may facilitate metastasis in colorectal carcinomas, *Int J Cancer* 2000; 89: 213–16.

45. Cheah PY, Cao X, Eu KW and Seow-Choen F. NM23-H1 immunostaining is inversely associated with tumor staging but not overall survival or disease recurrence in colorectal carcinomas, *Br J Cancer* 1998; 77: 1164–8.

46. He T, Sparks AB, Rago C *et al.* Identification of c-Myc as a target of the APC pathway, *Science* 1998; 281: 1509–12.

47. Tetsu O and McCormick F. *β*-catenin regulates expression of cyclin D1 in colon carcinoma cells, *Nature* 1999; 398: 422–6.

48. Shtutman M, Zhurinsky J, Simcha I *et al.* The cyclin D1 gene is a target of the *β*-catenin/LEF-1 pathway, *Proc Natl Acad Sci USA* 1999; 96: 5522–7.

49. Lin S, Xia W, Wang JC *et al.* *β*-catenin, a novel prognostic marker for breast cancer: its roles in cyclin D1 expression and cancer progression, *Proc Natl Acad Sci USA* 2000; 97: 4262–6.

50. Perez-Roger I, Kim S, Griffiths B, Sewing A and Land H. Cyclins D1 and D2 mediate Myc-induced proliferation via sequestration of p27kip1 and p21cip1, *EMBO J* 1999; 18: 5310–20.

51. Bouchard C, Thieke K, Maier A *et al.* Direct induction of cyclin D2 by Myc contributes to cell cycle progression and sequestration of p27, *EMBO J* 1999; 18: 5321–33.

52. Cheah PY, Choo PH, Yao J, Eu KW and Seow-Choen F. A survival-stratification model of human colorectal carcinomas with *β*-catenin and p27^{kip1}, *Cancer* 2002; 95: 2479–86.

53. Hoffman RM. *In vitro* sensitivity assays in cancer: a review, analysis, and prognosis, *J Clin Lab Anal* 1991; 5: 133–43.

54. Guadagni F, Roselli M and Hoffman RM. Maintenance of expression of tumor antigens in three-dimensional, *in vitro* human tumor gel-supported histoculture, *Anticancer Res* 1991; 11: 543–6.

55. Gura T. Systems for identifying new drugs are often faulty, *Science* 1997, 278: 1041–2.

56. Vescio RA, Redfern CH, Nelson TJ, Ugoretz S, Stern PH and Hoffman RM. *In-vivo*-like drug responses of human tumors growing in three-dimensional gel-supported primary culture, *Proc Natl Acad Sci USA* 1987; 84: 5029–33.

57. Freeman AE and Hoffman RM. *In-vivo*-like growth of human tumors *in vitro*, *Proc Natl Acad Sci USA* 1986; 83: 2694–8.

58. Hoffman RM, Connors KM, Meerson-Monosov AE, Herrana H and Price JH. A general native state method for determination of proliferation capacity of human normal and tumor tissues *in vitro*, *Proc Natl Acad Sci USA* 1989; 86: 2013–17.

59. Gan Y, Wientjes, MG, Schuller, DE and Au JLS. Pharmacodynamics of taxol in human head and neck tumors, *Cancer Res* 1996; 56: 2086–93.

60. Liu Y, Eu KW, Seow-Choen F, Cheah PY. Differential cytostatic effect of sodium salicylate in human colorectal cancers using an individualized histoculture system. Cancer Chemotherapy and Pharmacology 2002, DOI 10.1007/s00280-002-0441-7.

61. Au JLS, Wientjes MG, Rosol TJ, Koolemans-Beynen A, Goebel EA and Shuller DE. Histocultures of patient head and neck tumors for pharmacodynamics studies, *Pharmaceutical Res* 1993; 10: 1493–9.

62. Klampfer L, Cammenga J, Wisniewski HG and Nimer SD. Sodium salicylate activates caspases and induces apoptosis of myeloid leukemia cell lines, *Blood* 1999; 93: 2386–94.

63. BeDell LS (ed.). Physicians geneRx—the complete drug reference. Mosby, St Louis, 1996.

CHAPTER 28

Staging of Colorectal Carcinoma

JF Lim

Introduction

In recent years, there has been an explosion of interest in the molecular biology of cancer and many have attempted to link it to prognostication of the disease. However, this is still in its embryonic stage. The most reliable factor to date is still the pathological stage of disease, i.e. the depth of penetration of the tumour and the status of the lymph nodes.

Evolution of Staging

Lockhart-Mummery[1] was the first to stage rectal carcinoma in 1926, correlating stage with survival. He classified them into stages A, B and C based on depth of invasion and lymph nodal involvement. Dukes modified the staging in 1932 (Table 1) and subdivided stage C into C1 (perirectal node involvement only) and C2 (apical mesenteric node involvement).[2] Subsequently, several other authors have made attempts to modify the system with minimal change.

Astler and Coller extended the system with some modifications to include colon and rectal cancer.[3] In this system, the significant thing was that prognosis of stage C1 disease approximated that of stage B disease. Turnbull, in 1963, added stage D to Dukes' system for patients with metastasis or direct invasion of adjacent organs. Because of the confusion from having several staging systems, the American Joint Committee on Cancer and the Union Internationale Centre Cancer developed a TNM system for colorectal carcinoma.[4]

TNM Staging

Tx   Primary tumour cannot be assessed
T0   No evidence of primary tumour
Tis   Carcinoma *in situ*
T1   Tumour invades submucosa
T2   Tumour invades muscularis propria
T3   Tumour invades subserosa or nonperitonealized pericolic/perirectal tissue
T4   Tumour directly invades adjacent organ or perforates visceral peritoneum
Nx   Regional lymph nodes cannot be assessed
N0   No regional lymph node metastasis
N1   1–3 pericolic/perirectal lymph node involvement
N2   4 or more pericolic/perirectal lymph node involvement
N3   Metastasis in a lymph node along the course of a named vascular trunk and/or metastasis to apical node
Mx   Presence of distant metastasis cannot be assessed
M0   No distant metastasis
M1   Distant metastasis

The TNM staging undergoes regular reappraisal and the working group has come up with several issues which warrant discussion.

Table 1. Comparison of various staging systems used by different authors.

Maximal Depth of Invasion	Lockhart-Mummery 1926	Dukes 1932	Dukes 1935	Simpson 1939	Kirklin 1949	Astler-Coller 1954	Turnbull 1967	Pihl 1980
				Stage (% 5-Year Survival)				
Mucosa	A(73.7)			A(100)	A(100)	A(100)		
Submucosa		A(80)	A(91)					A1(90)
Muscularis propria	B(44.1)			B(61.9)	B1(75)	B1(66.6)	A(98.9)	A2(89)
Pericolic/rectal adipose tissue		B(73)	B(64)		B2(70)	B2(53.9)	B(84.9)	B(76)
Positive nodes	C(44.4)	C(7)	C(16)	C(49.4)	C(36.4)		C(67.3)	
Regional			C1			C1(43)		C1(43)
Apical			C2			C2(22.4)		C2(12)
Invades adjacent tissue or distant							D(14.3)	D1(11)
Spread								D2(0)

Carcinoembryonic Antigen

Serum CEA levels should preoperatively be added, as a raised preoperative CEA correlates with a poorer prognosis.[5,6] In a review of 261 patients with curative resection by surgeons of our department from 1989 to 1994 and a minimum follow-up of five years, we found the preoperative CEA level to be an important independent indicator of recurrence.[7] No patients with CEA <1 ng/ml had developed recurrence. When the cut-off of 5 ng/ml was taken, 23 and 37.2% of patients with raised preoperative CEA developed recurrence at two and five years, respectively. CEA of 15 ng/ml or more was an adverse prognostic indicator independent of Dukes' stage.

Peritoneal Surface Involvement

Shepherd *et al.*[8] studied a total of 412 patients and found that in 112 (27%) cases, the peritoneal surface was unequivocally infiltrated, and in a further 130 (32%) resections there was peritoneal ulceration and tumour cells lying freely in the peritoneum. Localized peritoneal involvement was found to have a strong independent prognostic influence in curative surgery patients.

Lymph Node Sampling

How many nodes should be sampled to provide a representative amount? How many sections should be taken from each node to ensure microscopic foci are not missed?

Mainprize *et al.*[9] in 1998 claimed that routine manual dissection without fat-clearing solutions could accurately diagnose up to 99% of Dukes C colorectal carcinomas. Koren *et al.*[10] employed lymph-node-revealing solutions in their colectomy specimens, upstaging from Dukes B to C occurred in 8 out of 30 specimens; Greenson *et al.*[11] found that in 50 cases originally node-negative (Dukes B), use of immunoperoxidase methods showed positive staining for cytokeratin in 14 patients, 6 of whom died of cancer within 66 months. Only 1 of the remaining 36 patients with cytokeratin-negative nodes died of cancer over the same period.

Conversely, Broll *et al.*[12] conducted a similar study and even though patients who were upstaged were more likely to develop local recurrence or distant metastasis, long term follow-up showed no difference in survival. To date, the clinical and prognostic significance of micrometastasis to lymph nodes needs more assessment before it can be widely accepted.

Histologic Grading of Tumour

The degree of tumour differentiation is an independent prognostic indicator. However, assessment is subjective and hence substantial interobserver variation and a lack of strict guidelines cloud the issue.

Lymphocytic Infiltrate

The inflammatory response to a tumour has traditionally been regarded as an indication of host resistance to neoplastic spread. Murray *et al.*[13] found that the five-year survival rate doubled when there was intense inflammatory response around the colorectal carcinoma. Jass[14] semiquantitated the degree of lymphocytic infiltration around the tumour into pronounced, moderate and little, with corresponding five-year survival rates of 92%, 65% and 36%.

Character of the Invasive Margin— Pushing or Invasive?

Cianchi *et al.*[15] found that in a series of 235 patients with colorectal cancer who had undergone radical resection, the prognosis for patients with pushing tumour margins was better in Dukes A and B patients. C1 and C2 patients with infiltrative margins had a worse prognosis.

Venous Invasion

While extramural venous invasion is accepted to have a poor prognosis, the importance of intramural venous involvement remains controversial. Talbot *et al.*[16] found that in their series of 703 cases, the corrected five-year survival rate of 108 cases with intramural venous invasion did not differ significantly from the 328 cases without venous invasion. Other authors have found a reduction in the survival rate with intramural venous involvement but not all have reached statistical significance.

At the AJCC consensus conference in 1998,[17] several other prognostic indicators were thought to be important but not sufficiently well established for use in a prognostic system, such as 18q/DCC, p53, Bcl-2/Bax, measures of proliferation and DNA content.

With time, more of these genetic markers will prove their worth in staging and prognostication but, until then, the final outcome in clinical practice would most aptly be summarized by the words of JR Jass, who stated: "Prognosis is influenced almost exclusively by the extent of spread of the tumour and the ability of the surgeon to achieve total clearance."

References

1. Lockhart-Mummery JP. Two hundred cases of cancer of the rectum treated by perineal excision, *Br J Surg* 1926; 14: 110.
2. Dukes CE and Bussey HJR. The spread of rectal cancer and its effect on prognosis, *Br J Cancer* 1958; 12: 1016.
3. Astler VB and Coller FA. The prognostic significance of direct extension of carcinoma of the colon and rectum, *Ann Surg* 1954; 139: 846.
4. Hutter RVP and Sobin LH. A universal staging system for cancer of the colon and rectum: let there be light, *Arch Pathol Lab Med* 1986; 110: 367.
5. Wanebo HJ, Rao B, Pinsky CM *et al*. Preoperative carcino-embryonic antigen levels as a prognostic indicator in colorectal cancer, *N Engl J Med* 1978; 299: 448.
6. Moertel CG, Judith R, Fallon O *et al*. The preoperative carcinoembryonic antigen test in the diagnosis, staging and prognosis of colorectal cancer, *Cancer* 1986; 58: 603.
7. Wiratkapun S, Kraemer M, Seow-Choen F *et al*. High preoperative serum carcinoembryonic antigen predicts metastatic recurrence in potentially curative colonic cancer: results of a 5-year study, *Dis Colon Rectum* 2001; 44: 231.
8. Shepherd NA, Baxter KJ and Love SB. The prognostic importance of peritoneal involvement in colonic cancer: a prospective evaluation, *Gastroenterol* 1997; 112: 1096.
9. Mainprize KS, Hewarisinthe J *et al*. How many lymph nodes to stage colorectal carcinoma? *J Clin Pathol* 1998; 51: 165.

10. Koven R, Siegel A *et al.* Lymph node revealing solution: simple new method for detecting minute lymph nodes in colon carcinoma, *Dis Colon Rectum* 1997; 40: 407.

11. Greenson JK, Isenhart CE *et al.* Identification of occult micrometastases in pericolic lymph nodes of Dukes B colorectal cancer patients using monoclonal antibodies against cytokeratin and CC49, *Cancer* 1994; 73: 563.

12. Broll R *et al.* Prognostic relevance of occult tumour cells in lymph nodes of colorectal carcinoma, *Dis Colon Rectum* 1997; 40: 1465.

13. Murray D *et al.* Prognosis in colon cancer: a pathological reassessment, *Arch Surg* 1975; 110: 908.

14. Jass JR. Lymphocytic infiltration and survival in rectal cancer, *J Clin Pathol* 1986; 39: 585.

15. Cianchi F *et al.* Character of the invasive margin in colorectal cancer: does it improve prognostic information of Dukes staging? *Dis Colon Rectum* 1997; 40: 1170.

16. Talbot IC, Ritchie S and Leighton M. Invasion of veins by carcinoma of rectum: method of detection, histological features and significance, *Histopathology* 1981; 5: 14.

17. Yarbro JW *et al.* American Joint Committee on Cancer prognostic factors consensus conference, *Cancer* 1999; 86: 2436.

Carcinoembryonic Antigen for Staging, Prognosis and Follow-up in Patients with Colorectal Cancer

SM Heah

Abstract

The carcinoembryonic antigen (CEA) is an intracellular glycoprotein. Its level in the serum may be raised in both benign and malignant conditions. Its role as a tumour marker is well established in colorectal malignancy. CEA levels are raised in proportion to the stage of disease and has also been used as an independent prognosticator of disease. It is a sensitive marker after colorectal resection for malignancy when raised levels usually mean that either residual tumour is present or recurrent disease has occurred.

Metastatic liver disease generally produces higher CEA levels than metastatic disease elsewhere and local recurrences tend to produce minimal or no rise in CEA levels. Early detection of recurrent disease by serum CEA, complemented by radiological techniques, may improve the curative resection rates and prognosis of patients with colorectal cancers.

Introduction

The serum carcinoembryonic antigen (CEA), discovered by Gold and Freeman in 1965,[1] is an intracellular gycoprotein normally found in low concentrations in the embryonic and fetal gut, pancreas and liver cells. It may be elevated in smokers and other benign gastrointestinal conditions, such as liver cirrhosis, pancreatitis, peptic ulcer disease and ulcerative colitis.[2] Although by no means specific, its role as a tumour marker arises from the fact that colorectal cancer cells secrete it in large quantities and can be detected in the serum. However, despite being one of the most extensively investigated tumour markers, the issues regarding its uses in staging, prognosis and follow-up of patients with colorectal cancer remain unsettled. Recently, tissue CEA was proposed to be a metastatic potentiator by modulating immune responses, facilitating intercellular adhesions and cellular migration.[3] Therefore tissue CEA could affect the invasiveness of colorectal cancer.[4] The distribution of CEA within cancer cells and surrounding tissue was closely correlated with invasiveness and metastatic behaviour in colorectal cancer, and CEA immune staining and localization within cancer cells were considered useful in determining patients at high risk of recurrence.[4] A recent study in Japan found that lymph nodes involved with metastatic colorectal cancer had a significantly higher CEA content than those without.[5] The authors suggested that this may provide an alternative tool for the diagnosis of metastasis even in the absence of positive histology. This has obvious implications for staging, prognosis and possibly even adjuvant therapy, and further studies are required. The objective of this review is to provide an updated synopsis of the clinical uses of CEA in the management of colorectal cancer patients that are currently available in the literature.

What Is CEA's Role in Screening?

CEA is of no value in colorectal cancer screening because of its lack of sensitivity and specificity[6,7] and is not recommended as a screening tool (clinical practice guidelines of the American Society of Clinical Oncology).[8] If a CEA level of 5 ng/ml is used as the upper limit of normal, more than 60% of potentially surgically curable disease (Dukes B, C) will be missed.[9–11] In spite of this, colorectal surgeons and gastroenterologists are likely to be continually confronted with referrals by primary health physicians request-ing colonoscopic evaluation as a result of "a raised CEA". This practice will continue as long as most health screening protocols incorporate CEA as part of its "culture" and will inevitably lead to many unnecessary colonoscopic examinations with implications for rising health costs.

What About Staging Disease?

Herrera *et al.*[12] showed in 1976 that preoperative CEA levels increased with the tumour stage. Several authors[11,14–16] have since suggested that preop-erative serum CEA levels correlated with the extent of colorectal cancers. When the CEA level exceeded 20 ng/ml, Wang *et al.*[11] found that 37% of patients had Dukes D cancer compared with only 4% of those whose value was below this. Moertel *et al.*,[9] in an earlier study, had confirmed the cor-relation between CEA levels and invasiveness of the primary tumour, and the presence of regional nodal and distant metastasis. In stage A and B lesions, the size of the primary tumour was significantly correlated with the elevation of CEA, suggesting that there is increased CEA production with greater tumour bulk.[9]

The ploidy status of stage B tumours was previously shown to be an independent prognostic marker of survival.[16] In one study,[17] 48% of patients with an aneuploid tumour had a raised preoperative CEA com-pared with 34% of patients with diploid tumorus ($P > 0.05$). It may be inferred that cells with abnormal nuclear DNA (aneuploid) produce abnor-mal quantities of CEA compared with cells containing a normal quantity of nuclear DNA (diploid). The same authors[17] found that, when stratified to the stage of disease, aneuploid tumours produced an elevated CEA in only 38% of stage A and B disease, compared to 61% in stages C and D, suggest-ing that even aneuploid tumours produce more CEA at a more advanced stage of disease.

The data relating to the levels of CEA in poorly differentiated tumours are conflicting, with some authors showing reduced production[9,15] and others showing either no correlation[11] or even increased production.[18] It is possible that some specimens labelled as "poorly differentiated" may comprise only a minor component and therefore the majority of cells may retain the ability to produce CEA.[11] Nevertheless one should bear in mind that poorly differentiated tumours at an advanced stage may not produce an elevated CEA.[9]

Does Raised CEA Indicate Greater Risks of Recurrence and Poorer Prognosis?

As pathological staging is the most important prognostic factor, it is hardly surprising that the majority of studies[13,14,19,20] show an adverse relationship of raised CEA to survival. However, this applies mainly to stage B and C tumours. Wanebo[13] reviewed 172 patients and reported higher recurrence rates amongst Dukes B and C patients with preoperative levels exceeding 5 ng/ml. The National Surgical Adjuvant Breast and Bowel Project[14] concluded that the relative risks of treatment failure in Dukes B for a preoperative CEA value >10 ng/ml was 3.24 times more than patients with CEA <2.5 ng/ml. In Dukes C patients, the equivalent risk was 1.76 times when the same two CEA cut-off values were used but the prognostic significance of CEA was independent of the number of positive nodes. In another study, Chu *et al.*[19] also found that preoperative CEA levels significantly affected survival rates of patients with TNM stage 2 and 3 disease. Others[15,21] have found only correlation between preoperative CEA and survival among Dukes C patients with CEA >10 ng/ml.[21]

The Gastrointestinal Tumor Study Group[10] was even more specific in concluding that only in colon cancer patients with one to four nodes involved was a preoperative CEA value of >5 ng/ml associated with significantly greater recurrence rates of 42%, compared with 14% for a value <5 ng/ml. In contrast, Moertel *et al.*[9] found that a raised preoperative CEA was an independent prognostic determinant in patients with four or more nodes involved. Of note in this group of patients is that if the CEA <10 ng/ml, the five-year survival rate was 37%, compared with none surviving when CEA >10 ng/ml. On the other hand, Stabb *et al.*,[22] using a CEA level cut-off at 5 ng/ml, found that the correlation with survival was seen only in stage 2 disease but not in node-positive patients.

Our department reviewed 261 patients with known preoperative CEA levels who had curative colonic carcinoma with a minimal follow-up of five years.[18] The cumulative disease-free survival of patients with a preoperative CEA level within the normal range was significantly better than of those whose levels were 5 ng/ml or more ($P = 0.001$). No patient with a CEA level of less than 1 ng/ml developed metastatic recurrence. Twenty-three per cent of all patients with a raised CEA above 5 ng/ml, compared with 2.1% of patients with levels below 5 ng/ml, developed metastases at two years. At five years, the differences remain at 37.2% and 7.5%, respectively. CEA levels were directly correlated with Dukes staging ($P < 0.001$). A CEA level of more than 15 ng/ml was a significant adverse prognostic indicator for disease-free survival in all Dukes stages ($P < 0.02$). Raised CEA levels predicted distant metastatic recurrence ($P < 0.001$) but not local recurrence ($P = 0.72$).[18] The authors concluded that CEA levels exceeding 15 ng/ml may indicate the presence of occult metastases and, hence, understaged disease.

In the light of the present available evidence, one may conclude that a strong inverse correlation exists between a raised preoperative CEA and survival among node-positive patients, and a somewhat weaker but similar correlation also exists among stage 2 (Dukes B) patients. Fit patients with stage 3 (Dukes C) disease will be sent for adjuvant treatment regardless of preoperative CEA levels. However, medically fit patients with stage 2 (Dukes B) disease and raised preoperative CEA may be selected to undergo adjuvant chemotherapy (and radiotherapy for rectal cancers). It is possible that in this group of "node-negative" patients, a more aggressive form of disease exists which may include lymphatic micrometastases undetected by conventional pathological techniques. This understaging may explaining the raised preoperative CEA levels in these "Dukes B" patients. Currently, data are insufficient to support the use of CEA to determine whether a patient should be treated with adjuvant therapy.[8] Perhaps future prospective randomized trials may seek to address this issue.

How Useful Is CEA in the Follow-up of Patients?

There is good evidence to suggest that in patients with raised preoperative CEA that returns to normal after surgery, a subsequent rise at follow-up is a sensitive (80%[7] to 97%[11]) indicator of recurrence. However, if preoperative CEA is normal and found to be raised at follow-up after surgery, the sensitivity is then diminished (40%[23] to 66%[11]).

The Eastern Cooperative Oncology Group followed patients after surgical resection for high risk stage B2 and C colon carcinoma.[24] Ninety-six of 421 patients with recurrent disease underwent surgical resection with curative intent. For those with resectable disease, the first test to detect recurrence was CEA, chest X-ray, colonoscopy, and other tests.[25] Physical examination was unsuccessful in detecting respectable disease. CEA was the most cost-effective test for detecting resectable colonic cancer metastases. Another study found that CEA first detected 64% of recurrences, far more than other tests used.[26] It was recently recommended that if resection of liver metastases would be clinically indicated, postoperative serum CEA testing should be done 2–3-monthly in patients with stage 2 or 3 disease for two or more years after diagnosis.[8] This guideline reflects compromise and cost savings in that only those regarded as fit enough for surgery should be monitored with CEA levels.

The half-life of CEA is 4–5 days.[27] After curative resection, serum CEA levels should return to normal in 6 weeks[7] to 4 months.[28] Persistently elevated postoperative CEA suggests the presence of residual tumour.[29] However, transient increases in CEA may occur after normalization in up to 14% of patients[30] and do not necessarily equate to recurrence. CEA levels that remain persistently elevated after apparent curative surgery usually suggest that residual disease has been left behind.[29] Wang *et al.*[11] reported that all patients with CEA that persisted above 5 ng/ml developed clinical recurrent disease within one year postoperatively.

Slowly rising serial CEA levels may indicate local recurrence, whereas a rapidly rising level may signify distant metastasis.[31,32] Liver metastases produce higher elevations of CEA when compared to lung and bone metastasis, and local recurrences produce the least CEA level elevations.[11,33]

Sensitivity of CEA levels for detecting recurrence is between 70%[10] and 80%[11,30] and specificity may be up to 90%.[11,34] The rise of CEA mat precede symptoms or radiological detection of recurrent disease by a median lead time of 30 weeks.[30] However, only a minority 23 will have localized disease. The trend of a rising CEA should alert the physician towards radiological and endoscopic investigations targeted at detecting localized or distant metastasis with the purpose of achieving curative re-resection. When conventional investigations fail to detect a recurrence, positron emission tomography with [^{18}F]-fluorodeoxyglucose (FDG-PET) has reportedly been a more sensitive (79%) test, with a positive predictive value of 89%.[35] It can detect disease at the resectable and potentially curative stage. However, it is expensive and as yet not widely available. Large multicentre trials with prospective and blinded study design in which FDG-PET is performed in parallel with conventional investigations are required to confirm the lead time and cost-effectiveness of FDG-PET in the postoperative follow-up of colorectal cancer.

There have been instances where a second look laparotomy was done on the basis of a raised CEA in the absence of radiological evidence of recurrence. About half of such second look surgery does not disclose resectable tumour, and in the best case only 3% of all patients monitored might be cured by the protocol.[7] In a multi-institutional study, Minton *et al.*[36]

reported that 37% of patients with CEA-directed second look operations were alive at five years after operation, compared with 28% of clinically directed laparotomy patients. However, there was no significant difference in survival between the two groups. The present recommendation is for surgeons to use conventional investigations such as CT scans, chest X-rays and colonoscopy to establish the presence and resectability of a recurrence before undertaking surgery in the light of a raised postoperative CEA. Such patients may then benefit from further surgery.[30]

In summary, CEA is a fairly sensitive and specific marker for relapse of colon cancer. Whilst there are no large randomized studies showing that monitoring asymptomatic patients with CEA after surgery results in improved survival, there is definite evidence that long term survival can result from resection of isolated metastases.[37] CEA monitoring remains the most effective method to date for achieving early detection.

Conclusion

It appears reasonable to consider preoperative CEA as a prognostic variable which may be partly independent of the pathological stage. A postoperative raised CEA is a sensitive indicator of recurrent disease and especially so if CEA is also raised preoperatively. Distant metastasis raises CEA to a larger extent than for local recurrence. Raised CEA levels frequently precede radiological detection of recurrent disease, although blind second look laparotomy without clinically detectable tumour has provided a low yield and is not recommended at the present time. CEA remains the best tumour marker available and may be an independent prognostic factor recommended as a monitor of recurrent disease after curative colorectal resection.

References

1. Gold P and Freeman SO. Demostration of tumor specific antigens in human colonic carcinomata by immunoogical tolerance and absorption techniques, *J Exp Med* 1965; 121: 439–62.
2. Gordon PH. Malignant neoplasm of the colon. In Gordon PH and Nivatvong S (eds.), *Principles and Practice of Surgery for the Colon, Rectum and Anus.* St Louis: Quality Medical Publishing, 1992, pp. 501–77.

3. Kim JC, Roh SA and Park KC. Adhesive function of carcinoembryonic antigen in the liver metastasis of KM-12c colon carcinoma cell line, *Dis Colon Rectum* 1997; 40: 946–53.

4. Kim JC, Hans MS, Lee HK *et al*. Distribution of carcinoembryonic antigen and biological behavior in colorectal carcinocer, *Dis Colon Rectum* 1999; 42: 640–8.

5. Kanoh T, Monden T, Tanaki Y, Ohnishi T *et al*. Extraction and analysis of carcinoembryonic antigen in lymph nodes: a new approach to the diagnosis of lymph node metastasis of colorectal cancer, *Dis Colon Rectum* 2002; 45(6): 757–63.

6. National Institutes of Health Consensus Development Conference. Carcinoembryonic antigen: its role as a marker in the management of cancer: *Cancer Res* 1981; 41: 2017–18.

7. Fletcher RH. Carcinoembroyonic antigen, *Ann Intern Med* 1986; 104: 66–73.

8. Bast RC, Ravdin P, Hayes DF, Bates S *et al*. 2000 update of recommendations for the use of tumor markers in breast and colorectal cancer: clinical practice guidelines of the American Society of Clinical Oncology, *J Clin Oncol* 2001; 19(6): 1865–78.

9. Moertel CG, O'Fallon JR, Go VL, O'Connell MJ and Thynne GS. The preoperative carcinoembryonic antigen test in the diagnosis, staging and prognosis of colorectal cancer, *Cancer* 1986; 58: 603–10.

10. Steele G Jr, Ellenberg S, Ramming K *et al*. (Gastrointestinal Tumour Study Group). Carcinoembryonic antigen monitoring among patients in multuinstitutional adjuvant GI: therapy protocols, *Ann Surg* 1982; 96: 162–9.

11. Wang JY, Tang R and Chiang JM. Value of carcinoembryonic antigen in the mangement of colorectal cancer, *Dis Colon Rectum* 1994; 37: 272–7.

12. Herrera MA, Chu TM. Pinsky CM *et al*. Preoperative carcinoembryonic antigen level as a prognostic indicator in colorectal cancer, *N Engl J Med* 1979; 299: 448–51.

13. Wanebo HJ, Rao B, Pinsky CM *et al*. Preoperative carcinoembryonic cancer, *N Engl J Med* 1978; 299: 448–51.

14. Wolmark N, Fisher B, Wieard HS *et al*. The prognostic significance of preoperative carcinoembryonic antigen levels in colorectal cancer—results from NSABP clinical trials, *Ang Surg* 1984; 199: 375–81.

15. Goslin R, O'Brien MJ, Steele G *et al*. Correlation of plasma CEA and CEA attaining in poorly differentiated colorectal cancer, *Am J Med* 1981; 71: 246–53.

16. Chapman MA, Hardcastle JD and Armitage NC. Five-year prospective study of DNA ploidy in colorectal cancer survival, *Cancer* 1995; 76: 383–7.

17. Kouri M, Pyrthonen S, Mecklin, JP *et al.* Serum carcinoembryonic antigen and DNA ploidy in colorectal carcinoma: a prospective study, *Scand J Gastroenterol* 1991; 26: 812–18.

18. Chapman MAS, Buckley D, Henson DB and Armitage NC. Preoperative carcinoembryonic antigen is related to tumour stage and long-term survival in colorectal cancer survival, *Br J Cancer* 1998; 78(10): 1346–9.

19. Chu DZ, Erickson CA, Russell MP *et al.* Prognostic significance of carcinoembryonic antigen in colorectal carcinoma: a prospective study, *Scand J Gastroenterol* 1991; 126: 3314–16.

20. Wiratkapun S, Kraemaer M, F Seow-Choen, Ho YH and Eu KW. High preoperative serum carcinoembryonic antigen predicts metastatic recurrence in potentially curative colonic cancer: results of a five-year study, *Dis Colon Rectum* 2001; 44: 231–5.

21. Lewi H, Blumgart LH, Carter DC *et al.* Preoperative carcinoembryonic antigen and survival in patients with colorectal cancer, *Br J Surg* 1984; 71: 206–8.

22. Staab HJ, Anderer FA, Brummendorf T, Stumpf E and Fischer P. Prognostic value of preoperative serum CEA level compared to clinical staging, *Br J Cancer* 1981; 44: 652–62.

23. Zeng Z, Cohen AM and Umacher C. Usefulness of carcinoembryonic antigen monitoring despite normal preoperative values in node-positive colon cancer patients, *Dis Colon Rectum* 1993; 36: 1063–8.

24. Graham RA, Wang S, Catalano PJ *et al.* Postsurgical surveillance of colon cancer: preliminary cost analysis of physical examination, carcinoembryonic antigen testing, chest x-ray, and colonoscopy, *Ann Surg* 1998; 228: 59–63.

25. American Society of Clinical Oncology: recommended colorectal cancer surveillance guidelines by the American Society of Clinical Oncology, *J Clin Oncol* 1999; 17: 1312–21.

26. Castells A, Bessa X, Daniels M *et al.* Value of postoperative surveillance after radical surgery for colorectal cancer, *Dis Colon Rectum* 1998; 41: 714–24.

27. Mai M and Takahashi Y. prediction of recurrence of gastrointestinal cancer from standpoint of biological malignancies tumor marker doubling time and its half life period line, *Hum Cell* 1993; 6: 82–7.

28. Mach JP, Vienny H, Jaeger P *et al.* Long-term follow-up of colorectal carcinoma patients by repeating CEA radio-immunoassay, *Cancer* 1978; 42: 1439–47.

29. Arnaud JP, Koehl C and Adloff M. Carcinoembryonic antigen (CEA) in diagnosis and prognosis of colorectal carcinoma, *Dis Colon Rectum* 1980; 23: 141–4.

30. Hine KR and Dykes PW. Serum CEA testing in the postoperative surveillance of colorectal carcinoma, *Br J Cancer* 1984; 49: 689–93.

31. Staab HJ, Anderer FA, Stumpf E and Fischer R. Carcinoembryonic antigen follow-up and selection of patients for second-look operation in management of gastrointestinal carcinoma, *J Surg Oncol* 1978; 10: 273–82.

32. Wood CB, Ratcliffe JG, Burt RW, Malcom AJ and Blumgart LH. The clinical significance of the pattern of elevated serum carcinoembryonic antigen (CEA) levels in recurrent colorectal cancer, *Br J Surg* 1980; 67: 46–8.

33. Staab HJ, Anderer FA, Stumpf E and Fischer R. Slope analysis of the postoperative CEA time course and its possible application as an aid in diagnosis of disease progression in gastrointestinal cancer, *Am J Surg* 1978; 136: 322–7.

34. Tate H. Plasma CEA in the post-surgical monitoring of colorectal carcinoma, *Br J Cancer* 1982; 46: 323–30.

35. Flamen P, Hoekstra OS, Homans F, Van Cutsem E *et al.* Unexplained rising carcinoembrtonic antigen (CEA) in the postoperative surveillance of colorectal cancer: the utility of positron emission tomography (PET), *Eur J Cancer* 2001; 37: 862–9.

36. Minton JP, Hoehn JL, Gerber DM *et al.* Results of a 400-patient carcinoembryonic antigen second-look colorectal cancer study, *Cancer* 1985; 55: 1284–90.

37. Canil CM and Tannock IF. Doctor's dilemma: incorporating tumor markers into clinical decision-making, *Semin Oncol* 2002; 29: 286–93.

CHAPTER 30

Management of Malignant Polyps in the Colon and Rectum

KH Ng, HM Quah and F Seow-Choen

Introduction

Invasive carcinoma is said to be present in a polyp when the carcinoma penetrates through the muscularis mucosa. This definition is used to distinguish a malignant polyp from one with carcinoma-*in-situ* or intraepithelial carcinoma. The latter two terms are used in some countries to denote malignant-looking cells, limited by the muscularis mucosa. The diagnosis is different from that of invasive carcinoma. In Singapore, the term "severe dysplasia" is preferred to carcinoma-*in-situ*. Cancer is only present when the muscularis mucosa is breached.

Factors Affecting Management

The key problem in the management of malignant polyps is whether polypectomy alone is sufficient or bowel resection is necessary. Review of the literature suggests that the following are important in deciding the likelihood of recurrence or lymphatic recurrence following polypectomy:

- Margins of resection
- Depth of invasion
- Degree of differentiation
- Vascular and lymphatic invasion

Margin of Resection

A clear margin of resection is synonymous with adequate cancer surgery and is no different in endoscopic removal of malignant polyps. What constitutes an adequate margin is controversial. In the absence of a universal definition of a clear margin, it is perhaps necessary to include in our analysis all papers in which authors have defined the margin of resection as clear and this may vary from 1 mm to 10 mm.

It is generally accepted that involved margins of resection are a marker of residual disease. Cranley[1] reported that 10 out of 22 patients with tumour involving or near the margin of resection had residual disease or died of carcinoma of the colon. Similarly, Wolff and Shinya[2] reported that all 5 of their patients with involved margins had residual disease. Cooper[3] reported that of 24 cases of carcinoma near or involving the margin of resection, 21 had lymph node involvement and 2 had liver metastases. Christie[4] reviewed 106 consecutively encountered malignant colorectal polyps over a 10-year period. Sixty-two lesions were removed by colonoscopic polypectomy alone. All patients in this group have done well, except for one patient who had tumour involvement at the margin of polyp transection, who was considered inoperable because of severe medical problems, and who died from hepatic metastases 5 months later. Christie also reviewed 122 patients in 11 studies on the subject, who had polypectomy followed by surgery due to involvement of margins. There was residual tumour in 27 cases, of which 18 had nodal involvement. It is clear that if involved margins are present, patients should undergo further bowel resection.

Depth of Invasion

Haggitt *et al.*[5] proposed a system of classification in which the depth of invasion is stratified into the following levels:

Level 0: above muscularis mucosa
Level 1: invades muscularis mucosa but limited to the head
Level 2: invades the neck
Level 3: invades the stalk
Level 4: invades the submucosa of the bowel wall below the polyp but
          above the muscularis propia

Based on this classification, Haggitt *et al.*[5] reported that 26 patients with level 1 and level 2 invasions did not develop recurrent disease or lymph node metastases, whereas 7 out of 28 patients with level 4 invasions had an adverse outcome. Nivatvongs *et al.*[6] reported that there was no incidence of lymph node involvement when the depth of invasion was limited to the head, neck and stalk (levels 1–3), but that lymph node metastases were present in 27% of patients with level 4 involvement. Thus, he concluded that invasion into the submucosa beyond the level of the base of the adenoma is associated with a higher incidence of lymphadenopathy. In conclusion, all level 4 tumours should undergo bowel resection whenever possible because of the high chance of lymph node metastases.

Degree of Differentiation

Many of the reports on the outcome of polypectomy based on the degree of differentiation involved only a small number of patients. Nevertheless, there is strong evidence that polyps with poorly differentiated carcinoma have a poorer prognosis. Coverlizza *et al.*[7] reported that of 6 patients with at least a focus of poorly differentiated tumour in a malignant polyp, 5 had lymph node metastases. Williams and Geraghty[8] described 3 patients with poorly differentiated adenocarcinoma in their polyps. Two had residual tumour at laparotomy and the third has died from metastatic disease despite negative lymph nodes and no residual tumour at the time of bowel resection. Standard operative resection is recommended for poorly differentiated carcinoma.

Vascular and Lymphatic Invasion

Venous and lymphatic invasion has been considered a risk factor for metastatic disease. Muller *et al.*[9] identified vascular invasion in 6 out of 34 patients. Of the 6 patients, 3 had recurrent disease or involved regional lymph nodes despite a clear margin of resection. In Cooper's series of 6 patients with lymphatic invasions, 1 (16%) had lymph node involvement.[3] Nivatvongs *et al.*[6] correlated vascular invasion with lymph node metastases and found that 11 out of 35 patients with vascular invasion had positive lymph nodes. Nevertheless, it is reasonable to consider that malignant polyps with vascular invasion should be treated as high-risk lesions.

Cooper *et al.*[10] later defined unfavorable polyp histology as tumour at or near 1.0 mm of the margin and/or grade III and/or lymphatic and/or venous invasion. Recurrence, local cancer and/or lymph node metastasis were found to be 19.7%, 8.6% and 0% when unfavourable histology was present, indefinite and absent, respectively. They therefore recommended that patients with unfavourable histology are probably best managed by resection postpolypectomy; whereas, in the absence of unfavourable histology, they recommended that it probably can be treated by polypectomy only. Volk *et al.*[11] reported similar results, with 16 out of 47 patients with malignant adenoma having favourable histology. None of these patients developed recurrence at 30-month follow-up. However, 10 out of 30 patients with unfavourable histology developed recurrence. A recent study by Nezter *et al.*[12] showed that incomplete polypectomy and a resection margin not clearly cancer-free were two independent risk factors associated with adverse outcome and recommended surgery. And lymphatic or venous invasion or grade III carcinoma was not associated with an adverse outcome when either of these was the sole risk factor. Operations in such cases should be individually assessed on the basis of surgical risk.

In our series of resected rectal tumours, we found that the presence of lymph vessel invasion is a strong indicator of lymph node metastases (positive predictive value of 98%). In addition, even for T1 rectal cancer (defined as tumour invasion of the submucosa only) young patients below the age of 45 have a much higher incidence of lymph node involvement than patients aged 45 years or above, 33.3% vs. 3.1% respectively.[13] We recommend that patients younger than 45 years of age with a T1 tumour be offered radical surgery.

Operative Considerations

A final consideration as to whether to proceed to a colectomy after endoscopic removal of a malignant polyp is the assessment of operative morbidity and mortality. Haggitt[5] described this dilemma as the choice between dying of residual malignant disease and dying of perioperative complications. An audit of a surgical unit's operative morbidity and mortality can provide a realistic assessment of operative risk. This can then be balanced against the patient's chance of an adverse outcome based on the malignant polyp's histological characteristics as well as his overall physiological status.

References

1. Cranley JP, Petras RE, Carey WD, Paradis K and Sivak MV. When is endoscopic polypectomy adequate therapy for colonic polyps containing invasive carcinoma? *Gastroenterology* 1986; 91: 419–27.
2. Wolff WI and Shinya H. Definitive treatment of "malignant" polyps of the colon, *Ann Surg* 1975; 182: 516–25.
3. Cooper HS. Surgical pathology of endoscopically removed malignant polyps of the colon and rectum, *Am J Surg Pathol* 1983; 7: 613–23.
4. Christie JP. Polypectomy or colectomy? Management of 106 consecutively encountered colorectal polyps, *Am Surg* 1988; 54: 93–9.
5. Haggitt RC, Glotzbach RE, Soffer EE and Wruble LD. Prognostic factors in colorectal carcinomas arising in adenomas: implications for lesions removed by endoscopic polypectomy, *Gastroenterology* 1985; 89: 328–36.
6. Nivatvongs S, Rojanasakul A, Reiman HM, Dozois RR, Wolff BG, Pemberton JH *et al.* The risk of lymph node metastasis in colorectal polyps with invasive adenocarcinoma, *Dis Colon Rectum* 1991; 34: 323–8.
7. Coverlizza S, Risio M, Ferrari A, Fenoglio P and Rossini FP. Colorectal adenomas containing invasive carcinoma: pathologic assessment of lymph node metastatic potential, *Cancer* 1989; 64: 1937–47.
8. Williams CB and Geraghty JM. The malignant polyp—when to operate: the St Mark's experience. *Can J Gastroenterol* 1990; 4: 549–53.

9. Muller S, Chesner IM, Egan MJ, Rowlands DC, Collard MJ, Swarbrick ET *et al*. Significance of venous and lymphatic invasion in malignant polyps of the colon and rectum, *Gut* 1989; 30: 1385–91.

10. Cooper HS, Deppisch LM, Gourley WK, Kahn EI, Lev R, Manley PN *et al*. Endoscopically removed malignant colorectal polyps: clinico-pathologic correlations, *Gastroenterology* 1995; 108: 1657–65.

11. Volk EE, Goldblum JR, Petras RE, Carey WD and Fazio VW. Management and outcome of patients with invasive carcinoma arising in colorectal polyps, *Gastroenterology* 1995; 109: 1801–7.

12. Netzer P, Forster C, Biral R, Ruchti C, Neuweiler J, Stauffer E *et al*. Risk factor assessment of endoscopically removed malignant colorectal polyps, *Gut* 1998; 43: 669–74.

13. Sitzler PJ, Seow-Choen F, Ho YH and Leong AFPK. Lymph node involvement and tumor depth in rectal cancers: an analysis of 805 patients, *Dis Colon Rectum* 1997; 40: 1472–6.

CHAPTER 31

Local Therapies in the Management of Rectal Cancer

C Barben

Introduction

Local therapies have been used in the management of rectal cancer for many years. It is a less morbid approach to radical resection, but its role as a curative therapy is unclear. The first, and most important, distinction that needs to be made is between therapies that are (i) curative, where the goal is eradication of all disease and the avoidance of recurrence, and (ii) palliative, where the goal is the relief of symptoms.

All the treatments discussed in this chapter can be used for the palliation of symptoms, as they are effective for this indication. The role of local therapy as a cure for rectal cancer, however, has some fundamental problems to overcome. The only other treatment modality with which local therapy as a cure can be compared is radical excision of a tumour, excised *en bloc* with its lymphovascular pedicle.

Curative Treatments

The main problem with local therapies for rectal cancers is that they cannot, by their very nature, assess lymph node involvement, which is a strong predictor of local recurrence.

Local excision of rectal cancer for cure

The rate of lymph node metastasis in T1 tumours varies from 6 to 27%,[1–6] and the factors that predicted lymph node metastases were lymphovascular invasion in the excised specimen, lesions invading to the deeper layers of the submucosa, poor differentiation, and lesions in the lower third of the rectum.[3] It is likely that local recurrence will occur from the presence of lymph node metastases. If the treatment of rectal cancer by local excision is to be justified, the local recurrence rates must be acceptable. Factors other than T-stage that lead to higher local recurrence rates after local excision include poor histologic grade, the presence of lymphovascular invasion, and positive margins.[7]

The local recurrence rate after local excision for rectal cancer increases from T1, progressively to T3 lesions. The rate in T1 lesions is around 10%, increasing to 25% in T2 lesions, and 38% in T3 lesions.[1,2] This means that although local excision for cure is used in T1 tumours, as long as there are no adverse factors on histology, inadequate clearance can be expected in about 10%. T3 and T4 tumours are contraindications to local excision for cure. Most surgeons would not resect T2 tumours at present, although postoperative adjuvant radiotherapy may reduce the incidence of local recurrence. There are arguments that either preoperative downstaging, or postoperative adjuvant therapy with radio- and/or chemotherapy can improve these results. Some patients, who show a complete pathologic response with T2 or T3 tumours, have local recurrence rates which are less than 10%,[5] although five-year recurrence rates after T2/T3 lesions in patients who had postoperative radiotherapy may be as high as 33%.[8] The guidelines suggested by Graham *et al.*,[6] shown below, are followed in most units:

Best indications

- Freely mobile tumour
- T1 on transrectal ultrasound

- Well- or moderately differentiated histology
- Size ≤3 cm

Contraindications

- Fixed tumour
- T3 on transrectal ultrasound
- Poorly differentiated histology

Other local operative treatment of rectal cancer for cure

Transanal endsocopic microsurgery (TEM) has been developed in the last 15 years, and it increases the distance from the anal margin by which tumours can be locally excised. Without TEM, tumours must be within 6 cm of the anal margin for local excision, but TEM has been reported to be able to remove tumours as high as 18 cm. The results from series of patients who have undergone TEM for cure for rectal cancer give similar local recurrence rates to those who underwent local excision.[9]

Low morbidity and mortality rates are also recorded for transsacral and transsphincteric excision of rectal cancers. The transsacral procedure is performed with the patient prone, and the approach is via an incision from the anal verge to the sacrum, excising the distal part of the sacrum, if necessary. Rectal mobilization from the posterior approach allows the tumour to be excised.[10] The transsphicnteric approach is performed with the patient prone, and the sphincter muscle is tagged with sutures, before being opened through a posterior, midline incision. Good exposure to the middle and lower rectum can be obtained from this approach.[11]

Radiation treatment of rectal cancer for cure

The use of intracavity radiation treatment with curative intent also has controversy attached to it. Added to the uncertainty of the presence of lymph node spread is the absence of a histological specimen from which to glean further information. Having said this, Papillon treated 310 patients with intracavity radiation, with curative intent.[12] The local treatment failure rate was only 5% for T1/T2 tumours. If more advanced (T2/T3) tumours are treated in this way, however, the local recurrence rate is over 20%. These recurrence rates are similar to those achieved with local excision, and need to follow the same strict selection criteria if good results are to be achieved.

External beam radiotherapy has been tried as primary therapy for rectal cancers by some. Cummings reported using 44–50 Gy as a sole treatment, but the five-year survival was only 22%, making it ineffective in this setting.[13]

Palliative Treatments

Local excision, TEM, and both intracavity and external beam radiation can be used in the palliation of the symptoms of rectal cancer. Rectal malignancy can give a variety of distressing symptoms, including bleeding, diarrhoea, per rectal discharge, and prolapse. Palliation is only intended to make life more palatable for the patient.

Ablative therapies for palliation

Strauss first published results of electrocoagulation for palliation of poor risk patients with rectal cancer, nearly 70 years ago.[14] The procedure is performed by applying coagulation to the tumour, with successive removal of the necrotic tissue and scar. This process is repeated until normal tissue is found, and may take over an hour. The most common complication is pyrexia, although late haemorrhage, stricturing and fistulization can occur.

Laser ablation, using the Nd-YAG laser, has been adopted for use in palliative cases. This can be performed via a flexible sigmoidoscope if necessary, although the normal precautions for laser therapy need to be observed. Multiple sessions may be required. Although symptom relief is adequate, if patients survive for longer than two years, they are likely to eventually require a loop colostomy.[15]

Cryotherapy involves the application of liquid nitrogen via a probe inserted through a proctoscope. Very low temperatures are achieved, but this procedure can be performed on an outpatient basis. Complications include haemorrhage, stenosis, occasional peritonitis, and a malodorous discharge. In a study of patients who were unfit for more invasive treatments, symptom control rates were almost 80%, although the success rate was lower in cirumferential tumours.[16]

Rectoscopic resection has been used to alleviate symptoms in large or recurrent rectal tumours. The procedure is similar to a transurethral resection of prostate tissue or bladder tumours. Symptom control can be achieved in nearly 90% of patients, with minimal morbidity.[17]

Radiotherapy for palliation

External beam radiotherapy can provide short-term palliation for irresectable rectal cancer in 70% of patients.[13,18,19] Not surprisingly, five-year survival in these patients is less than 5%, but symptom control is good.

Colonic stenting

Obstructive symptoms are a common presenting complaint, and in those who are unwilling or unfit to undergo a palliative resection, or have a proximal diverting colostomy, endoluminal stenting is one option for the relief of the obstructive symptoms. Lesions less than 5 cm from the anal verge are inappropriate for stenting, as a minimum overlap of 1.5 cm of the stent is advised, and avoidance of contact between the stent and the area at, or below, the dentate line is advisable to avoid the sensation of chronic tenesmus.[20] The proximal level of the disease is only an issue as far as the technical difficulty of the procedure is concerned, and lesions in all areas of the colon have been treated with endoluminal stenting.[21,22] Lesions less than 3 cm in length are technically easier to stent.[22]

The success rates for colonic stenting range from 64% to 100% in published series,[23,24] and the failure of stent deployment is usually due to the inability to pass a guidewire through the malignant stricture. Lesser complications of stenting include rectal bleeding, transient anorectal pain, temporary incontinence and faecal impaction. More severe complications are perforation, which occurs in up to 15% of cases, stent dislocation, and obstruction.[20] Obstruction due to tumour ingrowth can be treated with laser therapy.

Conclusion

The use of local surgical procedures, ablative therapies and radiotherapy for the palliation of symptoms in the treatment of rectal cancer is not in doubt. These are widely used, and are of great benefit. The newer technique of stenting still requires validation for rectal cancer, as cost, complications and long-term efficacy have yet to be determined.

The local treatment of rectal cancer for cure has engendered a great deal of writing and comment. This is primarily because the morbidity of the surgical procedure for locally excising a rectal tumor is significantly less than that of an abdominoperineal or low anterior resection. It is obvious from the published work that the prognosis is only acceptable when operating for cure, in T1 tumours. There are suggestions that the addition of pre- or postoperative adjuvant therapy can bring the local recurrence down to acceptable levels.

If local excision is undertaken for any tumour, which is more advanced than T1, it should be considered to be a palliative procedure. The question of whether T1 tumours should be treated by local excision is not so easy to answer. Local recurrence rates must be monitored, and compared with those patients undergoing radical resection with lymphovascular clearance. If the price of local excision is a reduction in the local control of the malignancy, then this needs to be considered with the patient when planning treatment.

References

1. Sitzler PJ, Seow-Choen F, Ho YH and Leong AP. Lymph node involvement and tumor depth in rectal cancers: an analysis of 805 patients, *Dis Colon Rectum* 1997; 40(12): 1472–6.
2. Nascimbeni R, Burgart LJ, Nivatvongs S and Larson DR. Risk of lymph node metastasis in T1 carcinoma of the colon and rectum, *Dis Colon Rectum* 2002; 45(2): 200–6.
3. Akasu T, Kondo H, Moriya Y, Sugihara K, Gotoda T, Fujita S *et al.* Endorectal ultrasonography and treatment of early stage rectal cancer, *World J Surg* 2000; 24(9): 1061–8.
4. Kim CJ, Yeatman TJ, Coppola D, Trotti A, Williams B, Barthel JS *et al.* Local excision of T2 and T3 rectal cancers after downstaging chemoradiation, *Ann Surg* 2001; 234(3): 352–8.
5. Graham RA, Garnsey L and Jessup JM. Local excision of rectal carcinoma, *Am J Surg* 1990; 160: 306–12.
6. Nivatvongs S, Rojanasakul A, Reiman HM, Dozois RR, Wolff BG, Pemberton JH *et al.* The risk of lymph node metastasis in colorectal polyps with invasive adenocarcinoma, *Dis Colon Rectum* 1991; 34(4): 323–8.

7. Sengupta S and Tjandra JJ. Local excision of rectal cancer: what is the evidence? *Dis Colon Rectum* 2001; 44(9): 1345–61.

8. Pigot F, Dernaoui M, Castinel A, Juguet F, Chaume JC and Faivre J. Local excision with postoperative radiotherapy for T2 or T3 distal rectal cancer: long-term results (*in French*), *Annales de Chirurgie* 2001: 126(7): 639–43.

9. Demartines N, von Flue MO and Harder FH. Transanal endoscopic microsurgical excision of rectal tumors: indications and results, *World J Surg* 2001; 25(7): 870–5.

10. Nambiar R. Transsacral approach to the rectum, *Annals Acad Med, Singapore* 1987; 16(3): 462–5.

11. Bergman L and Solhaug JH. Posterior trans-sphincteric resection for small tumours of the lower rectum, *Acta Chirurgica Scandinavica* 1986; 152: 313–16.

12. Papillon J. Present status of radiation therapy in the conservative management of rectal cancer, *Radiother Oncol* 1990; 17(4): 275–83.

13. Cummings BJ, Rider WB, Harwood AR, Keane TJ and Thomas GM. Radical external beam radiation therapy for adenocarcinoma of the rectum, *Dis Colon Rectum* 1983; 26: 30–6.

14. Strauss AA, Strauss SF, Crawford RA and Stauss HA. Surgical diathermy of carcinoma of the rectum: its clinical end results, *JAMA* 1935; 104: 1480–4.

15. Meijer S, Rahusen FD and van der Plas LG. Palliative cryosurgery for rectal carcinoma, *Int J Colorectal Dis* 1999; 14(3): 177–80.

16. Farouk R, Ratnaval CD, Monson JR and Lee PW. Staged delivery of Nd : YAG laser therapy for palliation of advanced rectal carcinoma, *Dis Colon Rectum* 1997; 40(2): 156–60.

17. Ziani M, Tuech JJ, Chautard D, Regenet N, Pessaux P, Randriamananjo S and Arnaud JP. Palliative treatment of rectal carcinoma using a urologic resectoscope (*in French*), *Gastroenterologie Clinique et Biologique* 2001; 25(11): 957–61.

18. Urdanetta-Lafee N, Kligerman MM and Knowlton AH. Evaluation of palliative irradiation in rectal carcinoma, *Radiology* 1972; 104: 673–7.

19. Brierley JD, Cummings BJ, Wong CS *et al.* Adenocarcinoma of the rectum treated by radical external radiation therapy, *Int J Radiat Oncol Biol Phys* 1995; 31: 225–9.

20. Harris GJC, Senagore AJ, Lavery IC and Fazio VW. The management of neoplastic colorectal obstruction with colonic endolumenal stenting devices, *Am J Surg* 2001; 181(6): 499–506.
21. Baron TH, Dean PA, Yates MR *et al.* Expandable metal stents for the treatment of colonic obstruction: techniques and outcomes, *Gastrointest Endoscopy* 1998; 47: 277–86.
22. Binkert CA, Ledermann H, Jost B *et al.* Acute colonic obstruction: clinical aspects and cost-effectiveness of preoperative and palliative treatment with self-expanding metallic stents: a preliminary report, *Radiology* 1998; 206: 199–204.
23. Dohmoto M, Hunerbein M and Schlag PM. Application of rectal stents for palliation of obstructing rectosigmoid cancer, *Surg Endosc* 1997; 11: 758–61.
24. Wright KC, Wallace S, Charnsangavej C *et al.* Percutaneous endovascular stents: an experimental evaluation, *Radiology* 1985, 156: 69–72.

CHAPTER 32

Colorectal Cancer in the Young

KW Eu and MH Kam

Introduction

Colorectal cancer is the second-commonest cancer among Singaporean males and females, with an age-standardized rate (per 100 000 per year) of 37.5 and 29.4, respectively. There have been a total of 4899 reported cases of colorectal cancer in the Singapore Cancer Registry from Jan 1993 to December 1997, making it the No. 1 cancer (combined) in Singapore. The incidence in the young, generally defined as those 40 years and below, is increasing.[1–12] Locally, they make up almost 4% of all colorectal cancers. Many studies have quoted no significant difference in the presentation of younger patients, and there has been no conclusive evidence that young age is a poor prognostic marker. Certainly, the incidence of familial cancers is markedly increased in this age group, and its role and impact warrants further discussion.[13–15]

Family History

There are four general categories of colorectal cancers as far as family history is concerned. They are familial adenomatous polyposis (FAP), hereditary nonpolyposis colorectal cancer (HNPCC), family history of colorectal cancer (not fulfilling strict criteria for the previous two), and sporadic cases.

Familial adenomatous polyposis

Screening of family members in those diagnosed with familial adenomatous polyposis (FAP) is well entrenched in medical practice. Carcinomas in otherwise asymptomatic patients are thus picked up, in young patients who otherwise would not have been screened. Timely proctocolectomy in such cases results in favourable long-term outcomes.

Hereditary nonpolyposis colorectal cancer

Patients in this group are defined by the Amsterdam criteria. A study[16] comparing features of hereditary nonpolyposis colorectal cancer (HNPCC) with sporadic cases showed that patients with HNPCC tended to be younger (31 vs 35 years) and had a higher incidence of metachronous cancers (27% vs 2%). They seemed to present at an earlier stage with fewer having nodal or metastatic spread (35% vs 65%), however.

Family history of colorectal cancer

Those who have a definite family history of colorectal cancer in a first-degree relative but do not fulfil the strict criteria for either FAP or HNPCC will belong to this group. Individuals with such a positive family history had a four-fold increase in the risk of developing colorectal cancer in their lifetime. This is especially true for cases of a young index patient or cancer affecting two or more first-degree relatives. In addition, the risk for gastric cancer in such relatives was also increased almost four-fold.

Sporadic cases

There are cases where there is no or only a very inconsequential family history of colorectal cancer.

Clinical Presentation

Rectal bleeding was the predominant presenting symptom, possibly because it is widely thought to be associated with cancer in the young. Routine colonoscopic screening for young patients presenting with only rectal bleeding showed significant findings in up to 20% of patients. These included polyps, colitis, diverticular disease and angiodysplastic lesions. Carcinoma, however, was detected in less than 0.5%.

Pain was the only symptom found more commonly in younger patients. All other symptoms listed in Table 1 were found in equal distributions for both young and older patients.

Diagnosis and Management

The most common diagnostic investigation would be colonoscopy. Other investigations included sigmoidoscopy, barium enema and CT scanning. Rarely, colorectal carcinoma may be the cause of intestinal obstruction or peritonitis, diagnosed only at the time of laparotomy.

Location of tumours in the young was no different from that for older patients. The commoner sites of occurrence remained the rectum and sigmoid. A higher incidence of mucinous and signet-cell tumours was associated with young patients. These histological subtypes of tumours generally had a poorer prognosis than other subtypes. However, they did not occur in numbers large enough to influence overall survival rates. Adenocarcinoma was still the predominant tumour type (80–90%) in all studies.

The majority of patients (60–70%) present late (Dukes C or D) and, correspondingly, five-year survival rates range from 20 to 50%. Management

Table 1. Common presenting symptoms.

Symptoms	Relative Percentage in Young Patients
Change in bowel habit	65–70
Bleeding per rectum	51–58
Weight loss	48–52
Abdominal pain	40–45
Mucus from rectum	15–17
Abdominal distension	10–13
Abdominal mass	2–4

depends on the stage and grade of tumours at diagnosis, the location of these lesions, and the general fitness of the patient to undergo surgery, though this is rarely a problem in patients under 40 years of age. Resection follows the basic principles of oncologic surgery, with up to 75% of patients undergoing curative resection. Adjuvant therapy is advocated for Dukes C and some Dukes B tumours.

Prognosis and Advances

Conventional wisdom had suggested that younger patients had a lower incidence of carcinoma but a poorer prognosis. Whether a result of delayed diagnosis or increased aggression of tumours in the young, they seem to present at a later stage. Recent studies, however, showed no difference in stage at presentation between the young and the older age group. This was attributed to the widespread use of endoscopy, and screening programmes targeted at familial polyposis syndromes.

Many studies have shown that young age per se does not account for a poorer prognosis. In both overall and stage-for-stage analysis, young patients have a comparable, if not better, outcome. In fact, the only independent predictor of a poor outcome was the stage at presentation. In Dukes A tumours, there were no deaths at five years. Correspondingly, there were no five-year survivors among Dukes D patients. Survival rates for Dukes B and C lesions were 86% and 65%, respectively.[1] The overall five-year survival was 55%.

Studies are now under way to investigate the use of gene therapy for treatment of colorectal cancer.[17] This represents the next big step forwards. With strategies like immune stimulation, mutant gene correction, prodrug activation and oncolytic virus therapy, this may well revolutionize the future of cancer treatment.

References

1. Chung YFA, Eu KW, Machin D, Ho JMS, Nyam DCNK, Leong AFPK, Ho YH and Seow-Choen F. Young age is not a poor prognostic marker in colorectal cancer, *Br J Surg* 1998; 85: 1255–9.
2. Minardi AJ Jr, Sittig KM, Zibari GB and McDonald JC. Colorectal cancer in the young patient, *Am Surg* 1998; 64(9): 849–53.

3. Parramore JB, Wei JP and Yeh KA. Colorectal cancer in patients under forty: presentation and outcome, *Am Surg* 1998; 64(6): 563–7; discussion 567–8.

4. Mitry E, Benhamiche AM, Jouve JL, Clinard F, Finn-Faivre C and Faivre J. Colorectal adenocarcinoma in patients under 45 years of age: comparison with older patients in a well-defined French population, *Dis Colon Rectum* 2001; 44(3): 380–7.

5. Cozart DT, Lang NP, Hauer-Jensen M *et al*. Colorectal cancer in patients under 30 years of age, *Am J Surg* 1993; 166(6): 764–7.

6. Chen LK, Hwang SJ, Li AF, Lin JK and Wu TC. Colorectal cancer in patients 20 years old or less in Taiwan, *South Med J* 2001; 94(12): 1202–5.

7. Moore PA, Dilawari RA and Fidler WJ. Adenocarcinoma of the colon and rectum in patients less than 40 years of age, *Am Surg* 1984; 50: 10–14.

8. Adloff M, Arnaud J-P, Schloegel M, Thibaud D and Bergamaschi R. Colorectal cancer in patients under 40 years of age, *Dis Colon Rectum* 1986; 29: 322–5.

9. Walton WW, Hagihara PF and Griffen WO. Colorectal adenocarcinoma in patients less than 40 years old, *Dis Colon Rectum* 1976; 19: 529–34.

10. Shahrudin MD and Noori SM. Cancer of the colon and rectum in the first three decades of life, *Hepatogastroenterology* 1997; 44(14): 441–4.

11. Rodriguez-Bigas MA, Mahoney MC, Weber TK and Petrelli NJ. Colorectal cancer in patients aged 30 years or younger, *Surg Oncol* 1996; 5(4): 189–94.

12. Parry BR, Tan BK, Parry S and Goh HS. Colorectal cancer in the young adult, *Singapore Med J* 1995; 36(3): 306–8.

13. Hall NR, Bishop DT, Stephenson BM and Finan PJ. Hereditary susceptibility to colorectal cancer: relatives of early onset cases are particularly at risk, *Dis Colon Rectum* 1996; 39(7): 739–43.

14. Chen MJ, Chung-Faye GA, Searle PF, Young LS and Kerr DJ. Gene therapy for colorectal cancer: therapeutic potential, *BioDrugs* 2001; 15(6): 357–67.

15. Karner-Hanusch J, Mittlbock M, Fillipitsch T and Herbst F. Family history as a marker of risk for colorectal cancer: Austrian experience, *World J Surg* 1997; 21(2): 205–9.

16. Guillem JG, Puig-La Calle J Jr, Cellini C, Murray M, Ng J, Fazzari M, Paty PB, Quan SH, Wong WD and Cohen AM. Varying features of early age-of-onset "sporadic" and hereditary nonpolyposis colorectal cancer patients, *Dis Colon Rectum* 1999; 42(1): 36–42.

17. Gryfe R, Kim H, Hsieh ET, Aronson MD, Holowaty EJ, Bull SB, Redston M and Gallinger S. Tumour microsatellite instability and clinical outcome in young patients with colorectal cancer, *N Engl J Med* 2000; 342(2): 69–77.

CHAPTER 33

Colorectal Cancer Involving the Bladder

KW Eu

Introduction

Despite the potential for early detection of colorectal cancer and public education efforts, some patients still seek medical attention only when their disease is locally advanced and requires treatment by radical surgical procedures. Adjacent organ involvement in colorectal cancer occurs in 5–12% of all colorectal cancers.[1–6] The organ most commonly involved in cancer of the colon and rectum is the urinary bladder. While most locally advanced colorectal cancers may be amenable to less radical resection, such as *en bloc* resection of the tumour with the bladder, some will require resection of greater magnitude, such as pelvic exenteration or abdominosacral resection.

Although these extensive surgical procedures present a formidable challenge to the surgeon and entail significant short-term risks and long-term

254

sequelae for the patients, they can result in long-term survival of a significant proportion of selected patients with locally advanced colorectal cancer. In addition, surgical removal of the locally advanced colorectal tumour has the potential to improve the quality of life by preventing the development of unrelenting symptomatology of uncontrolled pelvic malignancy, in particular intractable pelvic pain and tenesmus.

Long-term survival of between 32% and 80% has been reported when *en bloc* resection of the colorectal cancer with its involved adjacent structures was performed.

Bladder Involvement

As the bladder is the most commonly involved extracolonic organ in colorectal cancer, a study was conducted in the department to determine the accuracy of intraoperative assessment and prognosis of colorectal cancer with bladder involvement.[7]

Results

Twenty-seven (19 males) out of 542 patients treated over a two-year period were found to have tumour attachment to the urinary bladder and had undergone an *en bloc* partial cystectomy. Together with the partial cystectomy, 8 had sigmoid colectomy, 10 had anterior resection and 9 others. Only 7 patients had histological evidence of bladder invasion. Twenty had only inflammatory adhesions.

Urological symptoms were present in 9 of the 27 patients. Six (85%) of the 7 patients with malignant invasion had symptoms, while only 4 (20%) of the 20 patients with inflammatory adhesion had urinary symptoms.

Accuracy of intraoperative assessment was also analysed. A single consultant surgeon was present in all cases to determine if bladder involvement was malignant or inflammatory. Eight tumours were assessed to have invaded the bladder, while another eight were assessed to be due to inflammatory adhesions only. The nature of involvement was uncertain in the remaining 10 patients.

Bladder involvement was not found to affect survived in Dukes staging provided clear histological margins were obtained.

The median follow-up was 40 months. There were no urinary complaints postoperatively from any patients. At last follow-up, 20 patients (74%) were alive and had evidence of local or distant metastases. Five patients died—3 from metastases disease and 2 from unrelated causes.

Discussion

The urinary bladder remains the most often involved adjacent organ in colorectal cancer. *En bloc* resection may give good locoregional control of the cancer and offers the best chance for cure. The most important factor is the achievement of tumour-free margins.

Distinguishing between malignant infiltration and inflammatory adhesion during surgery is not easy. Finger fracturing or lysis of adherent adjacent organs should be discouraged as tumour spillage and recurrence almost invariably occurs and *en bloc* resection is recommended.

Also, five-year survival is markedly decreased by dissecting through tumour. Therefore, it is usually safer to assume malignant involvement rather than inflammatory when doubt exists.

Most patients with malignant involvement of the bladder had urinary symptoms compared to those with inflammatory adhesions. Therefore, preoperative genitourinary symptoms appeared to be an important question and perhaps an important prediction of malignant bladder invasion. Urinary symptoms due to malignant invasion may be due to the presence of a colovesicle fistula and thus further supports an *en bloc* resection during surgery.

Colorectal cancer patients with urinary symptoms should therefore be thoroughly assessed. Preoperative CT scans and cystoscopy may be helpful.

The overall prognosis of patients with bladder involvement is not different for patients without bladder involvement provided an *en bloc* resection was performed with clean margins.

References

1. Pittman MR, Thomton H and Ellis H. Survival after extended resection for locally advanced carcinomas of the colon and rectum, *Ann R Coll Surg Eng* 1984; 66: 81–4.

2. Sugarbaker PH and Corlew S. Influence of surgical techniques on survival in patients with colorectal cancer, *Dis Colon Rectum* 1982; 25: 545–57.

3. Heslor SF and Frast DB. Extended resection for primary colorectal carcinoma involving adjacent organs or structures, *Cancer* 1998; 62: 1637–40.

4. Boey J, Wong J and Ong GB. Pelvic exenteration for locally advanced colorectal carcinoma, *Ann Surg* 1982; 195: 513–18.

5. Lopez MJ, Kraybill WG, Downey RS, Johnston WD and Bricker EM. Exenterative surgery for locally advanced rectosigmoid cancers: is it worthwhile? *Surgery* 1987; 102: 644–51.

6. Gall FP, Tonak JA and Altendorf KA. Multivisceral resections in colorectal cancer, *Dis Colon Rectum* 1985; 30: 337–41.

7. Nyam DCNK, Seow-Choen F, Ho MS and Goh HS. Bladder involvement in patients with colorectal carcinoma, *Singapore Med J* 1995; 36: 525–6.

CHAPTER 34

Anastomotic Techniques in Intestinal Surgery

KW Eu

Introduction

The basic principles involved in the safe performance of an anastomosis remain the same regardless of the technique used. They would include an anastomosis which is well-vascularized, tension-free, an adequate lumen and an air/water-tight anastomotic line.

The art of joining one part of the bowel to another has advanced tremendously, especially over the last several years. The various techniques range from the time-tested traditional hand-suturing technique to stapling techniques and, more recently, the biofragmentable anastomotic ring.

Hand-Suturing Techniques

This technique is time-tested and has been found to be safe and effective, especially if performed by experienced surgeons. Indeed, there are multiple ways of performing hand-suturing anastomoses, and these include single-versus-double-layer anastomosis, seromuscular-versus-full-thickness anastomosis and interrupted-versus-continuous suturing. It is reasonable to believe that differences of opinion with respect to the various hand-suturing techniques and suture materials exist and are real. However, there is certainly no disagreement that an inverting anastomosis is the proper one for all intestinal anastomoses when a conventional hand-suturing technique is used.[1]

Stapling Techniques

Although numerous stapling devices were developed in the 1800s for wound closure and anastomosis, it was not until the 1900s that the first mechanical stapling device was invented. The evolution of the stapling device has since escalated immensely. At present, staplers are simple, light, reliable, reusable and, most importantly, reloadable. This therefore provides convenience for the surgeon and cost savings for the patient.

The use of staples for anastomosis in intestinal surgery is at least as safe as conventional suturing and in some circumstances offers distinct advantages. Clinical studies have shown that intestinal anastomosis using staples is faster than traditional suturing techniques, hence reducing operating time. Furthermore, stapling can reduce tissue trauma by minimizing tissue handling. Also, the availability of stapling instruments has enabled the development of operative techniques that was previously difficult or impossible with traditional techniques because of limited access, such as in an ultralow anterior resection with coloanal anastomosis.

Research into tissue healing has also shown that stapled tissue anastomoses heal as reliably and rapidly as sutured anastomoses.

The use of staplers for anastomosis, however, does not guarantee a successful outcome for a surgical procedure. Effective and safe use of a mechanical stapling device depends upon good basic surgical technique, including clean, atraumatic dissection, careful haemostasis, attention to tissue condition and blood supply, and creation of a tension-free anastomosis.[2,3]

Types of Stapling Devices

There are three types of stapling devices available for anastomosis: the linear stapler, which applies two staggered rows of staples; the linear cutting stapler, which applies two staggered rows of staples and divides the tissue by means of a contained knife; and the circular end-to-end anastomosis stapler, which secures two rows of staples from within the lumen of the bowel to produce an inverting anastomosis in a circular fashion.

Types of Stapling Anastomoses

Anastomoses of the bowel using staples can be accomplished by a number of methods. These include:

- Triangulation technique
- Side-to-side anastomosis
- Functional end-to-end anastomosis
- End-to-side anastomosis
- End-to-end circular anastomosis

Triangulation technique

This technique involves the creation of an anastomosis using the linear stapler by a triangulation technique. The two bowel lumens are brought together and held in place by three stay sutures inserted at three corners. Three firings of the linear stapler or linear cutting stapler are then applied with the staples crossing each other. This produces an everting anastomosis which, despite some criticism, does not seem to create a problem when compared to the hand-suturing technique.

Side-to-side anastomosis

This technique is usually adopted for quick creation of an intestinal bypass. This involves making two enterotomies in the two bowels placed side by side. A linear cutting stapler is then inserted into the two enterotomies and fired, thereby creating the anastomosis. The enterotomy can then be closed using a second firing of the stapler or sutures.

Functional end-to-end anastomosis

This anastomosis is technically a side-to-side anastomosis but functions as an end-to-end one. It involves placing the linear cutting stapler into two bowel lumens aligned together and fired. The bowel ends are then closed with a second application of the linear cutting stapler, thereby creating a functional end-to-end anastomosis.

End-to-side anastomosis

The circular stapling device can be used to effect an end-to-side anastomosis. This is particularly useful for an ileocolic anastomosis following an ileocaecal resection. The detachable anvil can be placed into the ileal luminal end and a previously inserted purse-string tied down. The stapling device is placed into the colonic lumen and the instrument is opened with the spike piercing through the antimesentric border of the bowel. The anvil is then inserted in place and the stapler closed and fired. The open colonic end can then be closed either by sutures or by a linear stapler.

End-to-end circular anastomosis

This anastomosis is created using the intraluminal circular stapler. This can be used for any colocolic anastomosis with the stapler inserted transanally. Usually, two purse-string sutures are placed in the bowel luminal ends and the stapler is inserted either transanally in a colorectal anastomosis or via a colotomy in a colocolic anastomosis. The anvil is then inserted into the other bowel end and the purse-string tied down. The instrument is then closed and fired.

Biofragmentable anastomotic ring

Hardy and colleagues described a biofragmentable ring for sutureless intestinal anastomosis in 1985.[4] The ring is composed of two segments containing polyglycolic acid (Dexon) and 12% barium sulphate. This device fragments during the third week following implantation and can be applied to all parts of the intestine. This device was also found to be as safe as other anastomotic alternatives.[5]

A purse-string suture is placed on the two bowel ends to be anastomosed, and preferably a monofilament absorbable suture is recommended.

The biofragmentable anastomotic ring (BAR) is then placed into one luminal end first and the suture tied down. The other bowel end is placed into the half of the device and the purse-string tied down. The ring is then snapped shut with an audible and tactile click, and an inverted serosa-to-serosa anastomosis is created.

Conclusion

Stapling instruments have replaced conventional suture techniques for many surgeons today. Not only is stapling faster, it also minimizes the risk of needle stick injuries. Other than this, it appears to have no superior advantage over conventional hand-suturing techniques for anastomosis. However, it must be re-emphasized that healing of an anastomosis does not depend on whether staples or suture material is used, but on good and safe surgical principles.

References

1. Mathesa M. Single-layer interrupted serosubmucosal anastomosis. In: Rob C and Smith A (eds.), *Operative surgery*, 3rd ed. Butterworth, London, 1977, p. 43.
2. Everett WG, Friend PJ and Forly J. Comparison of stapling and hand-suture for left-sided large bowel anastomosis, *Br J Surg* 1986; 73: 345.
3. Waxman BP. Large bowel anastomoses II: the circular staplers, *Br J Surg* 1983; 70: 64.
4. Hardy TG Jr, Pace WG and Maney JW. A biofragmentable ring for sutureless bowel anastomosis, *Dis Colon Rectum* 1985; 28: 484.
5. Seow-Choen F and Eu KW. Circular staplers versus the biofragmentable ring for colorectal anastomosis: a prospective randomized study, *Br J Surg* 1994; 81: 1790–1.

CHAPTER 35

Duodenal Involvement with Hepatic Flexure Cancer

BS Ooi

Introduction

Approximately 6–12% of all colorectal cancers involve adjacent structures without distant metastases.[1–3] Most of these are located in the left-sided colon and rectum due to the "close proximity" to the adjacent structures such as the bladder, ureter, uterus, ovary, fallopian tubes and iliac vessels. While it is relatively common for left-sided colonic cancers to invade adjacent pelvic organs, it is rare for locally advanced right-sided colonic cancers to be adherent to the surrounding neighbouring structures. The surgical management of locally advanced left-sided colorectal cancers, be it an *en-bloc* resection of tumour together with the involved structures or total pelvic exenteration, is quite well established and often undertaken when the need arises.[4,5] However, the management of advanced right-sided colonic cancers with adherence to the duodenum, pancreas or liver represents a great challenge to surgeons, with the perceived higher level of difficulty and magnitude. The extent of resection in order to achieve a tumour-free margin involving some vital organs remains a difficult problem during surgery. Furthermore, the role of extended resection for locally advanced right-sided colonic cancers (ascending colon or hepatic flexure) involving the duodenum is unclear. Is duodenectomy or pancreaticoduodenectomy (Whipple's operation) the optimum surgical therapy? The answer is unknown and remains to be seen even today.

In 1929, Grey Turner[6] first published a case of duodenectomy for an advanced carcinoma of the right colon, while Van Prohaska[7] first described pancreaticoduodenectomy for colonic cancer in 1956. However, resection of the duodenum or pancreas or both for colonic cancer was still rarely undertaken until about two decades later, when, in 1972, both Polk[2] of the United States and Ellis[8] of the United Kingdom showed that some locally invasive right-sided cancers were associated with a negative lymph node status. Both surgeons demonstrated that prolonged survival is possible in some cases following extended resection. Recent reports have also suggested that extended resection for locally advanced primary colonic cancer invading the duodenum can be undertaken safely and is associated with a prolonged survival time.[9,10] This form of radical surgery, nevertheless, remains an operation limited to centres with very special interests and support. The perceived radical nature of the procedure deters it from being offered to some patients, to whom it may be of definite benefit. In addition, there is little published evidence of the feasibility, morbidity and mortality of extended resection for locally advanced right-sided colonic cancers. Most publications are case reports, small case series or solitary cases from a large analysis of extended resections at all sites of the colon. To date, there are only 9 publications[2,3,8–14] with 27 cases of advanced right-sided colonic cancers treated with extended right hemicolectomy and duodenectomy, and only 5 publications[9,10,12,13,15] reporting a total of 14 patients who underwent pancreaticoduodenectomy.

Management of Hepatic Flexure Cancer with Duodenal Involvement

There are several key issues to consider in the management of hepatic flexure cancer involving the duodenum.

Preoperative diagnosis and assessment

Duodenal involvement from primary carcinoma of the colon can be difficult to define preoperatively. The presenting symptoms typically include those of right-sided colonic cancer, such as anaemia, epigastric pain and a palpable mass.[10] Some authors[2,16] found that many right-sided cancers with contiguous organ involvement are palpable preoperatively and that, when the tumour is palpable and immobile, involvement of adjacent structures should be suspected. However, a palpable tumour is not a consistent finding in all cases. In addition, Curley *et al.*[16] demonstrated that although 81 of 101 patients with colonic cancers who required extended resections had gastrointestinal tract symptomatology, there was no correlation between any one symptom or combination of symptoms and the presence of pathologic invasion of contiguous structures.

In the absence of reliable symptoms, a preoperative CT scan becomes an important imaging technique to further assess the tumour before surgery. A large colonic mass in the hepatic flexure area abutting the duodenum is suggestive of possible duodenal involvement.[17] The loss of a visible plane between the mass and the duodenum indicates tumour invasion of the duodenum. Particular attention should also be paid to any involvement of the pancreas by the tumour. Tumour involving the superior mesenteric vein and artery in this instance usually renders it unresectable.[10] Although a CT scan may provide some indications of the nature and extent of resection required, it may also be unreliable in certain instances in predicting duodenal or pancreatic involvement by colonic cancers.[10]

A thorough preoperative assessment is an important part of the management of this advanced hepatic flexure tumour involving the duodenum. Patients need to be reasonably fit, with favourable disease, which would enable them to recover satisfactorily from surgery and to have worthwhile disease-free survival thereafter. A careful patient selection is of the utmost importance, as radical surgery of this magnitude carries with it major morbidity and mortality. Patients with metastatic disease in the liver, lungs and bones have a very poor prognosis and should be excluded. Patients with multiple peritoneal or pelvic tumour implantations or carcinomatosis peritonei are also unlikely to benefit from radical surgery. In a study,[14] the mean survival time was less than one month for patients who underwent duodenal and pancreatic resection in the presence of peritoneal disease. Patients over the age of 70 years, unless remarkably fit, would also be unlikely candidates, although there is evidence to show that following extended resections for colorectal cancer, the mean survival time, morbidity and 30-day mortality in patients more than 70 years old were similar to those less than 70 years.[18] Lastly, it is important that the decision to proceed with surgery, and the risk of morbidity and mortality, are discussed thoroughly with the patient and his family. Their wishes must be clearly understood and respected by the surgical team. The expectation of the patient, his family and the surgeons must be realistic.

Intraoperative assessment

Thorough laparotomy

The first thing to do intraoperatively is to perform a full laparotomy. In the event that there is extensive carcinomatosis peritonei or peritoneal disease, extended resection should be abandoned, as it has been well shown that this group of patients has a very grave prognosis.[14] Bypass surgery to prevent colonic and duodenal obstruction should be performed instead. Some authors[10] have suggested performing a diagnostic laparoscopy to better assess for any peritoneal disease before proceeding to full laparotomy.

Assessment for resectability

Exploratory dissection to assess for resectability should be attempted. But this should be done with the condition that the tumour is not to be violated, or that a resection that is neither technically feasible nor biologically wise is not to be committed. The best approach to assessing for resectability is to employ the traditional Turnbull no-touch procedure.[19] This involves an initial incision along the left leaf of the small bowel mesentery up to the duodenum and jejunal junction. In the bloodless plane immediately inferior to the edge of the third part of the duodenum, posterior to the superior mesenteric vessels, a plane is developed with the left index finger (the surgeon standing to the left of the patient) and is mobilized beneath the junction of the second and third parts of the duodenum to the lower pole of the right kidney, which is then palpated. This manoeuvre will rapidly exclude fixation of right-sided colon lesions to the duodenum, pancreas, vena cava or aorta. At this point, a mesenteric window is made between the ileocolic artery and either the right colic artery (if present), or the right branch of the middle colic artery if the right colic artery is absent. This will enable rapid control of the ileocolic, the right colic and the right branch of the middle colic arteries, which are then divided and ligated. If the tumour is involving the superior mesenteric vessels, it is deemed unresectable for cure.

Assessment of tumour adherence

Adherence between tumour and duodenum as seen intraoperatively may not be direct tumour invasion. Some studies[15,20] have shown that in up to 40% of cases with tumour adherence to the duodenum or pancreas, the actual cause is due to inflammatory adhesions rather than malignant infiltration. Certainly, it is not easy to differentiate whether the adherence is due to inflammation or tumour infiltration without histopathologic confirmation intraoperatively. Furthermore, intraoperative biopsy and frozen section is not advocated as it may be inaccurate due to sampling error and carries a real risk of tumour cell implantation and spillage, which is known to result in recurrence rates of up to 90%.[7,15,21] Therefore, if tumour adherence is present, it should always be assumed to be caused by malignant infiltration.

Surgical reconstruction

Direct closure

If the duodenal defect is small and can be repaired without tension, a direct closure transversely in two layers, without injuring the ampulla of Vater, should suffice.

Jejunal serosal patch

If the duodenal defect is too large, a jejunal serosal patch can be safely used as suggested by Ellis *et al.*[8]

Roux-en-Y jejunoduodenostomy

A roux-en-Y jejunoduodenostomy to repair the duodenal defect can be performed if direct closure or a jejunal serosal patch proves to be unsafe.

Combined duodenal and pancreatic resection

A standard pancreaticoduodenectomy (Whipple's procedure) is performed if the pancreas is also involved by tumour. A pylorus-preserving pancreaticoduodenectomy (PPPD) is an alternative, as some authors[10] believe that dissection of the pyloric lymph nodes is not necessary for locally advanced right-sided colonic cancer.

Results of extended resection

Morbidity

The reported morbidity of extended resection for locally advanced right-sided colonic cancer is low.[9,10] This low incidence holds good even if multivisceral resection is undertaken for advanced colorectal cancers at all sites. The reported postoperative morbidity was 3–6%.[3,13,15]

Mortality

Gall *et al.*[20] found that the 30-day mortality rate for extended resections at all sites in the colon in nearly 2000 patients treated between 1969 and 1983 was 12%, in comparison to 6% for nonextended colonic resections. This indicates that the operative risk in patients undergoing extended resections is increased or may be due to a poor patient selection where patients with poor surgical risks were subjected to a more radical resection. Others have reported a lower postoperative mortality of 3–8%.[3,13,15] However, in a more recent study from a specialized centre,[10] the 30-day mortality rate for all 8 patients undergoing either duodenectomy ($n = 4$) or pancreatico-duodenectomy ($n = 4$) for locally advanced right-sided colonic cancer was zero.

Survival time

(a) *Completeness of en-bloc resection*
The performance of a complete en-bloc resection clearly influences survival time. In a study from the MD Anderson Cancer Center[16] involving 101 patients with locally advanced colorectal carcinoma, complete tumour resection with en-bloc removal of adjacent organs was associated with a mean survival time of 40 months. In contrast, palliative bypass is associated with a median survival time of only 9 months, and incomplete resection including organ separation, with a mean survival time of 11 months. The 5-year actuarial survival rate for the patients who underwent a curative extended resection was 54%. In another recent study, in Germany,[22] a total of 173 patients with advanced colorectal carcinoma who underwent a multivisceral resection, the 5-year survival rate of the subgroup undergoing

curative surgery was 51% while that of the subgroup receiving only palliative resection was a dismal 0%.

In the context of advanced right-sided colonic cancer involving the
duodenum or pancreas or both, this improved survival remains to be
true, as evidenced by the study from the Memorial Sloan-Kettering Cancer
Center.[10] Six of 8 patients remained alive and disease-free at a median
follow-up of 26 months, with 1 long-term survivor who was alive and
disease-free at 84 months after extended resection. This finding is supported by others.[9] At the MD Anderson Cancer Center, Curley *et al.*[9] found
that the median survival time for all 12 patients who underwent en-bloc
pancreaticoduodenectomy or duodenectomy for locally advanced right-
sided colonic cancer was 32 months. The median survival time for the
eight patients who are still alive and disease-free was 42 months.

(b) *Stage of tumour*

Survival is influenced by the stage of the primary tumour. In a recent
study by Izbicki *et al.*[18] 220 patients with locally advanced colorectal cancer
underwent either extended resections ($n = 83$) or nonextended resections
($n = 137$). In the extended resection group, there was no significant difference in mean survival between pT3 and pT4 stage patients within 46 and
38 months, respectively. In patients who underwent nonextended resections, however, there was a significant difference in mean survival within
48 months for pT3 and 28 months for pT4 patients ($p < 0.05$). Postoperative
morbidity and mortality were comparable between the extended resection
group and the nonextended resection group.[18] Because extended resections can achieve comparable results in locally more advanced colorectal
cancer to nonextended resections in less advanced cancer, an aggressive
surgical approach is advocated. More importantly, the survival rates for
extended resection for right-sided colonic cancer are the same as those of
node-negative T4 sigmoid and rectal cancers with en-bloc resection of adjacent organs.[10] The biologic behaviour of invasive colonic cancer is therefore not any more aggressive in the right colon and these cancers should
be managed as aggressively as their counterparts in the left colon.[10]

(c) *Tumour adherence*

Long-term survival is also improved if tumour adherence is caused by
inflammation rather than infiltration. In a study of 121 patients who
had had multivisceral organ involvement, necessitating extended multivisceral radical resection, tumour infiltration was proven histologically in

55%, while 45% had inflammatory adherence to the attached organ only.[18] The 5-year survival rate (postoperative mortality included) was 54% for patients with inflammatory adherence, 49% for patients with tumour infiltration resected en bloc without tumour rupture, and 17% when the surgeon had inadvertently torn or cut into tumour tissue during resection. This experience is shared by other authors.[13,15,20] It is important to realize that lymphocytic infiltrate around a colorectal primary is a favorable independent prognostic sign[23] and implies some degree of host immune response to the tumour. Malignant invasion of the duodenum or pancreas was confirmed in all 12 patients in a study, but only 3 (25%) had lymph node metastases.[9]

Conclusions

Locally advanced hepatic flexure cancer involving the duodenum is rare but potentially curable. In about 40% of cases, tumour adherence is caused by inflammatory response rather than malignant infiltration. Both radiological imaging and intraoperative assessment are unreliable as to the cause of tumour adherence. The survival of patients with locally advanced right-sided colonic cancer involving the duodenum is influenced by completeness of en-bloc resection of the duodenum, the tumour stage and the lymph nodal status, and not by the size or site of primary tumour. Extended resection of locally advanced right-sided colonic cancer can be undertaken safely in specialized centres, with minimum morbidity and a 30-day mortality of less than 5%.

References

1. Sugarbaker ED. Coincident removal of additional structures in resections for carcinoma of the colon and rectum, *Ann Surg* 1946; 123: 1036–46.
2. Polk HC Jr. Extended resection for selected adenocarcinomas of the large bowel, *Ann Surg* 1972; 175: 892–9.
3. Eldar S, Kemeny MM and Terz JJ. Extended resections for carcinomas of the colon and rectum, *Surg Gynecol Obstet* 1985; 161: 319–22.
4. Brunschwig A. Complete excision of pelvic viscera for advanced carcinoma, *Cancer* 1948; 1: 177–83.

5. Hafner GH, Herrera L and Petrelli NJ. Morbidity and mortality after pelvic exenteration for colorectal adenocarcinoma, *Ann Surg* 1992; 215: 63–7.
6. Grey Turner G. Cancer of the colon, *Lancet* 1929; 1: 1017–23.
7. Van Prohaska J, Govostis MC and Wasick M. Multiple organ resection for advanced carcinoma of the colon and rectum, *Surg Gynecol Obstet* 1956; 177–82.
8. Ellis H, Morgan HN and Wastell C. Curative surgery in carcinoma of the colon involving duodenum, *Br J Surg* 1972; 59: 932–5.
9. Curley SA, Evans DB and Ames FC. Resection for cure of carcinoma of the colon directly invading the duodenum or pancreatic head, *J Am Coll Surg* 1994; 179: 587–92.
10. Koea JB, Conlon K, Paty PB, Guillem JG and Cohen AM. Pancreatic or duodenal resection or both for advanced carcinoma of the right colon: is it justified? *Dis Colon Rectum* 2000; 43: 460–5.
11. Jensen HE, Balslev IB and Nielsen J. Extensive surgery in the treatment of carcinoma of the colon, *Acta Chir Scand* 1970; 136: 431–4.
12. Kroneman H, Castelein A and Jeekel J. En bloc resection of colon carcinoma adherent to other organs: an efficacious treatment? *Dis Colon Rectum* 1991; 34: 780–3.
13. Heslov SF and Frost DB. Extended resection for primary carcinoma involving adjacent organs or structures, *Cancer* 1988; 62: 1637–40.
14. Davies GC and Ellis H. Radical surgery in locally advanced cancer of the large bowel, *Clin Oncol* 1975; 1: 21–6.
15. McGlone TP, Bernie WA and Elliot DW. Survival following extended operations for extracolonic invasion by colon cancer, *Arch Surg* 1982; 117: 595–9.
16. Curley SA, Carlson GW, Shumate CR, Wishnow KI and Ames FC. Extended resection for locally advanced colorectal carcinoma, *Am J Surg* 1992; 163: 553–9.
17. Charnsangavej C and Whitley NO. Metastases to the pancreas and peripancreatic lymph nodes from carcinoma of the right side of the colon: CT findings in 12 patients, *AJR Am J Roentgenol* 1993; 160: 49–52.
18. Izbicki JR, Hosch SB, Knoefel WT, Passlick B, Bloechle C and Broelsch CE. Extended resections are beneficial for patients with locally advanced colorectal cancer, *Dis Colon Rectum* 1995; 38: 1251–6.
19. Turnbull RB Jr, Kyle K, Watson FR and Spratt J. Cancer of the colon: the influence of the no-touch isolation technic on survival rates, *Ann Surg* 1967; 166: 420–7.

20. Gall FP, Tonak J and Altendorf A. Multivisceral resections in colorectal cancer, *Dis Colon Rectum* 1987; 30: 337–41.

21. Hunter JA, Ryan JA and Schultz P. En bloc resection of colon cancer adherent to other organs, *Am J Surg* 1987; 154: 67–71.

22. Gebhardt C, Meyer W, Ruckriegel S and Meier U. Multivisceral resection of advanced colorectal carcinoma, *Langenbecks Arch Surg* 1999; 384: 194–9.

23. Jass JR, Love SB and Northover JM. A new prognostic classification of rectal cancer, *Lancet* 1987; 1: 1303–6.

CHAPTER 36

Keeping Recurrence Low After Rectal Cancer Surgery

F Seow-Choen

Introduction

The variability of results from rectal surgery suggests that a better surgical technique may reduce the indication for adjuvant treatment, although proponents of adjuvant therapy for rectal cancer argue that further improvements in survival and reduction in recurrence rates will come only from a combination of chemotherapy and radiotherapy. Departments with poorer surgical results show a more significant improvement with adjuvant therapy than departments with better surgical results. Centres that achieve low recurrence rates following rectal cancer surgery alone may find it difficult to accept a policy of routine adjuvant chemoradiation advocated by centres with unacceptably high rates of recurrence for surgery alone. Adjuvant therapy results in a 10–15% increase in 5-year survival rates, which is much less than the variation between different institutions and surgeons.

Optimizing Surgical Technique

Reducing distal spread

Both lymphogenous and venous routes are possible for widespread dissemination of tumour, and the latter may account for the presence of distant metastases without lymph node involvement.[1,2] Premobilization isolation of the lymphatic and vascular pedicles was first advocated by Barnes[3] and later by Turnbull.[4] This no-touch technique was said to decrease vascular dissemination of tumour cells. Fisher and Turnbull[5] demonstrated cancer cells in the portal blood of 32% of their patients with colorectal cancer and theorized that early lymphovascular ligation before tumour manipulation might decrease metastases. They reported crude 5- and 10-year survival rates of 51% and 40% versus 35% and 29% with the no-touch versus conventional techniques, respectively. Wiggers *et al.*[6] conducted an eight-centre trial recruiting 236 patients randomized into conventional or no-touch groups. Although crude and corrected patient survival figures between the groups did not reach statistical significance, the data for liver recurrence was superior (41% vs 55%), with a longer tumour free interval (22.4 mths vs 12.6 mths) as well. The largest benefit was shown in the subset of patients with angioinvasive Dukes C carcinoma. However, these studies were performed on patients with colonic carcinoma and the significance and applicability to rectal cancer is uncertain.

High ligation of the inferior mesenteric vessels was designed to allow a more radical excision of the draining lymphatics and therefore decrease distant recurrence.[7] However, no definite advantage in the reduction of distant disease and improvement of survival has been demonstrated.[8]

Reducing Local Recurrence

A proportion of distant metastases may arise from local recurrence that were not present at the time of initial surgery. Some distant spread therefore may be reduced by reducing local recurrence through adequate radical surgery.

Implantation

Local recurrence following curative resection may be due to viable implantation of exfoliated tumour cells.[9,10] Transperitoneal tumour implantation may result from spillage of intestinal contents into the peritoneal cavity from divided or perforated bowel. Viable malignant cells scattered onto a freshly dissected pelvis are probably more dangerous than those scattered onto intact peritoneal surfaces. Disruption of the tumour intraoperatively during bowel resection or iatrogenic perforation is associated with decreased long term survival.[11] Tumours which have breached the serosal layer of the colorectum may also shed cells spontaneously during surgical manipulation into the perineal cavity by exfoliation. Peritoneal washing before and after rectal surgery has shown the presence of tumour cells. Viable tumour cells may be shed intraluminally and are capable of growth under favourable conditions.[13] Minimal and gentle manipulation of the tumour during surgery is important, as rough handling of the rectum may lead to tumour perforation and release of tumour cells into the operative field. Proper irrigation of the rectal stump is therefore important if suture line recurrence is to be prevented. Chlorhexidine, cetrimide, providone-iodine, water and mecuric perchloride have also been used for this purpose.[14] Normal saline should not be used, as it has no tumoricidal effect. Viable tumour cells within the rectal stump exfoliated during surgery may be washed out by irrigation below the rectal cross clamp before division of the bowel or performance of the anastomosis.

Development of an anastomotic leak has also been significantly associated with an increased incidence of local recurrence and poorer survival rates.[15] Better surgical techniques are therefore mandatory if leaks and recurrence are to be decreased.[16]

Digital extraction, finger fracture or trial dissection in areas of possible tumour infiltration will result in tumour cell exfoliation. Positive cytological smears of the tumour bed are associated with a higher likelihood of tumour recurrence.[17] Surgeons who are wont to perform such dissection must change their practice. Locally invasive tumours do not affect survival or local recurrence adversely compared to similarly staged tumour without local invasion provided that tumour-free margins are achieved with en-bloc extended rectal resection. Rectal cancer involving the bladder, seminal vesicles or female genital tract without distant metastases should be resected en-bloc where possible to maximize the chance of cure, as long term survival is influenced only by the stage and completeness of cancer incision.[18]

A careful and gentle surgical technique also decreases blood loss, leading to a decreased incidence of unnecessary blood transfusion, which had been thought to increase local and systemic recurrence. A review of 20 papers representing 5236 patients showed that perioperative blood transfusion was associated with an increased risk of recurrence of colorectal cancer and death,[19] possibly due to the immune-suppressive effects of allogenic blood transfusion.

Cancer recurrence may also be caused by implantation of viable tumour cells at the anastomotic site. Protein-based and mulifilament sutures had been shown to attract the most malignant cells, whereas stainless steel and monofilament polydioxanone have the smallest number of adherent tumour cells.[20] Sutureless anastomoses also had the lowest crypt cell proliferation rate, which might indicate a decreased susceptibility to anastomotic carcinogenesis.

A major contributor of local recurrence is inadequate local resection of the rectal tumour. Distal intramural spread is rare and extends for less than 1 cm beyond the macroscopic edge of the tumour in potentially curable tumours.[21] In cases where the distal intramural spread is greater than 1 cm, death from distant metastases usually occurred before local recurrence. Routine application of the 5 cm rule of distal excision below a rectal tumour is unnecessary. A distal margin less than 2 cm below a rectal carcinoma does not affect survival or local recurrence adversely.[21] A sufficient distal margin as judged by the ability to place a clamp below the palpable edge of tumour did not lead to local recurrence provided the distal bowel lumen was washed out. Indications that an abdominoperineal resection is necessary are fixation of the tumour to the anal sphincter or a tumour less than 1 cm above the anal sphincter.[22] Poorly differentiated tumours do not benefit from a wider distal margin of resection.

Total mesorectal excision is associated with a low rate of local recurrence. This was thought to be due to the enclosing effect of fascia propria, which is an avascular plane crossed only by a minimal number of small vessels as the rectum passes through the levators sealing the entire lymphatic system of the rectum. Involved lymph nodes, or tumours with lymphatic, blood vessel or fat involvement are commonly found within the mesorectum and may be left behind with conventional anterior or abdominoperineal resection, and this had been offered to explain the high intersurgeon variability of local recurrence following these operations.[23] A less skillful surgeon may cone down or bevel towards the rectal wall as the levator ani are approached and therefore leave substantial mesorectal deposits leading to recurrence. Conventional hand dissection of the rectum from the presacral fascia may tear along the edge of the tumour, and this method also causes haemorrhage with possible extravasation of viable tumour cells. Diathermy dissection, however, tends to seal vessels and lymphatics as it cuts and may decrease tumour cell implantation. Total mesorectal excision should be performed with sharp dissection gives a crude and cumulative risk of local recurrence at 5 years of only 2.5% and 3.5% following curative surgery for rectal cancer.[24] Upon adoption of total mesorectal excision, Swedish surgeons significantly decreased their local recurrence rates from 14.2% to 6.3% and increased their crude survival rates at four years ($P < 0.03$). McCall reviewed the literature and found an 18.5% local recurrence rate in 10 465 patients overall, but in 1033 with total mesorectal excision the local recurrence rate was 7.1%.[26] In more recent times, use of this technique for rectal cancer without radiotherapy or chemotherapy has been shown to result in very low median local recurrence rates of 3% (range 0–5) and 6% (range 0–7) at 2 and 5 years of follow-up respectively for six surgeons in our unit.[21]

Spread to the lateral pelvic wall including the iliac lymph nodes is another key determinant for an increased risk of local recurrence. Lateral spread is often underestimated by surgeons and pathologists and may be the main cause of local recurrence. Deddish and Stearns[27] therefore developed a policy of extended pelvic lymphadenectomy, but abandoned this when they observed that though 12% of their 122 patients had pelvic lymph node involvement, only 2 patients had enhanced survival. The Japanese are now the main proponents of extended pelvic lymphadenectomy in which high ligation of the inferior mesenteric vessels is performed, followed by an extended periaortic and pelvic lymphadenectomy beginning as high as the duodenum. Such surgery is very extensive and time-consuming. Blood loss averaged 2 litres, micturation disorders occurred in almost all patients and sexual dysfunction was seen in 100% of all males. Enker *et al.*[28] found that few patients survived 5 years or more if carcinoma had spread to the pelvic nodes. Very few surgeons outside of Japan therefore perform routine extended pelvic or preaortic lymphadenectomy for this reason.

Conclusion

Much of the intersurgeon variability may be found in the surgical technique and the extent and adequacy of local surgical clearance. It would appear that in some units specializing in colorectal cancer, rates of local recurrence and survival are comparable to or better than those obtained with adjuvant therapy. The results of trials investigating a combination of chemotherapy and radiotherapy for high-risk rectal cancers are not better than those observed at other centres following surgery alone. Chemotherapy and radiotherapy are associated with significant side effects and the remedy for surgical failure must therefore be to improve surgical technique as a first priority.[29]

References

1. Weiss L, Grundmann E, Torhorst J, Hartveit F, Moberg I *et al*. Haematogeneous metastatic patterns in colonic carcinoma: an analysis of 1541 patients, *J Pathol* 1986; 150: 195–203.
2. Taylor FW. Cancer of the colon and rectum: a study of routes of metastases and death. *Surgery* 1962; 52: 305–8.
3. Barnes JP. Physiologic resection of the right colon, *Surg Gynaecol Obstet* 1952; 94: 722–4.
4. Turnbull RB Jr, Kyle K and Watson FR. Cancer of the colon—the influence of the no-touch isolation technique on survival rates, *Ann Surg* 1967; 166: 420.
5. Fisher ER and Turnbull RB. The cytologic demonstration and significance of tumour cells in the mesenteric venous blood in patients with colorectal carcinoma, *Surg Gynecol Obstet* 1955; 100: 102–4.
6. Wiggers T, Jeekel J, Arends JW *et al*. No touch isolation technique in colon cancer: a controlled prospective trial, *Br J Surg* 1988; 75: 409–14.
7. McElwain JW, Bacon HE and Trimpi HD. Lymph node metastases: experience with aortic ligation of inferior mesenteric artery in cancer of the rectum, *Surgery* 1954; 35: 513–31.
8. Surtees P, Ritchie JK and Phillips RKS. High vs low ligation of the inferior mesenteric artery in rectal cancer, *Br J Surg* 1990; 77: 618–21.
9. Long RTL and Edwards RH. Implantation metastasis as a cause of local recurrence of colorectal carcinoma, *Am J Surg* 1989; 157: 194–201.
10. Umpleby HC and Williamson RC. Anastomotic recurrence in large bowel cancer, *Br J Surg* 1987; 74: 873–8.
11. Stanetz CA Jr. The effect of inadvertent intra-operative perforation on survival and recurrence in colorectal cancer, *Dis Colon Rectum* 1984; 27: 792–7.
12. Leather AJM, Kocjan G, Savage F, Hu W, Yiu CY, Boulos PB, Northover JMA and Phillips RKS. Detection of free malignant cells in the peritoneal cavity before and after resection of colorectal cancer, *Dis Colon Rectum* 1994; 37: 814–19.
13. Seow-Choen F. Irrigation of the rectal stump decreases the chance of exfoliated cells on staplers, *Dis Colon Rectum* 1992; 35: 1108.

14. Umpleby HC and Williamson RC. Efficacy of agents employed to prevent anastomotic recurrence in colorectal carcinoma, *Ann R Coll Surg Engl* 1984; 66: 192–4.

15. Akyol AM, McGregor JR, Galloway DJ, Murray GD and George WD. Anastomotic leaks in colorectal cancer surgery: a risk factor for recurrence, *Int J Colorect Dis* 1991; 6: 179–83.

16. Seow-Choen F. Function of the distal rectum after low anterior resection for carcinoma, *Br J Surg* 1992; 79: 1248.

17. Wilwerman SH, Moore J, Thompson H and Keighley MRB. Preoperative detection of patients with rectal cancer at high risk of local recurrence, *Ann Coll Surg Engl* 1985; 76: 164–6.

18. Nyam DCNK, Seow-Choen F and Ho MS. Bladder involvement in patients with colorectal carcinoma, *Sing Med J* 1995; 36: 525–6.

19. Chung M, Steinmetz OK and Gordon PH. Perioperative blood transfusion and outcome after resection for colorectal carcinoma, *Br J Surg* 1993; 80: 427–32.

20. Uff CR, Yiu CY, Boulos PB and Phillips RKS. Influence of suture physicochemical and surface topographic and surface topographic structure on tumour adherent, *Dis Colon Rectum* 1993; 36: 850–4.

21. Kraemer M, Wiratkapun S, Seow-Choen F, Ho YH, Eu KW and Nyam D. Stratifying risk factors follow-up: a comparison of recurrent and non recurrent colorectal cancer, *Dis Colon Rectum* 2001; 44: 815–21.

22. Seow-Choen F. Colonic pouch after low anterior resection of the distal third of the rectum, *Ann Acad Med* 1993; 22: 229–32.

23. Heald RJ and Ryall RD. Recurrence and survival after total mesorectal excision for rectal cancer, *Lancet* 1986; i, 1479: 82.

24. Heald RJ, Husband EM and Ryall RDH. The mesorectum in rectal cancer surgery the clue to pelvic recurrence? *Br J Surg* 1982; 69: 613.

25. Arbman G, Nilsson E, Hallbrook O and Sjodahl R. Local recurrence following total mesorectal excision for cancer, *Br J Surg* 1996; 83: 375–9.

26. McCall JL, Cox MR *et al.* Analysis of local recurrence rates after surgery for rectal cancer, *Int J Colorect Dis* 1995; 10: 126–32.

27. Deddish MR and Stearns MW. Surgical procedures for carcinoma of the left colon and rectum with 5-year results following abdomino-pelvic dissection of lymph nodes, *Ann J Surg* 1960; 99: 188–92.

28. Enker WE, Laffer UT and Block GE. Enhanced survival of patients' with colon and rectal cancer is based upon wide anatomic resection, *Ann J Surg* 1979; 193: 350.

29. Seow-Choen F. Adjuvant therapy for rectal cancer cannot be based on the results of other surgeons. *Br J Surg* 2002; 89: 946–7.

CHAPTER 37

Pelvic Exenteration

C Barben

Introduction

Pelvic exenteration, for the treatment of advanced pelvic malignancy, was first reported by Brunschwig in 1948.[1] Many authors have reported their experience of using this procedure in a wide range of tumours, including advanced carcinoma of the cervix, vagina, colon, rectum, bladder, uterus, prostate and urethra.[2] Although the morbidity and mortality were originally thought to be prohibitively high to make this a viable treatment option, improvements in perioperative care, and the use of specialist centres employing multidisciplinary teams, have reduced the mortality from almost one quarter[1] to around 10%.[3] The 5-year survival figures of around 50% make this a reasonable option for patients with advanced pelvic malignancy.

Definition

Total pelvic exenteration (TPE) is defined as removal of the rectum, distal colon, bladder, lower ureters, internal reproductive organs, draining lymph nodes and pelvic peritoneum. This operation may be indicated when there is involvement of the trigone of the urinary bladder by a primary or recurrent tumor, without metastatic disease elsewhere. In men, involvement of the prostate gland by a rectal carcinoma could be an indication for TPE.

Modifications of TPE have been described. They include anterior pelvic exenteration (APE), which involves removing the bladder, lower ureters, reproductive organs, draining lymph nodes and pelvic peritoneum. This operation is indicated in similar situations to TPE, but when the malignancy has not involved the rectum. Posterior pelvic exenteration (PPE) removes the rectum, distal colon, internal reproductive organs, draining lymph nodes and pelvic peritoneum. This is usually indicated in rectal adenocarcinomas involving the uterus or vagina, or when the primary rectal tumor is anteriorly located or involves the entire circumference of the bowel wall, without bladder involvement. A further modification is supralevator pelvic exenteration (SPE), for tumours of the cervix, upper vagina, urinary bladder and/or the upper rectum, where an adequate distal margin of resection can be achieved, allowing primary anastomosis of the bowel after removal of the affected structures.

Indications and Contraindications

Pelvic exenteration can be used for the treatment of primary or recurrent colorectal cancer. Approximately 10% of newly diagnosed colonic tumours are adherent to adjacent organs, without metastases.[4] Whilst not all of these adhesions will be malignant, the incidence of histologically proven malignant adhesions has been reported to range from 40 to 89%.[4–11] It is imperative that en bloc excision of the tumor and adjacent organs be performed, in order not to compromise the curative nature of the surgery. Less than an en bloc resection compromises survival, and increases the recurrence rate.[12] Even in the presence of regional lymph node metastases, which is the most important prognostic factor after "curative" resection, and adjacent organ involvement, an en bloc resection is justified, since at least a quarter of these patients will be alive at five years.[4] Rectal carcinoma most often involves the uterus, ovaries, posterior vaginal wall, and bladder.[13]

The commonest gynaecological indication for pelvic exenteration is recurrent or persistent cervical carcinoma that is limited to the central pelvis. Other indications are vaginal, vulvar, and endometrial and ovarian tumours.[14]

Some authors have used pelvic exenteration for palliation,[15–17] for pelvic pain, tumor abscess with drainage, urinary incontinence, recurrent haemorrhage, ureteral or bowel obstruction, and rectovesical, vesicovaginal and rectovaginal fistulas. Others, however, claim that the high morbidity and mortality of the operation renders it unsuitable for palliation.[18] Certainly, the presence of distant metastasis is a contraindication to pelvic exenteration.

The contraindications are set out below, noting the slight difference between primary and recurrent disease:

Absolute contraindications:
- Pelvic sidewall involvement
- Sacral bone involvement*
- Involvement of major vessels or nerves
- Distant metastases

Relative contraindications:
- Unilateral or bilateral hydronephrosis*
- Inability to care for stomas
- Major systemic disease
- Senility

*Only in recurrent disease

Preoperative Evaluation

A full history and examination should be performed in every patient. Preoperative evaluation is designed to exclude the presence of all contraindications, especially distant metastases. Attention to symptoms may reveal those that give clues to the tumour being unresectable. Pelvic pain in a pattern similar to sciatica suggests nerve root involvement. Rectal and/or vaginal examination may reveal fixity of the tumor and even perineal spread.

Computerized tomography (CT) scanning and magnetic resonance imaging (MRI) can be used to assess the neoplasm itself, adjacent organ involvement, and pelvic side wall and vessel/nerve invasion. The use of

MRI in predicting resectability was poor at distinguishing tumour involvement from radiation or postoperative changes in those with abnormalities on the side wall.[19]

Fixation of the tumour is an ominous sign, but not necessarily a contraindication to exenteration.[20,21] Some authors suggest that sacral involvement is only a contraindication in recurrent disease.[2]

Tumours may grow and invade the ureters, producing unilateral or bilateral hydronephrosis. Patients who undergo exenteration for cervical carcinoma have poorer survival with ureteral obstruction.[22] In recurrent rectal carcinoma, unilateral or bilateral hydronephrosis is an indicator of nonresectability for cure.[23]

Surgical Technique

The initial focus should be on ensuring that the cancer can be removed safely, and that the exenteration will be of benefit to the patient in terms of cure and control of local disease. A thorough laparotomy is undertaken to look for distant metastases, and frozen section histology is used where necessary. The tumour is then assessed to rule out involvement of lateral pelvic sidewalls, the sacrum (if recurrent disease is present), and involvement of the major nerves or vessels.

Once resectability is confirmed, the dissection begins with the ureters, which are divided above the pelvic brim. The sigmoid colon is divided, and then mobilized, with the presacral dissection continuing into the pelvis. From this point, further dissection must be tailored to the location of the tumour mass to determine the structures that need to be removed to perform an en bloc resection.

Reconstruction

After the specimen has been removed, reconstruction takes place, and this will obviously differ, depending on which tissues have been removed. The reconstruction is the aspect of the exenterative procedure that is a major source of postoperative morbidity, and must be done in a systematic, meticulous fashion, by an experienced surgical team.

As far as the faecal stream is concerned, the two options are permanent end colostomy, and restoration of colonic continuity if the pelvic floor has not been resected, as in a supralevator pelvic exenteration. After restoration of colonic continuity, a temporary, defunctioning colostomy may be used, especially if there has been previous irradiation. Those with a rectal stump longer than 6 cm have a better functional outcome than those with a shorter stump.[24] A colonic J-pouch may also be constructed, which improves early postoperative bowel function.[21]

After removal of the bladder, there is a need for urinary diversion. The ideal requirements for bladder diversion are continence, antireflux, and minimal life-style implications for the patient. The simplest diversion is an ileal conduit, which has the disadvantage of not being continent, but is associated with fewer complications.[2] The creation of a continent urinary reservoir is better for the patient, and, although the experience in some centres is extensive, complications can occur in over 20% of cases,[25] requiring reoperation for urinary leakage in 15% of patients.[26] Another option is the continent ileocolonic urinary reservoir, which is reported to have around 90% continence rates, and also provides bulk for tissue coverage in the pelvis.[27,28] A newer procedure is the creation of an ileal neo-bladder, which allows continence and passage of urine via the urethra.[29]

After TPE, there remains a bed of poorly vascularized tissue, which may have been previously irradiated. This area heals poorly, and is prone to infection. There is also the possibility of small bowel entrapment, leading to adhesions, exposing the small bowel to radiation injury, and perineal hernias.

Occasionally, the pelvic defect can be primarily repaired. However, more often than not, autologous tissues must be brought into the pelvis, or an absorbable mesh used.[30] Methods to close this defect include an omental flap based on the left gastroepiploic vessels, or a rectus abdominis flap. Reconstruction of pelvic organs will also bring in vascularized tissue, and occupy space in the pelvis. Vaginal reconstruction can be performed at the time of surgery, or as a delayed procedure. If only part of the vagina has been resected, it can be primarily repaired. Otherwise, several alternatives, including split-thickness skin grafts, transpositional skin flaps omental flaps and myocutaneous flaps, can be performed.[31,32]

Primary closure of the perineal wound is the preferred method. The trade-off is the increased incidence of perineal wound infection. After abdominoperineal resection, the primary healing rate of the perineal wound is around 40%, and closing the wound rather than leaving it open is associated with a shorter hospital stay.[33] However, when a septic wound complication occurs in a closed perineal wound, the time to healing is no different than that in an open wound.[34,35] Options for closing large perineal defects include an inerior gluteal flap and a rectus abdominis flap.[36]

Complications

The in-hospital mortality for pelvic exenteration ranges from 0 to 14%.[3,4,14,18,37–42] The advent of better preoperative and postoperative care, as well as better patient selection, has accounted for the decrease in mortality to its present level. Most mortalities are associated with a major complication, such as an anastomotic leak.

Morbidity rates range from 32 to 84%.[3,4,14,18,37–42] The major morbidities include ureterointestinal leaks, pelvic haemorrhage and pelvic abscess. Predictive factors for the development of complications include the use of previous irradiation and the lack of pelvic floor reconstruction.[43] This poses some difficulty, as prior irradiation can improve the chance of resectability in some colorectal and bladder cancers.[44]

The short-term and long-term complications of pelvic exenteration are summarized in Table 1. The 5-year survival after pelvic exenteration ranges from 23 to 68% in the large, reported series.[3,4,14,18,37–42] TNM staging is the only independent factor identified for survival.[45] The recurrence rates are worse in those operated on for recurrent disease, when compared to those with locally advanced primary cancer.[46] The 5-year survival for recurrent disease is less than one-third.[47,48] The reasons for this include the fact that recurrent cancers are more aggressive than primary, locally advanced disease,[3] and the fact that most will have undergone radiotherapy, adding to the technical difficulties and complications.[43,49]

Conclusion

Pelvic exenteration is a complex surgical procedure, undertaken for locally advanced primary, or recurrent, pelvic tumours, from which good results can be obtained. Those selected for the procedure should be medically fit to tolerate the extended procedure, and free of metastatic disease. Patients should be warned that complication rates are high, and that disease-free survival is not guaranteed. However, pelvic exenteration is the only curative option for the treatment of advanced pelvic malignancy.

Table 1. Short- and long-term complications of pelvic exenteration.

Short-Term Complications	Long-Term Complications
Intestine	*Intestine*
• Colostomy retraction	• Parastomal hernia
• Prolonged ileus	• Small bowel obstruction
• Perineal hernia	• Perineal fistula
• Upper GI haemorrhage	• Perineal hernia
	• Upper GI haemorrhage
Conduit and urinary tract	*Conduit and urinary tract*
• Anastomotic leak	• Ureteral obstruction
• Conduit infarction	• Staghorn calculi
• Urinary retention	• Urinary tract sepsis
Vascular	*Vascular*
• Renal cortical abscess	• Deep vein thrombosis
• Iliac artery thrombosis	
• Pulmonary embolus	
• Pelvic haemorrhage	
General	*General*
• Intraoperative myocardial infarct	• Pelvic abscess
• Wound infection	
• Pelvic abscess	
• Pneumonia	
• Depression	

References

1. Brunschwig A. Complete excision of pelvic viscera for advanced carcinoma, *Cancer* 1948; 1: 177–83.
2. Rodriguez-Bigas MA and Petrelli NJ. Pelvic exenteration and its modifications, *Am J Surg* 1996; 17: 293–301.
3. Hafner GH, Herrera L and Petrelli NJ. Morbidity and mortality after pelvic exenteration for colorectal adenocarcinoma, *Ann Surg* 1992; 15: 63–7.
4. Lopez MJ and Monafo WW. Role of extended resection in the initial treatment of locally advanced colorectal carcinoma, *Surgery* 1993; 113: 365–72.
5. Eisenberg SB, Kraybill WG and Lopez MJ. Long-term results of locally advanced colorectal adenocarcinomas, *Surgery* 1990; 108: 779–86.
6. Gall FP, Tonak J and Altendort A. Multivisceral resections in colorectal cancer, *Dis Colon Rectum* 1987; 30: 337–41.

7. Glass RE, Fazio VW, Jagelman DJ *et al.* The results of surgical treatment of cancer of the colon at the Cleveland Clinic from 1965–1975: classification of the spread of colon cancer and long term survival, *Int J Colorectal Dis* 1986; 1: 33–9.

8. Heslov SF and Frost DB. Extended resection for primary colorectal carcinoma involving adjacent organs or structures, *Cancer* 1988; 62: 1637–40.

9. Jensen HE, Balslev IB and Nielsen J. Extenseive surgery in the treatment of carcinoma of the colon, *Acta Chir Scand* 1970; 136: 431–4.

10. McGlone TP, Bernie WA and Ellit DW. Survival following extended operations for extracolonic invasion by colon cancer, *Arch Surg* 1982; 117: 595–9.

11. Sugarbaker ED and Wiley HM. The significance of fixation in operable carcinoma of the large bowel, *Surgery* 1990; 27: 343–7.

12. Hunter JA, Ryan JA Jr and Schultz P. En bloc resection of colon cancer adherent to other organs, *Am J Surg* 1987; 154: 67–71.

13. Bonfanti G, Bozzetti F, Doci R *et al.* Results of extended surgery for cancer of the rectum and sigmoid, *Br J Surg* 1982; 69: 305–7.

14. Lawhead RA Jr, Clark GC, Smith DH *et al.* Pelvic exenteration for recurrent or persistent gynaecological malignancies: a 10-year review of the Memorial Sloan-Kettering Cancer Center experience (1972–1981), *Gynecol Oncol* 1989; 33: 279–82.

15. Lopez MJ, Kraybill WG, Downey RS *et al.* Exenterative surgery for locally advanced rectosigmoid cancers: is it worthwhile? *Surgery* 1987; 102: 644–51.

16. Deckers PJ, Olsson C, Williams LA *et al.* Pelvic exenteration as palliation of malignant disease, *Am J Surg* 1976; 131: 509–15.

17. Brophy PF, Hoffman JP and Eisenberg BL. The role of pelvic exenteration, *Am J Surg* 1994; 167: 386–90.

18. Anthapoulos AP, Manetta A, Larson JE *et al.* Pelvic exenteration: a morbidity and mortality analysis of a seven-year experience, *Gynecol Oncol* 1989; 35: 219–23.

19. Popovich M, Hricak H, Sugimura K *et al.* The role of MR imaging in determining surgical eligibility for pelvic exenteration, *Am J Radiol* 1993; 160: 525–31.

20. Takagi H, Morimoto T, Kato T *et al.* Pelvic exenteration combined with sacral resection for recurrent rectal cancer, *J Surg Oncol* 1983; 24: 161–6.

21. Wanebo HJ, Gaker DL, Whitehill R *et al*. Pelvic recurrence of rectal cancer: options for curative resection, *Ann Surg* 1987; 205: 482–95.

22. Barber HRK, Roberts S and Brunschwig A. Prognostic significance of preoperative non-visualizing kidney in patients receiving pelvic exenteration, *Cancer* 1963; 16: 1614–15.

23. Rodriguez-Bigas MA, Herrera L and Petrelli NJ. Surgery for recurrent rectal adenocarcinoma in the presence of hydronephrosis, *Am J Surg* 1992; 164: 18–21.

24. Hatch KD, Shingleton HM, Potter ME *et al*. Low rectal resection and anastomosis at the time of pelvic exenteration, *Gynecol Oncol* 1988; 32: 262–7.

25. Skinner DG, Lieskovsky G and Boyd S. Continent urinary diversion, *J Urol* 1989; 141: 1323–7.

26. Ehrlich RM. An improved method of creating an ileal conduit: the importance of a better vascular supply, *J Urol* 1973; 109: 993–5.

27. Pearlman NW, Donohue RE, Wettlaufer JN *et al*. Continent ileocolonic urinary reservoirs for filling and lining the post-exenteration pelvis, *Am J Surg* 1990; 160: 634–7.

28. Penalver MA, Bejany D, Donato DM *et al*. Functional characteristics and follow-up of the continent ileal colonic urinary reservoir: Miami pouch. *Cancer* 1993; 71: 1667–72.

29. Yamamoto S, Yamanaka N, Maeda T, Uchida Y, Yabe S, Nakano M, Sakano S, Yamada Y, Takenaka A and Yamamoto M. Ileal neobladder for urinary bladder replacement following total pelvic exenteration for rectal carcinoma, *Digestive Surgery* 2001; 18(1): 67–72.

30. Dasmahapatra KS and Swaminathan AP. The use of a biodegradable mesh to prevent radiation-associated small bowel injury, *Arch Surg* 1991; 126: 366–9.

31. Benson C, Soisson AP, Carlson J *et al*. Neovaginal reconstruction with a rectus abdominis myocutaneous flap, *Obstet Gynecol* 1993; 81: 871–5.

32. Hatch KD. Neovaginal reconstruction, *Cancer* 1993; 71: 1660–3.

33. Robles Campos R, Garcia Ayllon J, Paricio P *et al*. Management of the perineal wound after abdominoperineal resection: prospective study of three methods, *Br J Surg* 1992; 79: 29–31.

34. Petrelli NJ, Rosenfield L, Herrera L and Mittelman A. The morbidity of perineal wounds following abdominoperineal resection for rectal carcinoma, *J Surg Oncol* 1986; 32: 138–40.

35. Patrick Mazier W, Surrell JA and Senagore AJ. The bottom end: handling of the perineal wound after abdominoperineal resection, *Am Surg* 1991; 57: 454–8.

36. Waterhouse N and Northover JMA. Reconstructive surgery of the groin and perineum. In: Phillips R, Northover J (eds.), *Modern Coloproctology: Surgical Grand Rounds from St Mark's Hospital*. London: Edward Arnold, 1993, pp. 10–22.

37. Kiselow M, Butcher HR Jr and Bricker EM. Results of the radical surgical treatment of advanced pelvic cancer, *Ann Surg* 1967; 166: 428–36.

38. Rutledge FN, Smith JP, Wharton JT *et al.* Pelvic exenteration: analysis of 296 patients, *Am J Obstet Gynecol* 1977; 129: 881–92.

39. Kraybill WG, Lopez MJ and Bricker EM. Total pelvic exenteration as a therapeutic option in advanced malignant disease of the pelvis, *Surg Gynecol Obstet* 1988; 166: 259–63.

40. Hatch KD, Gelder MS and Soong SJ. Pelvic exenteration with low rectal anastomosis: survival, complications, and prognostic factors, *Gynecol Oncol* 1990; 38: 462–7.

41. Shingleton HM, Soong S-J, Getter MS *et al.* Clinical and histopathological factors predicting recurrence and survival after pelvic exenteration for cancer of the cervix, *Obstet Gynecol* 1989; 73: 1027–34.

42. Soper JT, Berchuk A and Creasman WT. Pelvic exenteration: factors associated with major surgical morbidity, *Gynecol Oncol* 1989; 35: 93–8.

43. Jakowatz JG, Porudominski D, Riihimaki DU *et al.* Complications of pelvic exenteration, *Arch Surg* 1985; 120: 1261–5.

44. Sombeck MD, Mendenhall WM, Parsions JT and Copeland EM III. Preoperative irradiation for advanced pelvic cancer, *Surg Oncol Clin North Am* 1994; 3: 247–56.

45. Yamada K, Ishizawa T, Niwa K, Chuman Y, Akiba S and Aikou T. Patterns of pelvic invasion are prognostic in the treatment of locally recurrent rectal cancer, *Br J Surg* 2001; 88(7): 988–93.

46. Law WL, Chu KW and Choi HK. Total pelvic exenteration for locally advanced rectal cancer, *J Am Coll Surg* 2000; 190: 78–83.

47. Wanebo HJ, Antoniuk P, Koness RJ, Levy A, Vezeridis M, Cohen SI *et al.* Pelvic resection of recurrent colorectal cancer: technical considerations and outcomes, *Dis Colon Rectum* 1999; 42: 1438–48.

48. Adachi W, Nishio A, Watanabe H, Igarashi J, Yazawa K, Nimura Y *et al.* Reresection for local recurrence of rectal cancer, *Surg Today* 1999; 29: 999–1003.

49. Takagi H, Morimoto T, Yasue M, Kato K, Yamada E and Suzuki R. Total pelvic exenteration for advanced carcinoma of the lower colon, *J Surg Oncol* 1985; 8: 59–62.

Laparoscopic Rectal Cancer Surgery

KW Eu

Introduction

Laparoscopic surgery for colorectal diseases is now widely used for the treatment of various benign lesions, such as polyps, diverticular disease, rectal prolapse and inflammatory bowel disease. Furthermore, recent advances in laparoscopic-surgical techniques and instrumentation have now made it feasible to resect and anastomose almost all parts of the large and the small intestine without the conventional laparotomy incision.[1–3]

However, as the most common indication for surgery in colorectal surgery is cancer, naturally the most common indication for laparoscopic colorectal surgery is cancer, as reported in many series.[4–11]

However, the role of laparoscopic surgery for the treatment of colorectal surgery, particularly rectal cancer, remains controversial. Furthermore, the safety and applicability of laparoscopic approaches to potentially curable colorectal cancer have been the subject of great concern as colorectal cancer is a disease that may be cured surgically in up to 50% of cases.

Benefits of Laparoscopic Rectal Cancer Surgery

The theoretical advantages of laparoscopic over conventional techniques for rectal cancer include decreased pain, a smaller incision, a shorter postoperative ileus, earlier discharge from the hospital, and a more rapid return to work or normal activity.

Franklin found that patients who underwent laparoscopically assisted resection returned to full activity within two weeks, compared to the conventional group, which took five weeks longer.

The other major benefit of laparoscopic surgery is the faster return of intestinal function after operation. This was attributed to the reduction in the opiate analgesic requirement. It is also possible that the reduction in the postoperative ileus may be due to the fact that the small intestine and the colon remain in a warm and moist environment in the abdominal cavity and are not exposed to the environment as in conventional surgery. Furthermore, tissue trauma is reduced to a bare minimum in laparoscopic surgery, thereby encouraging an earlier return of bowel function.

Concerns and Issues in Laparoscopic Rectal Cancer

Although there are many theoretical advantages to laparoscopic surgery, these benefits may be nullified if an inadequate cancer operation is performed. The main concerns therefore are: (1) the oncologic issue, (2) adequacy of lymhadenectomy, (3) tumour cell shedding and (4) port-site recurrence.

Oncologic Resection

The definition of an oncologic resection remains varied, although most authorities will define it as: (1) resection of the whole known extent of cancer in the bowel wall and adjacent soft tissue; (2) resection of a suitable margin of bowel wall above and below the cancer; (3) resection of draining lymph nodes accompanying the major vascular pedicle to the involved bowel (mesocolon/mesorectum).

There are several recent reports stating the feasibility of a laparoscopic oncologic resection (using an anatomical criterion) of colon and rectal cancer in the cadaver model. However, the correlation of this with the live patient is being questioned, with the absence of the potential problem of haemorrhage and the tissues being more turgid and less friable in the cadaver model.

The adequacy of margins of resection in laparoscopic rectal cancer surgery had also stirred some debate, as this is probably the single most important factor in anastomotic recurrence. Generally, most colorectal surgeons would agree that a 2–5 cm margin of resection is adequate, depending on tumour size, location and differentiation. Most series have found comparable margins and specimen lengths when comparing laparoscopic and conventional resections for cancer.

Adequacy of Lymphadenectomy

The next issue in laparoscopic rectal cancer surgery is the adequacy of lymphadenectomy. Colorectal surgeons would normally adopt a generous excision of lymph-node-bearing tissue in the conventional open surgery for cancer. Therefore it would be logical to compare the lymph node harvest between laparoscopic and nonlaparoscopic cancer operations. To date, major series have found lymph nodal yields similar in both laparoscopic and nonlaparoscopic groups. However, the number of lymph nodes reported may be more dependent upon the pathologist's enthusiasm in searching for them in the pathological specimen than upon surgical technique. Scott *et al.*[12] have reported that accurate staging of colorectal cancers depends on retrieval of at least 13 lymph nodes from the specimen. A specific number of lymph nodes excised, however, does not ensure that an oncologic resection has been performed successfully. This only allows the pathologist and surgeon to stage the tumour more accurately. Some would argue that the only number of lymph nodes which would prove that an oncologic resection has been accomplished is the number of lymph nodes remaining at the base of the mesenteric vessels which were ligated and not the number of lymph nodes that were removed!

Tumour Cell Shedding

Next is the issue of the potential risk of cancer cell shedding and subsequent implantation from the lumen of the bowel. Therefore, in the conventional open surgical setting, before transecting the rectum in surgery for cancer of the rectum, a rectal irrigation usually performed with a tumouricidal solution below a clamp applied distal to the tumour prior to firing the staples. This manoeuvre is, however, virtually impossible in the laparoscopic setting and to date has not been adequately addressed in most reported series in the literature.[13,14]

Port and Wound Site Recurrence

A recent concern is the possibility of port and wound site recurrence following laparoscopic resection for colorectal cancer.[15–18] To date, less than 20 cases of port site recurrence of cancer have been reported. The majority of these port site recurrences did not involve colorectal cancer patients. Also, these recurrences did not occur at the site of specimen retrieval. Additionally, most of these patients had advanced disease at the time of initial laparoscopy or at the time of recurrence. The explanation for port site recurrence remains unclear, and why recurrence should occur at the site of a distant port rather than at the wound site used for delivery of the specimen is not fully understood. One possible mechanism for port site recurrence is the transfer of exfoliated tumour cells via repetitive extraction and insertion of laparoscopic instruments. The small skin incision may provide a so-called "fertile ground" for tumour cell implantation and multiplication. Yet another possible mechanism may lie in the effects of the carbon-dioxide-induced pneumoperitoneum on tissue cell concentration, activation and spread. To date, there is no specific and convincing data to strongly refute or reinforce these theories. Suffice it to say that a tremendous amount of research is currently being performed to determine the causative mechanism of this phenomenon. Certainly, therefore, widespread acceptance of laparoscopic surgery for the potential cure of rectal cancer should not occur till these recognized problems are resolved.

Results of Comparative Studies

Several studies have been performed in the Department of Colorectal Surgery at the Singapore General Hospital comparing laparoscopic and conventional surgery for rectal cancer.

Laparoscopic Abdominoperineal Resection

A consecutive series of patients who underwent laparoscopic abdominoperineal resection (LAPR) were compared to patients who underwent conventional open abdominoperineal resection (CAPR).[19] Sixteen patients (8 females) and 11 patients (4 females) underwent LAPR and CAPR, respectively. There was no significant difference in the median operative time and amount of blood loss between the two groups. There was also no difference in the need for postoperative analgesics and time first stoma function, but the LAPR group showed significant improvement in starting fluids, diet, ambulation and discharge from hospital. Therefore, we concluded that the laparoscopic technique may be an acceptable alternative to conventional abdominoperineal resection for the patient requiring anal resection for rectal cancer.

Laparoscopic Anterior Resection

This study compared postoperative laparoscopic (LAR) with open anterior resection (OAR) in patients with rectosigmoid cancers.[20] Twenty patients (9 males) were allocated to the LAR group and 20 patients (6 males) to the OAR group. The median length of the distal margin of clearance beyond the tumour was similar in the two groups. The median numbers of lymph nodes harvested in the two groups were also similar. There was no significant difference in median operating time, blood loss and complication between the two groups. There were also no significant differences between LAR and OAR with regard to duration of parenteral analgesia, starting of fluids and solid diet after surgery, or time to first bowel movement and time to discharge from the hospital. The only significant difference was the length of incision in the two groups—5.5 (4–13) cm in the LAR group versus 18 (8–25) cm in the OAR group.

Systemic Immunity After Laparoscopic Cancer Surgery

Laparoscopic surgery is believed to produce an attenuated metabolic stress response and has a lower dampening effect on the immune response. We therefore performed a randomized controlled trial to study the impact of laparoscopic compared to conventional open surgery on the immune response in colorectal cancer.[21] Systemic immunity assessed by the T- and B-cell counts, the CD4/CD8 ratio, the NK cell counts, the IgG, IgM and IgA levels, the C3 and C4 levels and the white cell phagocytic activity (NBT test) were studied preoperatively and on the third postoperative day. Two hundred and thirty-six patients were randomized in the immune study. There was no difference in the mean response between the two surgical groups for each of the immune parameters studied. Our conclusion was therefore that there was no difference in the systemic immune response in laparoscopic colectomy when compared to open conventional surgery for colorectal cancer.

Conclusion

The primary goal in the surgical treatment of rectal cancer remains long term cure, low locoregional recurrence, low anastomotic problems and good functional outcome, and these goals should not be compromised when adopting laparoscopic techniques for the cure of rectal cancer.

The role of laparoscopic surgery for rectal cancer remains to be determined. The use of intraoperative laparoscopic ultrasound may help to better stage the disease and compensate for the lack of tactile sensation. A major hurdle is also the issue of specimen retrieval, which at present still necessitates the making of an incision. The possibility of tissue morcellation, which would avert an incision altogether, is also being researched into at the moment.

The adequacy of laparoscopic resection for cancer is obviously of paramount importance. Long term follow-up will be needed to determine if laparoscopic resection gives rise to the same morbidity, local recurrence, cure rate and overall mortality as open surgery.

Therefore, until some of these questions are answered, it is difficult at present to advocate routine laparoscopic surgery for cure of rectal cancer, unless it lies within the domain of a prospective randomized trial. The future of laparoscopic surgery for the treatment of benign diseases looks encouraging but, for cancer, it remains uncertain.

References

1. Philips EH, Franklin M, Carroll BJ, Fallas MJ, Ramos R and Rosenthal D. Laparoscopic colectomy, *Ann Surg* 1992; 216: 703–7.
2. Jacobs M, Verdeja JC and Goldstein HS. Minimally invasive colon resection (laparoscopic colectomy), *Surg Laparosc Endosc* 1991; 1: 144–50.
3. Monson JR, Darzi A, Carey PD and Guillou PJ. Prospective evaluation of laparoscopic assisted colectomy in an unselected group of patients, *Lancet* 1992; 340: 831–3.
4. Corbitt J. Preliminary results with laparoscopic guided colectomy, *Surg Laparosc Endosc* 1992; 2: 79–81.
5. Fowler DL and White SA. Laparoscopic assisted sigmoid resection, *Surg Laparosc Endosc* 1991; 1: 183–8.
6. Turnbull RB, Kyle K, Watson Fr and Spratt J. Cancer of the colon: the influence of the no-touch isolation technique on survival rates, *Ann Surg* 1967; 166: 420–5.
7. Goligher JC. *Surgery of the Anus, Rectum and Colon.* London: Balliere Tindall, 1975.
8. Eu KW, Milsom JW, Bohm B and Fazio VW. Is laparoscopic oncologic right colectomy feasible? (*abstract*). Society of American Gastrointestinal Endoscopic Surgeons (SAGES) Annual Scientific Meeting, 1995.
9. Decanini C, Milsom JW, Bohm B and Fazio VW. Laparoscopic oncologic abdomino-perineal resection, *Dis Colon Rectum* 1994; 37: 552–8.
10. Hoffman GC, Baker JW, Claibourne WF and Vansant JH. Laparoscopic assisted colectomy, *Dis Colon Rectum* 1993; 36: 28–34.
11. Falk PM, Beart RW Jr and Wexner SD. Laparoscopic colectomy: a critical appraisal, *Dis Colon Rectum* 1993; 36: 28–34.
12. Scott KW and Grace RH. Detection of lymph node metastasis in colorectal carcinoma before and after fat clearance, *Br J Surg* 1989; 76: 1165–7.
13. Umpleby HC, Fermon B, Symes MO and Williamson RCN. Viability of exfoliated colorectal carcinoma cells, *Br J Surg* 1984; 71: 659–63.

14. Skippes D, Jeffrey MJ, Cooper AJ, Alexander P and Taylor I. Enhanced growth of tumour cells in healing colonic anastomoses and laparotomy wounds, *Int J Colorect Dis* 1989; 4: 172–7.

15. Alexander RJT, Jaques BC and Mitchell KG. Laparoscopically assisted colectomy and wound recurrence, *Lancet* 1993; 341: 249–50.

16. Fusco MA and Paluzzi MW. Abdominal wall recurrence after laparoscopic assisted colectomy for adenocarcinoma of the colon—report of a case, *Dis Colon Rectum* 1993; 36: 858–61.

17. Nudka CC, Monson JRT, Menzies GWN and Darzi A. Abdominal wall metastases following laparoscopy, *Br J Surg* 1994; 81: 648–52.

18. Eu KW and Seow Choen F. Technical tips for preventing cancer cell shedding and spillage in laparoscopic anterior resection and colorectal anastomosis for cancer, *Techniq Coloproctol* 1997; 1: 90–2.

19. Seow-Choen F, Eu KW, Ho YH and Leong AFPK. A preliminary comparison of a consecutive series of open versus laparoscopic abdominoperineal resection for rectal adenocarcinoma, *Int J Colorect Dis* 1997; 12: 88–90.

20. Goh YC, Eu KW and Seow-Choen F. Early postoperative results of a prospective series of laparoscopic vs open anterior resection for rectosigmoid cancers, *Dis Colon Rectum* 1997; 40: 776–80.

21. Tang CL, Eu KW, Tai BC, Soh JGS, Machin D and Seow-Choen F. Randomised clinical trial of the effect of open versus laparoscopically assisted colectomy on systemic immunity in patients with colorectal cancer, *Br J Surg* 2001; 88: 801–7.

CHAPTER 39

Techniques of Colonic Pouch Construction

SR Brown and F Seow-Choen

Introduction

Sphincter-preserving surgery decreases the physical and psychological morbidity associated with a stoma. However, the re-establishment of intestinal continuity is not without its problems, with faecal incontinence, urgency and increased frequency of defecation—the so-called "anterior resection syndrome".

Is it possible to optimize anal function following anterior resection? Some aspects can be altered easily, while others cannot. Direct anal sphincter damage may be minimized by avoiding digital anal dilation, performing a rectal washout with a small proctoscope and using an appropriately sized stapler introduced gently into the anal canal.[1] Where possible oncologically, preservation of a minimal length of rectum will maintain function, possibly by retaining the normal rectoanal reflex pathways[2] but also by avoiding inclusion of the internal anal sphincter in the anastomosis. Meticulous surgical technique will minimize inadvertent damage to both the parasympathetic nerves of the anus and the rectum. Careful dissection must be carried out not only during mesorectal excision but also during division of the inferior mesenteric artery, where damage to the sympathetic plexus may occur. Finally, and most significantly, rectal compliance may be improved by formation of a colonic pouch. This has been said to act as a reservoir. However, it is more like a "pressure sump" dissipating any high intraluminal pressure waves generated within the noncompliant colon before they reach the anal canal and resulting in improved anal function.

The Colonic J-Pouch

In 1986, two French centres were the first to report the use of a colonic J-pouch after low anterior resection.[3,4] J-pouch construction reduces the severity of some of the symptoms of "anterior resection syndrome". Five randomized controlled trials comparing straight with pouch construction to date have shown that the frequency of defecation and the use of antidiarrhoeal medication at one-year postoperatively are reduced with a J-pouch.[5–10] Improvements of other symptoms of "anterior resection syndrome" are less obvious. Although urgency (or the inability to delay defecation by at least 15 minutes) is more frequent in the straight coloanal anastomosis patients, only one randomized controlled study has shown a statistically significant difference.[8] The pouch probably reduces incontinence by decreasing the stress on the anal sphincter by decreasing neorectal pressures.

Several studies have also alluded to evacuation difficulty, with 25% of patients with a pouch complaining of inadequate evacuation, requiring suppositories on alternate days to help evacuation.[6,11,12] Evacuation difficulties have been variously described as the inability to evacuate the pouch within 15 minutes, the sensation of incomplete evacuation or the necessity to use suppositories or enemas regularly to elicit defecation. Time since surgery may influence the proportion of patients with evacuation difficulties; an incidence of 15% was seen 1 month after surgery, increasing to 25% after 1 year. Because of these variations, the reported incidence of difficulties after pouch construction has ranged from 0% to as high as 78%.[9]

Technical Considerations

Despite the use of a colonic pouch, there remain problems with function after an anterior resection. However, function can be improved further by incorporating recent technical innovations.

Firstly, what size should the J-pouch be? Pouch sizes have varied from the more recent smaller 5 cm[13] to 12 cm.[3] The controversy concerns evacuation difficulties, implying that the incidence is higher with large colonic pouches. Evacuation difficulties may be avoided therefore by construction of a smaller pouch. Hida *et al.*[13] were the first to show that a smaller pouch evacuated more efficiently. In a later study, the same group reported that, one year after surgery, no patients with a 5 cm pouch complained of evacuation difficulty (defined as greater than 15 minutes spent on the toilet) and 98% were able to completely evacuate their bowels in one or two trips to the toilet.[14] Lazorthes *et al.*[15] compared 6 cm and 10 cm pouches in a prospective randomized study and found that the smaller pouch group required fewer laxatives and enemas for constipation and evacuation of the bowel. Interestingly, this difference was only seen 2 years after operation. This may be due to enlargement of the pouch with time. Using pouchography, Hida *et al.*[16] measured the width of the pouch at varying times after operation. Both the 5 cm pouch and 10 cm pouch groups increased in size with time, but the increase was substantially greater in the larger pouch group (1.9 times bigger at 1 year than at 3 months postoperatively, compared with 1.4 times bigger for the 5 cm pouch group). This group also showed that many pouch patients who experienced difficult evacuation also tended to have "floppy" pouches (shown by a decreased pouch-horizontal angle).[17] It is our experience that evacuation difficulties occur in pouches as they increase in size and become "baggy and floppy", which may be due to excessive intrapouch eddy currents. These would tend to dilate the pouch and would dilate a large pouch more easily than a small pouch (Laplace's law). With regard to "floppy" pouches it is relevant to point out that care must always be taken when tailoring the length of colon used for sacralization, as redundant loops proximal to the anastomosis may lead to problems of angulation.

Whether the sigmoid colon or the descending colon is to be used for the pouch is limited sometimes by vascular and other operative factors, particularly the presence of sigmoid diverticulosis restricting the use of the sigmoid colon. It used to be our opinion that the sigmoid colon should not be used if the functional outcome was to be optimized in colonic pouches.[18] This was for three reasons. Firstly, the sigmoid colon is a more propulsive organ than the descending colon and it was felt that a sigmoid pouch resulted in more motility dysfunction compared with the descending colon.[5,8] Secondly, a fatty sigmoid mesentery may occupy a significant proportion of a narrow pelvis, thereby limiting pouch expansion. Finally, sigmoid diverticulosis may limit the usefulness of the sigmoid colon as a pouch. Despite these theoretical disadvantages of using the sigmoid colon, a recently completed prospective randomized trial in our unit comparing sigmoid and descending colon pouches has shown no difference between the short- and the long-term functional outcome.[19] The sigmoid colon may therefore be used, provided it is healthy, as this avoids routine splenic flexure mobilization and simplifies the operation.

Although hand-sewn pouches may be made, the simplest method involves the use of a linear cutting stapler introduced through a colotomy at the apex of the "J" to form a side-to-side colonic anastomosis. The distal end is then used for the pouch-anal anastomosis.

Lazorthes *et al.*[3] described an abdominotrans-sphincteric approach whereby a synchronous abdominal resection is carried out along with mobilization of the lower rectum through a midline anosacral incision. Mobilization of the lower rectum was facilitated by dividing the sphincters posteriorly. These were then repaired after a stapled or hand-sewn ileoanal anastomosis had been carried out. Although the reported functional outcome after these procedures is good, we feel that a double-stapled coloanal anastomosis is technically simpler and quicker to carry out while giving comparable functional results.

We have recently reported the outcome after a laparoscopic assisted technique of ultralow anterior resection and pouch formation.[20] This technique results in a significantly shorter incision and lower analgesic requirements postoperatively while maintaining comparable functional and oncological outcomes. The disadvantage of prolonged operating times may not be an issue as experience with the procedure increases.

Advantages and Disadvantages of a J-Pouch

The colon J-pouch improves the functional outcome, most notably reducing bowel frequency and the need for antidiarrhoeal medication. But is this advantage over a straight anastomosis maintained over the long term? It is known that bowel dysfunction improves with time after a straight anastomosis.[9,10] This is presumably a result of the recovery of neorectal capacity as well as anal sphincter function and rectoanal reflexes. Studies looking at long-term function after straight and J-pouch construction agree that the incidence of incontinence is equal in the two groups after the first postoperative year.[9,10,21–23] With regard to frequency, all show an improvement with time in both groups. However, in some patients no significantly difference was seen after two years,[10,22,23] whereas a sustained difference was seen in the others.[9,21] Lazorthes *et al.*[9] pointed out that the term "frequency" does not reflect adequately the troublesome "fragmentation" or "clustering" associated with bowel evacuation. This interferes with both the employment and the social lifestyle of the patient. They found that fragmentation occurred in over 50% of straight coloanal anastomoses up to 24 months postoperatively, in contrast to only a minority in the pouch group. The numbers with two years' follow-up in this study were very small and it is difficult to draw accurate conclusions about long-term improved function. Nevertheless, the superior function within one year is without question. This in itself justifies pouch formation over straight coloanal anastomosis, as most patients undergoing such procedures have cancer and many will have a limited longevity. The quality of this limited lifespan therefore becomes paramount for the affected patient.

Another frequently cited advantage of a colonic J-pouch is the reduced anastomotic leak rate. The reported leak rates in studies that have compared the J-pouch and straight anastomosis range from 0 to 15% for the J-pouch patients and 5–27% for those with a straight anastomosis.[6,10] Anastomosis integrity and healing is dependent on several factors, the most important being tension, technique and vascular supply of the ends to be anastomosed. Although the first two factors cannot be investigated easily, the blood supply to the anastomotic ends can be measured using Doppler flowmetry. It is unlikely that the blood supply at the top of the anal canal is the critical factor. Unaffected blood flow to the site of the anastomosis of the pouch may be a favourable factor for anastomotic healing compared to decreased flow at the distal end of the straight colon. Other theoretical benefits of a pouch in reducing anastomotic leaks include the reduction in the pelvic dead space by the volume of the colonic pouch, preventing pelvic collections, and the extrapelvic position of the coloanal anastomosis allowing spontaneous evacuation of any fistulas via the anal canal, thereby minimizing pelvic sepsis. The only study comparing straight and pouch procedures that showed a significant difference in leak rates was by Hallböök *et al.*[6] They were not clear about who had temporary faecal diversion but the data given suggests that many of the leaks occurred in patients with straight anastomoses who were not defunctioned. Where all anastomoses were defunctioned there was no difference in leak rates between the groups.[11] With the existing data it is difficult to know whether the reduced leak rate after pouch formation compared with a straight anastomosis is due to the improved blood supply to the proximal bowel or due to the increased use of faecal diversion. However, no one can dispute that a pouch procedure with temporary faecal diversion will reduce the incidence of anastomotic complications.

Conclusion

The existing data allows several conclusions to be drawn. Certainly, the functional superiority of the J-pouch over the straight coloanal anastomosis is without doubt. However, this functional superiority is limited mainly to a reduction in the frequency of defecation and the J-pouch probably only remains superior for one to two years after operation, by which time the straight coloanal neorectum has adapted and symptoms have subsided in the majority of patients. This period is nevertheless the most critical in a large proportion of patients who may have a limited lifespan and in whom the quality of life during the early postoperative period is paramount. Although evacuation difficulties are a potential drawback of pouch formation, the incidence is reduced with smaller pouches. The optimum pouch size appears to be 5–6 cm. There is strong evidence that a J-pouch reduces the incidence of anastomotic complications compared with a straight coloanal anastomosis, although the data also suggests there that should be a period of temporary faecal diversion. Finally, recent evidence suggests that there is no functional difference when either the sigmoid or the descending colon is used in formation of the pouch. We would advocate the sigmoid colon if feasible, as this makes the operation simpler.

We feel that, until statistically sound large comparative studies are carried out that show clinically relevant results and significantly better function, a temporarily defunctioned small stapled colonic J-pouch-anal anastomosis using the sigmoid colon should be carried out after all total mesorectal excisions.

References

1. Ho YH, Tsang C, Tang CL, Eu KW and Seow-Choen F. Anal sphincter injuries from stapling instruments introduced transanally: randomized, controlled study with endoanal ultrasound and anorectal manometry, *Dis Colon Rectum* 2000; 43: 169–73.
2. Williams N and Seow-Choen F. Physiological and functional outcome following ultra-low anterior resection with colon pouch-anal anastomosis, *Br J Surg* 1998; 85: 1029–35.
3. Lazorthes F, Fages P, Chiotasso P *et al*. Resection of the rectum with construction of a colonic reservoir and colo-anal anastomosis for carcinoma of the rectum, *Br J Surg* 1986; 73: 136–8.
4. Parc R, Tiret E, Frileux P *et al*. Resection and coloanal anastomosis with colonic reservoir for rectal carcinoma, *Br J Surg* 1986; 73: 139–41.
5. Seow-Choen F and Goh HS. Prospective randomized trial comparing J colonic pouch-anal anastomosis and straight coloanal reconstruction, *Br J Surg* 82: 608–10.
6. Hallböök O, Pahlman L, Krog M *et al*. Randomized comparison of straight and colonic J pouch anastomosis after low anterior resection, *Ann Surg* 1996; 224: 58–65.
7. Hida J, Yasutomi M, Fujimoto K *et al*. Functional outcome after low anterior resection with low anastomosis for rectal cancer using the colonic J-pouch, *Dis Colon Rectum* 1996; 39: 986–91.
8. Ho YH, Tan M and Seow-Choen F. Prospective randomized controlled study of clinical function and anorectal physiology after low anterior resection: comparison of straight and colonic J pouch anastomosis, *Br J Surg* 1996; 83: 978–80.
9. Lazorthes F, Chiotasso P, Gamagani R *et al*. Late clinical outcome in a randomised prospective comparison of colonic J pouch and straight coloanal anastomosis, *Br J Surg* 1997; 84: 1449.
10. Joo JS, Latulippe JF, Alabaz O *et al*. Log-term functional evaluation of straight coloanal anastomosis and colonic J-pouch: is the fuctional superiority of the colonic J-pouch sustained? *Dis Colon Rectum* 1998; 41: 740–6.
11. Hallböök O, Nyström P and Sjödahl R. Physiological characteristics of straight and colonic J-pouch anastomoses after rectal excision for cancer, *Dis Colon Rectum* 1997; 40: 332–8.

12. Hallböök O and Sjödahl R. Comparison between the colonic J pouch-anal anastomosis and healthy rectum: clinical and physiological function, *Br J Surg* 1997; 84: 1437–41.

13. Hida J, Yasutomi M, Maruyama T *et al*. Functional outcome after low anterior resection with low anastomosis for rectal cancer using the colonic J-pouch: prospective randomized study for determination of optimum pouch size, *Dis Colon Rectum* 1996; 39: 986–91.

14. Hida J, Yasutomi M, Maruyama T *et al*. Indications for colonic J-pouch reconstruction after anterior resection for rectal cancer: determining the optimum level of anastomosis, *Dis Colon Rectum* 1998; 41: 559–63.

15. Lazorthes F, Gamagami R, Chiotasso P *et al*. Prospective randomized study comparing clinical results between small and large colonic J-pouch following coloanal anastomosis, *Dis Colon Rectum* 1997; 40: 1409–13.

16. Hida J, Yasutomi M, Maruyama T *et al*. Enlargement of colonic pouch after proctectomy and coloanal anastomosis: potential cause for evacuation difficulty, *Dis Colon Rectum* 1999; 42: 1181–8.

17. Hida J, Yasutomi M, Maruyama T *et al*. Horizontal inclination of the longitudinal axis of the colonic J-pouch: defining causes of evacuation difficulty, *Dis Colon Rectum* 1999; 42: 1560–8.

18. Seow-Choen F. Colonic pouches in the treatment of low rectal cancer, *Br J Surg* 1996; 83: 881–2.

19. Heah SM, Seow-Choen F, Eu KW, Ho YH and Tang CL. Randomized trial comparing using a sigmoid versus descending colonic J-pouch after total rectal resection, *Dis Colon Rectum* 2002; 45: 322–8.

20. Pasupathy S, Eu KW, Ho YH and Seow-Choen F. A comparison between a novel open versus laparoscopic assisted colonic pouches for rectal cancer, *Tech Coloproc* 2001; 5: 19–22.

21. Dehni N, Tiret E, Singland JD *et al*. Long-term functional outcome after low anterior resection: comparison of low colorectal anastomosis and colonic J-pouch-anal anastomosis, *Dis Colon Rectum* 1998; 41: 740–6.

22. Barrier A, Martel P, Gallot D *et al*. Long-term functional results of colonic J-pouch verses straight coloanal anastomosis, *Br J Surg* 1999; 86: 1176–9.

23. Ho YH, Seow-Choen F and Tan M. Colonic J-pouch function at six months versus straight coloanal anastomosis at 2 years: randomized controlled trial, *World J Surg* 2001; 25: 876–81.

CHAPTER 40

"Making It" as a Colorectal Surgeon

PL Roberts

When Professor Seow-Choen asked me to give this talk, I was not sure what I would tell a successful group of surgeons regarding how to achieve success. In fact, it seemed a bit like bringing coals to Newcastle or, to use a more modern analogy, after the most recent Masters tournament, a bit like giving Tiger Woods some tips on his short game.[1] Nevertheless I will attempt to discuss what it takes to "make it" as a colorectal surgeon.

I will assume that "making it" is synonymous with achieving "true success", which is synonymous with "personal satisfaction or happiness". A simple formula for satisfaction or happiness is to identify something more important than yourself and "go for it!" True happiness is also dependent on some degree of balance between family, career and outside interests. This balance is rarely achieved on a daily or weekly basis; but hopefully, over the course of a lifetime, we will have achieved some balance between these three competing elements.

We all have additional external constraints, including the fact that death is inevitable, the day is only 24 hours long, and with aging there is an inevitable decline in surgical skills. In our daily practice we all have increasing demands in the operating room, office and endoscopy suite. There has been a logarithmic increase in new technology and surgical techniques. There are increasing administrative tasks, increasing amounts of paperwork which encroach on teaching time, research time and other activities.

Peter Drucker, the management guru, has looked at the challenges faced by what he terms "knowledge workers".[2] Knowledge workers (such as doctors) have postponed entry into the workforce, joining it in their late 20s or early 30s. They have a life expectancy into the late 70s or early 80s and an average working life of up to 50 years, even though the average life expectancy of a successful business is generally only 30 years.

"Making it" then, according to Mr Drucker, depends on "managing oneself", which begins with a simple self-assessment:

- Who am I?
- What are my strengths?
- How do I work/perform?
- Where do I belong?
- What are my values?
- What is my contribution?

He suggests that we should concentrate on strengths, work on improving strengths, and waste little effort on improving areas of low competence since if takes far more work and energy to improve from incompetence to low mediocrity than it takes to improve from first-rate to excellent. Thus, if you are a great teacher, concentrate your efforts in a teaching institution teaching residents, students and fellows. If you are a gifted endoscopist, structure your practice around this. Mr Drucker suggests that we examine how we learn; in general, there are readers and listeners. John F. Kennedy was a "reader" and he surrounded himself with a large group of gifted writers such as Arthur Schlesinger Jr and Bill Moyers. These men would send extensive written documents to Mr Kennedy, who would read them prior to meeting with his staff. Upon assuming the presidency, Lyndon Johnson kept the same practice, and the results were disastrous for Mr Johnson's presidency as he was a listener, having come from the Senate, where his talents were as a legislator, a parliamentarian and a listener. Thus, if you learn best by reading, read journals, textbooks, etc., and if you learn best by listening, attend workshops, meetings, etc.

In addition to "managing oneself" I believe that our success and survival also depend on our response to change. We have all seen striking change in our practices, in the health care delivery system and in the practice of colorectal surgery itself. While adapting to change we should all maintain our commitment to the 3 Ps—our patients, our partners and professionalism.[3]

How do we apply these things to the field of colorectal surgery, including our office practice, endoscopy practice and the operating room in addition to research and writing, teaching responsibilities and membership in various professional societies and organizations? To apply these principles we must first look at the definition of "What is a surgeon?". The *Webster's* 1913 dictionary defined a surgeon as "one whose profession or occupation is to cure diseases or injuries of the body by manual operation".[4] In 1998 the definition had changed to "a medical specialist who practices surgery (a branch of medicine concerned with disease and conditions requiring or amenable to operative or manual procedure).[5] Thus there was a shift from a manual operation to a disease that could potentially require operation. And therefore there was a shift from a technician to a physician who treats a disease or, in more colloquial language, a shift from "cut 'n' cure" to disease management. This is perhaps most evident in the current treatment of rectal cancer, where the surgeon often makes the diagnosis, determines the applicability of neoadjuvant treatment, performs the operation and then performs the perioperative management and the subsequent follow-up. The surgeon is thus not just the "captain of the ship" in the operating room but the "captain of the ship" at large. The buck stops with the surgeon (to paraphrase Harry Truman, the 33rd president of the United States).

Well then, what makes an excellent surgeon? I believe the excellent surgeon has sound technical skills, safe judgment, a regard for patients' safety and high moral character. The latter may be defined as conscientiousness and dedication as reflected by the "mirror test"—that is, every morning, upon looking in the mirror to shave or put on lipstick, can the surgeon live with his or her decisions of the previous day? With respect to technical skills, Malcolm Gladwell, in an article in *The New Yorker* entitled "The Physical Genius", defines technical skills as being dependent on natural ability, practice and imagination.[6] Technical skills in surgery depend on hand–eye coordination and dexterity, but also on what the sociologist Bosk has called a "practical-minded obsession with the possibility and consequences of failure".[7] Bosk interviewed neurosurgery residents who were considered good residents and those who had been "cut from their training program". The good residents were concerned with the frequency of their mistakes, while the residents who had been terminated showed little insight into errors and blamed others or the system itself for any untoward events. While we all may not have the innate ability of Yo-Yo Ma, Wayne Gretsky or Michael Jordan, practice and the performance of repetitive events or tasks leads to competence. In surgery, I believe we must move away from "see one, do one, teach one" and more to training, as other industries such as the airline industry have done on simulators. The feasibility of transfer of skills from the bench to the cadaver model has been well documented.[8] In the field of laparoscopic surgery, concentrated didactic training in laparoscopy has improved skills. Imagination has been defined by Malcolm Gladwell as the ability to improvise, to cope skilfully with novel situations and be able to "feel the game". While sports analogies abound, innovators such as Sir Alan Parks in the development of the ileoanal pouch procedure have been able to apply a novel operation and to see possibilities where many others have not.

In surgery and in all fields of medicine, we must recognize that we function not so much as an individual but as a complex system and we need to understand the operation of the system to achieve success and provide the best outcome. It has been well documented that surgical outcomes improve with a higher surgical volume. We need to be aware of our results. To quote Peter Drucker: "If you can't measure it, you can't manage it." We must insist on and demand simple accurate contemporary data collection. And we need to measure both process and outcome.

Using the above, we may apply these principles and manage ourselves in the office, endoscopy suite and operating room. With respect to the other facets of our profession, particularly research and writing, the most important element is time. One must set aside or carve out a time for these activities. Self-imposed deadlines are very helpful. An optimal work environment should be identified, whether it is at home with a lined pad of paper, in the office early in the morning on the computer or during long airline trips to meetings. We must critically appraise the literature and be ruthlessly honest in the conduct of studies and reviews. While writing may be difficult at times, writer's block may not be all bad as some state it "inhibits the generation of ill-considered spontaneous rubbish".[10] Teaching and mentoring is extremely important. Working with medical students, residents and trainees helps to "keep us on our toes". Our membership in professional organizations and societies fosters collegiality, exchange of ideas in a noncompetitive collegial environment.

In summary, "making it" depends on self-knowledge and assessment and on concentrating on one's strengths. We must respond by being proactive and not reactive to change. We must maintain our commitment to patients, partnership and professionalism. It is only by doing this that we will create and not just experience the future.

References

1. Gawande AA. Creating the educated surgeon in the 21st century, *Am J Surg* 2001; 181: 551–6.
2. Drucker P. *Management Challenges for the 21st Century.*
3. Rothenberger DA. Mission impossible? Respond to the challenge, *Dis Colon Rectum* 1998; 41: 1083–6.
4. Porter N (ed.). *Webster's Revised Unabridged Dictionary.* Springfield, MA, 1913.
5. *Merriam-Webster's Collegiate Dictionary*, 10th ed. Springfield, MA, 1998.
6. Gladwell M. The physical genius, *The New Yorker*, Aug. 2, 1999.
7. Bosk C. *Forgive and Remember: Managing Medical Failure.* University of Chicago, 1979.
8. Reznich. *Am J Surg* 1999; 177: 167–70.
9. Rosser JC, Rosser LE and Salvagi RS. Objective evaluation of a laparoscopic surgical skill program for residents and senior surgeons, *Arch Surg* 1998; 133: 657–61.
10. Alderson D. On getting started, *Br J Surg* 2000; 87: 532–3.

CHAPTER 41

Managing Squamous Cell Carcinoma of the Anus

SM Heah

Introduction

Squamous cell carcinoma (SCC) of the anus is an uncommon tumour of the distal gastrointestinal tract and makes up 1.5% of all digestive system cancers.[1] Patients with SCC prior to the 1970s had an abdominoperineal resection (APR) leaving behind a permanent colostomy. Over the last three decades, first line management has progressed from surgery to radiation to combined chemoradiation therapy. This allows preservation of the anus, resorting to surgery only as a salvage procedure. Presently anal SCC remains the only gastrointestinal malignancy to be curable without definitive surgery.

Anatomy

The anus is divided into the anal canal and the anal margin. The anal canal extends from the junction of the levator ani muscle with the external anal sphincter (anorectal angle), proximally, to the intersphincteric groove (anal verge), which lies 1–2 cm distal to the dentate line.[2] The dentate line (white) is a visually identifiable border separating between squamous mucosa distally and a transitional area of squamous and nonsquamous mucosa. The lining of the anal canal is endodermal in origin, containing several types of epithelium. At its proximal extent, there is columnar epithelium. Moving distally towards the dentate line, there is transitional epithelium containing squamous and nonsquamous mucosa, followed by squamous epithelium only, once past the dentate line. Tumours arising distal to the dentate line are keratinizing SCC, whereas those appearing in the transitional zone above the dentate line are nonkeratizing SCC. Terms such as "junctional," "basaloid" and "cloacogenic" have caused confusion in the past and are now abandoned. The prognosis and management are similar for these two histological variants. Adenocarcinomas arise from the proximally located columnar epithelium and are treated in a similar fashion to rectal cancers.

Lymphatic spread of tumours above the dentate line is to the perirectal, para-aortic and internal iliac nodes (as in rectal cancers). Below the dentate line, tumour spreads to the inguinal and external iliac nodes.[3] It is thus mandatory to examine the anal region of patients presenting with inguinal lymphadenopathy.

The anal margin extends from the intersphincteric groove to an approximate 5 cm radius distally on the perineum.[4] This doughnut-shaped area is covered by nonkeratinizing squamous epithelium of ectodermal origin which changes to keratinizing squamous epithelium at its outer border at the perineal skin. Metastatic anal margin lesions usually spread to the inguinal nodes, but when these are obstructed they may be redirected to the pelvic nodes.

Presentation and Characteristics

Rectal bleeding occurring in half the patients is the most common symptom. The bleeding may be fresh and frequently attributed erroneously to haemorrhoidal bleeding. A third of patients present with either pain or the sensation of a rectal mass. However, up to a fifth are completely asymptomatic.[3] A history of anal warts is present in 50% of homosexual men but is found in only 20% of women and nonhomosexual men with anal cancer.[5]

Spread of tumor is by local extension, lymphatic and haematogenous dissemination. Involvement of sphincteric muscles is common at presentation. Adjacent structures most commonly involved are the prostate, seminal vesicles, bladder, and especially the vagina in women. Haematogenous spread occurs via the portal and systemic venous systems. Up to 8% of patients may have liver metastases, mostly involving tumours above the dentate line which drain via the portal system. Metastases to lung and bone are less frequent. Lymphatic spread is via inguinal (15%), pelvic and mesenteric nodes.

Staging

The size of the tumour is the most important prognostic feature. Eighty per cent of lesions less than 2 cm are cured, compared to less than 50% for those larger than 5 cm.[6] The probability of nodal involvement is also directly related to the size of the tumour, but it occurs more frequently in anal canal SCC compared to their anal margin counterparts. When dissection with or without radiotherapy was used to control nodal disease, Frost *et al.* demonstrated a 5-year survival rate of 44% for node-positive patients, compared to 74% for node negative patients.[7] Staging is based on the TNM system given below.

Primary tumor (T)

TX   Primary tumour cannot be assessed
T0   No evidence of primary tumour
Tis Carcinoma *in situ*
T1   Tumour 2 cm or less in greatest dimension
T2   Tumour more than 2 cm but not more than 5 cm in greatest dimension
T3   Tumour more than 5 cm in greatest dimension
T4   Tumor of any size invades adjacent organ(s), e.g. vagina, urethra, bladder (involvement of the sphincter muscles alone is not classified as T4)

Regional lymph nodes (N)

NX   Regional lymph nodes cannot be assessed
N0   No regional lymph node metastasis
N1   Metastasis in perirectal lymph node(s)
N2   Metastasis in unilateral internal iliac and or inguinal lymph
node(s) N3   Metastasis in perirectal and inguinal lymph nodes and/or
             bilateral internal iliac and/or inguinal lymph nodes

Distant metastasis (M)

MX   Distant metastasis cannot be assessed
M0   No distant metastasis
M1   Distant metastasis

Stage grouping

Stage 0	Tis	N0	M0
Stage I	T1	N0	M0
Stage II	T2	N0	M0
	T3	N0	M0
Stage IIIA	T1	N1	M0
	T2	N1	M0
	T3	N1	M0
	T4	N0	M0
Stage IIIB	T4	N1	M0
	Any T	N2	M0
	Any T	N3	M0
Stage IV	Any T	Any N	M1

Other Prognostic Factors

One study reported DNA ploidy to be an independent prognostic factor.[8] However, two other studies failed to support this.[9,10] Patients with low-grade tumours had 75% 5-year survival compared with 24% of cases with high-grade malignancy.[9] In a recent trial the female gender carried a favourable prognosis for improved local control and survival.[11]

Epidemiology

Perianal inflammation

It was previously believed that chronic irritation from anal fistulas, fissures haemorrhoids and inflammatory bowel disease, specifically Crohn's colitis,[12] could predispose one to anal SCC. However, recent studies have shown no relationship between the two.[5,13]

Sexual activity

The results of recent case control studies have shown that the vast majority of anal SCCs are due to human papillomavirus (HPV) infection. These studies demonstrated an increased risk for homosexual men and heterosexual men and women with multiple sexual partners, as well as those with sexually transmitted diseases like anal condylomata or gonorrhoea.[13,14] Women with cervical cancer which is linked with HPV infection have increased risks of developing anal SCC.[15] In a Danish study using polymerase chain reaction, HPV was found to be present in 88% of 394 anal cancers but not in any of the 20 cases with rectal adenocarcinoma.[16] Most often detected was HPV-16, the same strain linked to causation of cervical cancer. Anal cancers are frequently observed to arise from areas with anal intraepithelial neoplasm (AIN) with a well-established association with HPV infection. AINs with high grade appearance are especially at risk.[17]

The relationship of anal cancers to HIV infection and Aids is controversial, with some reporting an increased risk in men with Aids[18] and others showing no difference.[19] Nonetheless, HIV patients are frequently infected with HPV and AIN even without anal receptive intercourse.[14] Prospective trials are needed to determine if screening HIV seropositive patients with the Papanicolaou test to identify high grade dysplasia will be cost-effective in preventing anal cancers.

Smoking

Smoking increases anal cancer risk by 2–5 times and is independent of sexual practices.[20] This is further supported by the increased incidence of lung cancer in patients with anal cancer, occurring twice as frequently as those in the general population.[21]

Surgical Management

Due to the advancement in nonsurgical combined modality treatment of anal cancer, primary surgical management is now of historical interest. Three decades ago, abdominoperineal resection (APR) was the treatment of choice. APR involved the excision of the entire anorectum and necessitated the construction of a permanent colostomy. Initially, at the time of APR, a prophylactic formal inguinal nodal dissection was also performed. However, this was abandoned when found to be of limited benefit and was associated with high morbidity. Local recurrence in the pelvis or regional lymph node areas was as high as 40%.[22,23] Distant metastases occurred in 30% of cases.[23] Median survival was less than a year after either local or distant recurrence.[23] Five-year survival after APR depended on tumour and patient factors and ranged from 40 to 70%.[3,24,25]

Nonsurgical Management

Preliminary results

Nigro was the first to report (in 1974) that using preoperative chemoradiotherapy followed by APR could improve local control and overall survival.[26] Fluoropyrimidines, which potentiated the therapeutic effects of radiation on gastrointestinal cancers[27] and mitomycin with known anti-tumor effects against squamous cell tumors, were used in the initial Nigro protocol. Three patients underwent a radiation dose of 30 Gy in 15 fractions with a cobalt-60 source and concurrent chemotherapy consisting of 5-fluorouracil (5-FU) at 1000 mg/m^2 by continuous infusion on days 1–4, and mitomycin C at 15 mg/m^2 in an intravenous bolus on day 1. APR was carried out 6 weeks later in 2 of 3 patients and no tumour was found in the resected specimen. The third patient refused surgery but remained disease-free. When the data on 10 patients was updated in 1977, there was complete clinical disappearance of tumour in 60% and all cases had at least 50% tumour regression. Nine patients had APR and 6 specimens were found to be free of tumour. The treatment was well tolerated, with no cases interrupted by haematological toxicity.[28]

Michaelson *et al.*[29] used the Nigro protocol for 37 anal cancer patients. Fifty-two per cent had complete clinical response and 42% had at least a 50% decrease in tumour size. More than half the resected specimens had no evidence of tumour, with a fifth of the specimens showing only microscopic disease. The results prompted the conduct of many phase II studies.

Radiotherapy alone

Although a multimodality approach was used in the Nigro protocol, the role of chemotherapy was not yet established. In an effort to cut down the potential toxic effects of chemotherapy, radiotherapy by itself (60–65 Gy) was tried at many centres. Overall, these studies reveal local control rates between 56 and 100% and 5-year survival rates of 50–94%.[30–33] Complications included anal ulcers and strictures, with up to 15% requiring surgical correction. The results compare well with surgical series done in the past and most patients had a normal anorectal function.

Combined modality therapy

Phase II trials

The Eastern Cooperative Oncology Group (ECOG)[34] reported on 50 patients receiving 40 Gy of radiation to the anus and pelvis, followed by a 10–13 Gy tumour boost. Infusion of 5-FU and mitomycin C began with radiation on day 1, and a second infusion of 5-FU was given 28 days later. After 6–8 weeks, biopsy was performed, with the positive patients undergoing APR. Of the 46 patients evaluated, 34 (74%) had complete response and 11 had partial response. At a follow-up of 7 years, 80% had locoregional control and an overall survival of 58%. Severe toxic effects occurred in 37%, including 4% with life-threatening haematological toxicity. There were, however, no treatment-related deaths.

The RTOG/ECOG[35] reported on 79 patients treated with combined chemoradiation. The total dose was 40.8 Gy to the pelvis and perineum. Residual disease occurred in only 8 patients, who went on to receive an APR. Overall survival and local control rates at 3 years exceeded 70%. Acute side effects included skin reaction (86%), with mild nausea (25%) and diarrhoea (66%) making up the gastrointestinal effects. Severe neutropenia occurred in 3% but anal strictures were uncommon.

The Memorial Sloan Kettering Cancer Centre reported on 42 patients, each receiving mitomycin and 5-FU followed by a radiation dose of up to 30 Gy.[36] Five-year survival was 82%. Subsequent updates in this series reported that in 18 patients who had a positive biopsy after completion of chemoradiation, but did not undergo further treatment, half had no evidence of disease at the latest follow-up.[36,37] This important finding suggested that a positive biopsy at a short time posttreatment does not necessarily mean that recurrence will occur. It remains to be clarified as to the suitable interval after treatment whereby a positive biopsy would suggest recurrence and additional treatment recommended.

Randomized phase III trials

Whilst phase II trials demonstrated the efficacy and feasibility of combined modality treatment, the role of chemotherapy remained unproven. Three large recently conducted randomized trials convincingly proved the value of using concurrent chemotherapy.

1. The United Kingdom Coordinating Committee on Cancer Research (UKCCCR) Anal Cancer Trial Working Party randomized 585 patients into receiving 45 Gy of radiotherapy alone or in addition to concurrent 5-FU and mitomycin.[38] Good initial responders received a radiotherapy boost and poor responders underwent salvage surgery. This regime was accompanied with local failure of 36 versus 59% in the combined therapy and radiotherapy-only arms, respectively ($P < 0.0001$). Cancer-related death was significantly reduced in the combined arm (RR 0.71; $P = 0.02$), although overall survival was similar. Side effects were commoner in the combined arm but late morbidity was similar.

2. The European Organization for Research and Treatment of Cancer (EORTC) reported on 110 patients with locally advanced (T3-4, node-positive, or both) anal cancer.[11] Randomization was made to receiving radiotherapy alone (45 Gy plus a boost of 15–20 Gy) versus radiotherapy and concurrent 5-FU/mitomycin C. With chemotherapy, the remission rate increased from 54 to 80%. Local recurrence was 18% lower ($P = 0.02$), and a 32% higher colostomy-free interval rate could be achieved in the combined modality arm. Apart from an increased incidence of anal ulcers, the acute and late side effects were comparable in the two arms. However, the rates of metastases and overall survival (56%, 5 years) were similar in the two arms.

These studies provided clear and irrefutable evidence that the addition of chemotherapy was beneficial in the primary treatment of anal cancers.

However, two further issues remain:

The role of mitomycin

In one study of 291 patients,[39] each received radiotherapy (45–50.4 Gy) in addition to either 5-FU alone or 5-FU with mitomycin C. At 4 years' follow-up, patients in the mitomycin arm had lower colostomy rates (9% versus 22%, $P = 0.002$), higher colostomy-free survival (71% versus 59%, $P = 0.014$), and higher disease-free survival (73% versus 51%, $P = 0.0003$). Overall survival was similar. However, sepsis from neutropenia was more frequent in the mitomycin group (23% versus 7%, $P < 0.001$). A more recent update on this study shows that although the locoregional control remains superior, the colostomy-free survival no longer holds good for the mitomycin arm at 5 years' follow-up.[40]

The role of chemoradiotherapy for residual tumour

Salvage treatment consisting of pelvic radiotherapy (9 Gy) and 5-FU and cisplatin (100 mg/m^2) was used in treating 24 patients with residual disease after initial chemoradiotherapy.[39] Half the number of patients were rendered tumour-free, suggesting that salvage chemoradiotherapy can be tried first before salvage surgery with permanent colostomy. However, it remains unclear as to which patients with residual disease will require treatment.[36]

Therefore, the evidence is conclusive that combined modality treatment, consisting of radiotherapy with 5-FU and mitomycin, is the current standard of care. The management of patients with a positive biopsy but without clinical disease remains unsettled. One approach is to closely follow up these patients and implement salvage treatment only when clinical disease occurs.[41] However, further investigations are required to determine the optimal dose, timing and techniques before any particular strategy can be routinely recommended in this group of patients.

APR remains the surgical resection of choice for patients with recurrent disease.[42] In two recent studies, APR after locoregional recurrence produced 3-year and 5-year survival of 58[43] and 45%,[44] respectively.

Chemotherapy with cisplatin

Mitomycin causes significant haematological toxicity and has been associated with damage to the lungs, kidneys and bone marrow. A recent trial combined the use of radiotherapy with 5-FU and cisplatin in 35 patients, producing a 94% complete response and a low 14% requiring colostomy at 37 months' follow-up.[45] This was supported by a similar 95% response rate in another phase II ECOG study.[46] Further randomized trials comparing the use of 5-FU and mitomycin versus 5-FU and cisplatin in conjunction with radiotherapy are in progress and will hopefully clarify the benefits in terms of efficacy and reduced toxicity of cisplatin.

Radiotherapy dose and timing

Initial radiation fields include the primary tumour with an adequate margin and the regional nodes. The clinically-node-negative patient then receives additional radiotherapy to the primary tumour for eradication of the disease. The dose required that brings about the best results in terms of local recurrence, colostomy-free and overall survival is in the region of 55 Gy or greater.[47–49]

When a 2-week break was given between radiation treatments, a higher local failure and colostomy rate (23%)[50] resulted when compared to another study (11% colostomy rate) where there was no interval.[51] Therefore, radiation should not be interrupted within the confines of patient tolerance, as this may affect tumour control.

Managing HIV-positive patients

Generally, lower doses of combined therapy should be given and are relatively well tolerated. Radiotherapy includes a dose of 30 Gy in 15 fractions, along with $10 \, mg/m^2$ of mitomycin C and standard doses of 5-FU.[52] A clinical response of 100% can be achieved.[52] One can predict a decreased tolerance to treatment if the CD4 count drops below $200/mm^3$.

Metastatic disease

The liver is the most common site of distant metastatic disease. A combination of 5-FU and cisplatin has been used with mixed results although long term survival is possible.[53] However, relapse is common and prognosis is generally dismal.

Follow-up

Close clinical follow-up is essential, as salvage treatment has been associated with cure in a significant number of patients with locoregional recurrence. The patient should be seen at three-monthly intervals for the first three years after treatment.[41] No routine blood or radiological testing has ever been proven to be of benefit in the follow-up of these patients.

Anal margin cancer

The anal margin extends from the anal verge and includes the perianal tissues surrounding the anal canal. The incidence of malignant anal margin tumours is one fifth that of anal canal cancers. Squamous cell cancers here are staged as skin cancers elsewhere with a similarly favourable prognosis. Mostly they are well-differentiated, keratinized variants of squamous cell carcinoma. Metastases to distant sites and regional lymph nodes are less common than for anal canal cancers. Management depends on location, extent and patient factors, and options include local excision, APR and radiotherapy.[41]

Local excision

Local excision with at least a 1 cm margin will be sufficient to provide satisfactory local control and overall survival rates. A report from MSKCC[23] on 51 patients produced a 5-year disease specific survival rate of 88%. When locoregional recurrence occurred, they were managed satisfactorily by re-resection and inguinal lymphadenectomy. Results from patients who had APR were similar to those with local excision. The most important prognostic factors included tumour size and microscopic infiltration.[23]

Radiotherapy

The management of a tumour near the anal verge is less clearly defined. If adequate tumour excision involves removal of a significant amount of the anal sphincter that may cause incontinence, some will advocate an APR to ensure adequate tumour removal.[3] Others have used radiotherapy (50 Gy over 4 weeks or an 8-week split course), some with additional chemotherapy, to treat 29 patients with tumours within 5 cm of the anal verge.[54] Local control was achieved in 100% of tumours less than 5 cm, 70% of those between 5 and 10 cm, and 40% of those larger than 10 cm.

These good results led to the recommendation that radiotherapy be given as a first option before considering an APR. When tumour size exceeds 5 cm, the inguinal region should also be irradiated.

The current recommendations[41] are:

T1 and T2 tumours: radiotherapy and local excision.

More advanced tumours: combined radiotherapy (including the inguinal regions) and chemotherapy.

Locally recurrent tumour after radiotherapy may be treated by local excision with clear 1 cm margins. APR is reserved for tumours close to the anal verge involving the anal sphincters.

Radiotherapy is a suitable alternative to APR and can be part of a sphincter-sparing regimen when tumours lie close to the anal verge.

Summary

Malignant cancers of the anal canal and margin are rare but important tumours to detect, as the prognosis is good with appropriate treatment. There has been significant progress in the epidemiology and identification of high risk populations. The understanding of disease pathogenesis has enabled treatment strategies to be tuned towards sphincter-sparing techniques, thereby making significant improvements in the quality of life and prognosis of anal cancers. Future advances can be directed at studies designed to optimize the timing of administrating current techniques to manage such tumours.

References

1. Greenlee RT, Murray T, Bolden S *et al*. Cancer statistics, 1999, *CA Cancer J Clin* 2000; 50: 7–33.
2. Beck DE and Wexner SD. Anal neoplasms. In: Beck DE and Wexner SD (eds.), *Fundamentals of Anorectal Surgery*. New York: McGraw-Hill, 1992, pp. 222–37.
3. Beahrs OH and Wilson SM. Carcinoma of the anus, *Ann Surg* 1976; 184: 422–8.
4. Beck DE. Malignancies of the colon, rectum and anus. In: Beck DE (ed.), *Handbook of Colon and Rectal Surgery*. St Louis: Quality Medical Publishing, 1997, pp. 421–30.

5. Frisch M, Olsen JH, Bautz A and Melbye M. Benign anal lesions and the risk of anal cancers, *N Engl J Med* 1994; 331: 300–2.
6. Touboul E, Schlienger M, Buffat L *et al.* Epidermoid carcinoma of the anal canal: results of curative-intent radiation therapy in a series of 270 patients, *Cancer* 1994; 73: 1569–79.
7. Frost DB, Richards PC, Montague ED *et al.* Epidermoid cancer of the anorectum, *Cancer* 1984; 53: 1285–93.
8. Shepherd NA, Scholefield JH, Love SB *et al.* Prognostic factors in anal squamous carcinoma: a multivariate analysis of clinical, pathological, and flow cytometric parameters in 235 cases, *Histopathology* 1990; 16: 545–55.
9. Goldman S, Auer G, Erhardt K *et al.* Prognostic significance of clinical stage, histologic grade, and nuclear DNA content in squamous-cell carcinoma of the anus, *Dis Colon Rectum* 1987; 30: 444–8.
10. Scott NA, Beart RW Jr, Weiland LH *et al.* Carcinoma of the anal canal and flow cytometric analysis, *Br J Cancer* 1989; 60: 56–8.
11. Bartelink H, Roelofsen F, Eschwege F *et al.* Concomitant radiotherapy and chemotherapy is superior to radiotherapy alone in the treatment of local advanced anal cancer: results of a phase III randomized trial of the European Organisation for Reseach and Treatment of Cancer Radiotherapy and Gastrointestinal Cooperative Groups, *J Clin Oncol* 1997; 15: 2040–9.
12. Slater G, Greenstein A and Aufses AH Jr. Anal carcinoma in patients with Crohn's disease, *Ann Surg* 1984; 199: 348–50.
13. Holly EA, Whittemore AS, Aston DA, Ahn DK, Nickoloff BJ and Kristiansen JJ. Anal cancer incidence: genital warts, anal fissure or fistula, haemorrhoids, and smoking, *J Natl Cancer Inst* 1989; 81: 1726–31.
14. Critchlow CW, Surawicz CM, Holmes KK *et al.* Prospective study of high grade anal squamous neoplasia in a cohort of homosexual men: influence of HIV infection, immunosuppression and human papillomavirus infection, *AIDS* 1995; 9: 1255–62.
15. Rabkin CS, Biggar RJ, Melbye M *et al.* Second primary cancers following anal and cervical carcinoma: evidence of shared etiological factors, *Am J Epidemiol* 1992; 136: 54–8.
16. Frisch M, Glimelius B, van den Brule AJ *et al.* Sexually transmitted infection as a cause of anal cancer, *N Engl J Med* 1997; 337: 1350–8.
17. Tilston P. Anal human papillomavirus and anal cancer, *J Clin Pathol* 1997; 50: 625–34.

18. Melbye M, Cote TR, Kessler L *et al.* High incidence of anal cancer among AIDS patients; the AIDS/Cancer Working Group, *Lancet* 1994, 343: 636–9.

19. Goedert JJ, Cote TR, Virgo P *et al.* Spectrum of AIDS-associated malignant disorders, *Lancet* 1998; 351: 1833–9.

20. Daling JR, Sherman KJ, Hislop TG *et al.* Cigarette smoking and the risk of anogenital cancer, *Am J Epidemiol* 1992; 135: 180–9.

21. Frisch M, Olsen JH and Melbye M. Malignancies that occur before and after anal cancer: clues to their etiology, *Am J Epidemiol* 1994; 140: 12–19.

22. Clark J, Petrelli N, Herrera L *et al.* Epidermoid carcinoma of the anal canal, *Cancer* 1986; 57: 400–6.

23. Greenall MJ, Quan SHQ, Urmacher C *et al.* Treatment of epidermoid carcinoma of the anal canal, *Surg Gynecol Obstet* 1985; 161: 509–17.

24. Boman BM, Moertel CG, O'Connell MJ *et al.* Carcinoma of the anal canal: a clinical and pathological study of 188 cases, *Cancer* 1984; 54: 114–25.

25. Singh R, Nime F and Mittelman A. Malignant epithelial tumors of the anal canal, *Cancer* 1981; 48: 411–15.

26. Nigro ND, Vaitkevicius VK and Considine B Jr. Combined therapy for cancer of the anal canal: a preliminary report, *Dis Colon Rectum* 1974; 17: 354–6.

27. Childs DS Jr, Moertel CG, Holbrook MA *et al.* Treatment of unresectable carcinoma of the stomach with a combination of 5-fluorouracil and radiation, *AIR Am J Roentgenol* 1968; 102: 541–4.

28. Buroker TR, Nigro N and Bradley G. Combined therapy for cancer of the anal canal: a follow-up report, *Dis Colon Rectum* 1977; 20: 677–8.

29. Michaelson RA, Magill GB, Quan SHQ, Leaming RH, Nikrui M and Stearns MW. Preoperative chemotherapy and radiation therapy in the management of anal epidermoid carcinoma, *Cancer* 1983; 51: 390–5.

30. Cummings BJ, Keane TJ, O'Sullivan B, Wong CS and Catton CN. Epidermoid anal cancer: treatment by radiation alone or by radiation and 5-fluorouracil with and without mitomycin C, *Int J Radiat Oncol Biol Phys* 1991; 21: 1115–25.

31. Martenson JA Jr and Gunderson LL. External radiation therapy without chemotherapy in the management of anal cancer, *Cancer* 1993; 71: 1736–40.

32. Salmon RJ, Fenton J, Asselain B *et al.* Treatment of epidermoid anal canal cancer, *Am J Surg* 1984; 147: 43–8.

33. Touboul E, Schlienger M, Buffat L *et al.* Conservative versus nonconservative treatment of epidermoid carcinoma of the anal canal for tumors longer than or equal to 5 centimeters: a retrospective comparison, *Cancer* 1995; 75: 786–93.

34. Martenson JA, Lipsitz SR, Lefkopoulou M *et al.* Results of combined modality therapy therapy for patients with anal cancer (E7283): an Eastern Cooperative Oncology Group study, *Cancer* 1995; 76: 1731–6.

35. Sischy B, Doggett RL, Krall JM *et al.* Definitive irradiation and chemotherapy for radiosensitization in the management of anal carcinoma: interim report on radiation therapy; Oncology Group Study No. 8314, *J Natl Cancer Institute* 1989; 81: 850–6.

36. Miller EJ, Quan SH, Thaler T *et al.* Treatment of squamous cell carcinoma of the anal canal, *Cancer* 1991; 67: 2038–41.

37. Enker WE, Heilweil M, Janov AJ *et al.* Improved survival in epidermoid carcinoma of the anus in association with preoperative multidisciplinary therapy, *Arch Surg* 1986; 121: 1386–90.

38. UKCCCR Anal Cancer Trial Working Party. Epidermoid anal cancer: results from the UKCCCR randomized trial of radiotherapy alone versus radiotherapy, 5-fluorouracil, and mitomycin, *Lancet* 1996; 348: 1049–54.

39. Flam M, John M, Pajak TF *et al.* Role of mitomycin in combination with fluorouracil and radiotherapy, and of salvage chemoradiation in the definitive nonsurgical treatment of epidermoid carcinoma of the anal canal: results of phase III randomized intergroup study, *J Clin Oncol* 1996; 14: 2527–39.

40. Flam M, John M, Pajak TF *et al.* Role of mitomycin in combination with fluorouracil and radiotherapy, and of salvage chemoradiation in the definitive nonsurgical treatment of epidermoid carcinoma of the anal canal: results of a phase III randomized intergroup study, *Classic Papers Curr Comm Highlights Gastrointestinal Cancer Res* 1999; 3: 539–52.

41. Chawla AK and Willett CG. Squamous cell carcinoma of the anal canal and anal margin, *Hematol Oncol Clin North Am* 2001 Apr; 15(2): 321–44.

42. Ryan DP and Mayer RJ. Anal carcinoma: histology, staging, epidemiology, treatment, *Curr Opin Oncol* 2000; 12: 345–52.

43. Pocard M, Tiret E, Nugent K, Dehni N and Parc R. Results of salvage abdominoperineal resection for anal cancer after radiotherapy, *Dis Colon Rectum* 1998; 41: 1488–93.

44. Allal AS, Laurencet FM, Reymond MA, Kurtz JM and Marti MC. Effectiveness of surgical salvage therapy for patients with locally uncontrolled anal carcinoma after sphincter-conserving treatment, *Cancer* 1999; 86: 405–9.

45. Doci R, Zucali R, La Monica G *et al*. Primary chemoradiation therapy with fluorouracil and cisplatin for cancer of the anus: results in 35 consecutive patients, *J Clin Oncol* 1996; 14: 3121–315.

46. Martenson JA, Lipstitz SR, Wagner H Jr *et al*. Initial results of phase II trial of high dose radiation therapy, 5-fluorouracil, and cisplatin for patients with anal cancer (E4292): an Eastern Coorperative Oncology Group study, *Int J Radiat Oncol Biol Phys* 1996; 35: 745–9.

47. Constantinou EC, Daly W, Fung CY, Willet CG, Kaufman DS and DeLaney TF. Time dose considerations in the treatment of anal cancer, *Int J Radiat Oncol Biol Phys* 1997; 39: 651–7.

48. Hughes LL, Rich TA, Delclos L *et al*. Radiotherapy for anal cancer: experience from 1979–1987, *Int J Radiat Oncol Biol Phys* 1989; 17: 1153–60.

49. Myerson RJ, Shapiro SJ, Lacey D *et al*. Carcinoma of the anal canal, *Am J Clin Oncol* 1995; 18: 32–9.

50. John M, Pajak T, Flam M *et al*. Dose acceleration in chemoradiation for anal cancer: preliminary results of RTOG 9208, *Cancer J Sci Am* 1996; 2: 205.

51. John M. Dose escalation without split-course chemoradiation for anal cancer: results of a phase II RTOG study, *Proceedings of the American Society of Theurapeutic Radiology and Oncology*. Orlando, 1997.

52. Peddada AV, Smith DE, Rao AR, Frost DB and Kagan AR. Chemotherapy and low dose radiotherapy in the treatment of HIV-infected patients with carcinoma of the anal canal, *Int J Radiat Oncol Biol Phys* 1997; 37: 1101–5.

53. Jaiyesimi IA and Pazdur R. Cisplatin and 5-fluorouracil as salvage therapy for recurrent metastatic squamous cell carcinoma of the anal canal, *Am J Clin Oncol* 1993; 16: 536–40.

54. Cummings BJ, Keane TJ, Hawkins NV *et al*. Treatment of perianal carcinoma by radiation (RT) or radiation plus chemotherapy (RTCT) (*abstract*), *Int J Radiat Oncol Biol Phys* 1986; 12: 170.

CHAPTER 42

Fibre and Colorectal Neoplasia: What Is the Truth?

A Skandarajah, S Sengupta, P Gibson and JJ Tjandra

Abstract

Dietary risk factors, including fibre intake, are thought to be pre-eminent in the pathogenesis of colorectal cancer (CRC). The evidence regarding the role of dietary fibre in CRC is confusing, and the aim of this review is to summarize the current state of knowledge. English language publications on dietary fibre and CRC were identified by MEDLINE search. Epidemiological evidence in the form of case control studies was found to provide some evidence in favour of a protective role of fibre, but longitudinal studies and randomized controlled studies failed to confirm this. Animal studies suggest that fibre may vary in its effect, depending on what physical or chemical subtype is being studied. In summary, current evidence suggests that fibre supplementation cannot be recommended for the prevention of CRC. However, the lifelong consumption of a "high-fibre" non-Western diet may be protective, and may also provide other health benefits. Future efforts may identify patient subgroups that may have particular abnormalities in their colonic luminal environment that may be amenable to correction by the addition of dietary fibre.

Introduction

Colorectal cancer is a highly prevalent malignancy, with significant health costs. Preventive efforts have focused on dietary risk factors, most notably dietary fibre. Burkitt's original postulate[1] about the protective role of fibre in colorectal carcinogenesis appears to be intuitive and is supported by epidemiological data. Recent negative clinical trials, however, have cast doubts on this premise. The aim of this review is to examine the current evidence regarding fibre and colorectal neoplasia.

Defining Fibre and Proposed Mechanisms of Action in Preventing Colorectal Neoplasia

One of the difficulties in evaluating data regarding fibre lies in its definition. In terms of colorectal neoplasia prevention, a functional definition of fibre lies in its "indigestibility".[2] Hence, this may include anything from resistant starch to nonstarch polysaccharides and nonpolysaccharide plant wall components (such as lignins, cutin and suberin).[3]

Few studies define the specific fibre type used and, in many instances, no differentiation is made between dietary fibre and fibre-rich foods. The latter contain substances such as antioxidants and vitamins, which may have a confounding role in colorectal neoplasia. For the purposes of evaluating a protective role of fibre, there may also be differences between fibre supplementation to a "high-risk Western" processed diet and a fibre-rich "low-risk primitive" diet containing unprocessed foods.

Dietary fibre results in decreased transit time and increased stool bulk,[4] potentially decreasing the concentration and contact time of putative carcinogens that the colonic mucosa is exposed to. Adsorption of bile salts[5,6] and other mutagens such as those present in charred meat[7] are other postulated protective actions of fibre. In addition, fermentation of fibre by colonic bacteria produces substances such as the short chain fatty acid, butyrate, which promotes apoptosis and induces differentiation *in vitro*.[8–13]

Epidemiological Studies

The majority of the data regarding fibre has been collected from epidemiological rather than interventional studies. Although this is the data that best supports fibre's protective role in colorectal neoplasia, these studies are also the least reliable in determining the nature of the fibre type, the amount ingested and the presence of confounding factors.

Population-based correlation studies generally suggest a negative correlation between fibre intake and colorectal cancer but are frequently weakened by adjustment for variables such as meat or fat intake.[14–18] Simple chronological assessments correlated a decline in fibre intake with mortality incidence secondary to colorectal cancer in various populations.

Case control studies have involved identifying incident cases of colorectal neoplasia and examining dietary exposures using food frequency questionnaires and composition tables and comparing demographically matched controls over defined time periods. Being retrospective, recall bias is inherent in these studies and may artificially create a false association. Recent case control studies are summarized in Table 1. Most studies support a protective role of fibre and, when classified according to source, vegetable fibre generally has the lowest odds ratios. However, the role of other substances in vegetables in colorectal neoplasia means that they must

Table 1. Case control studies investigating the effect of dietary fibre on colorectal neoplasia (1990–2002).

Reference	Finding
Levi *et al.*, 2001[19]	P
Breuer-Katschincki *et al.*, 2001[20]	P
Ghadiran *et al.*, 1997[21]	P
Slattery *et al.*, 1997[22]	P
Almendingen *et al.*, 1995[23]	P
Kampman *et al.*, 1995[24]	P
Kono *et al.*, 1993[25]	Nil
Little *et al.*, 1993[26]	P
Neugut *et al.*, 1993[27]	P
Sandler *et al.*, 1993[28]	Nil
Steinmetz and Potter, 1993[29]	Nil
Zaridze *et al.*, 1992[30]	P
Arbman *et al.*, 1992[31]	P
Iscovich *et al.*, 1992[32,33]	P
Hu *et al.*, 1991[34]	P
Benito *et al.*, 1990/1991[35,36]	P/E
Freudenheim *et al.*, 1990[37]	P
Gerhardsson de Verdier *et al.*, 1990[38]	P
Whittlemore *et al.*, 1990[39]	P

P = protective; E = enhances; Nil = no effect of fibre

Table 2. Longitudinal studies investigating the effect of dietary fibre on colorectal neoplasia (1990–2002).

Reference	Finding
Fuchs *et al.*, 1999[42]	Nil
Kato *et al.*, 1997[43]	Nil
Gaard *et al.*, 1996[44]	Nil
Giovanucci *et al.*,1996[45]	Nil
Goldbohm *et al.*, 1994[46]	Nil
Steinmetz *et al.*, 1994[47]	Nil
Giovanucci *et al.*, 1992[48]	Nil
Shibata *et al.*, 1992[49]	Nil
Thun *et al.*, 1992[50]	P
Willet *et al.*, 1990[51]	Nil

Nil = no effect of fibre; P = protective

be considered as potential confounders. There are also studies that show benefit for dietary fibre and cereal fibre but not for vegetable fibre.

Two meta-analyses reviewing case control studies suggested an overall protective benefit of fibre in the prevention of colorectal neoplasia. Trock *et al.*[40] evaluated 12 case control studies and estimated a combined odds ratio of 0.57 (CI 95% = 0.50–0.64) for those who had a high fibre and vegetable intake. Howe *et al.*,[41] who analysed 13 case control studies, initially concluded a risk of 0.53 (0.47–0.61) but the quality of the individual studies was not considered and reanalysis revealed an odds ratio close to 1, implying no protective effect.

Longitudinal studies have the benefit of being prospective and hence eliminate recall bias, but the larger numbers and prolonged follow-up make these studies more difficult to run. Accurate assessment of dietary fibre intake is also a problem, as the food frequency questionnaires and food composition tables employed may become outdated over the time course of the study. Table 2 summarizes the more recent longitudinal studies, which generally are equivocal or nonsupportive of fibre protecting against colorectal neoplasia.

Interventional Studies

Randomized controlled trials provide the most reliable clinical data as interventions are clearly defined, and confounding factors are controlled for.

Table 3. Randomized controlled trials investigating the effect of fibre on colorectal neoplasia (1989–2002).

Reference	Finding
Schatzkin et al., 2000[52]	Nil
Alberts et al., 2000[53]	Nil
Bonithon-Kopp et al., 2000[54]	E
Maclennan et al., 1995[55]	Nil
McKeown-Eyssen et al., 1994[56]	Nil
DeCosse et al., 1989[57]	Nil

E = enhanced; Nil = no effect of fibre

However, human trials have several limitations. They evaluate groups that are already at high risk for carcinogenesis (postpolypectomy, familial adenomatous polyposis and older patients) and, to date, have had relatively short durations of follow-up with small numbers of patients studied (58–2079). Compliance in the intervention group and contamination in the control group are other potential problems that may lead to a falsely negative result. Adenoma recurrence is usually used as the end point rather than the perhaps more pertinent carcinoma incidence, but the latter has the inherent ethical issues regarding nonintervention with adenomas.

To date, six randomized control trials have been published, and they are summarized in Table 3. All trials generally indicate that increased dietary fibre in high-risk groups is not effective in reducing adenoma recurrence. It must also be noted that some intervention groups coupled fibre and vitamin supplementation or fat intake reduction, which complicates interpretation.

In a recent large trial, Schatzkin et al.[52] recruited 2079 patients aged 35 years or older. The intervention group was counselled to increase their dietary fibre to a mean of 17.4 g/100 kcal and decrease fat intake to 23.8%. Changes of similar but decreased magnitude occurred amongst the control group. With adenoma recurrence as the end point, 90% were compliant with follow-up colonoscopy and recurrence at 4 years was shown to be 39.7% in the intervention group compared with 39.5% in the control group.

A similar study by Alberts et al.[53] recruited 1429 patients aged 40–80 years and employed high (13.5 g) and low (2 g) wheat bran supplements daily in the intervention and control groups, respectively. Compliance with supplements (defined as 75% or more of the dietary supplements) was lower in the intervention group at 70%, compared to 80% amongst the controls. Recurrent adenomas were demonstrated in 35.9% in the intervention group versus 36.3% in the controls, with a lower recurrence rate of statistical significance amongst men on subgroup analysis.

The most recent trial, reported by Bonithon-Kopp[54] *et al.*, employed 3.5 g of ispaghula husk supplementation as the intervention and calculated an adjusted odds ratio of 1.67 (1.01–2.76; $p = 0.042$). The statistical power of the implied deleterious effect of fibre is reduced by low recruitment numbers ($n = 198$) but nonetheless raises the issue of potential harm caused by supplemental fibre added to a pre-existing Westernized diet.

The only trial to demonstrate any protective effect of fibre supplementation was the Australian Polyp Prevention Project,[55] which on subgroup analysis showed a lower recurrence of large polyps in the high-fat high-fibre intervention group. The exact significance of this finding is difficult to interpret in the context of the other negative results.

Animal

Animal studies have the benefit of being able to analyze individual dietary components by means of well-designed interventional diets, and have less ethical and time constraints compared to human interventions. However, it is difficult to assess the validity of extrapolating results of such studies, given the differences from humans in terms of the gastrointestinal physiology, the chemical induction of colorectal neoplasia and the artificial interventional diets used. Additionally, the diversity of design, intervention and end points make comparisons difficult.

Recent animal studies suggest a generally protective trend for fibre.[58–73] However, interventions involve varying fibre types, with some studies demonstrating more specifically protection from poorly fermented fibres such as wheat bran and cellulose, while an enhancement of neoplasia was seen with resistant starch and oat bran. This suggests that the effects of dietary fibres on colorectal neoplasia risk may depend upon specific physicochemical characteristics.

Studies in our laboratory using a chronic colonic intubation model[74] have assessed the effects of luminal interventions on early tumorigenic events. These experiments (Sengupta, unpublished results) demonstrated a protective effect of infusions per se, suggesting a physical basis such as dilution or mucosal cleansing. In addition, luminal infusions of butyrate led to a greater protective effect. Taken together, these studies reinforce the view that fibres that replicate these luminal alterations in the colon may be the most protective. Conversely, some fibre types may have luminal effects that are ineffective, or perhaps even procarcinogenic.

Current Recommendations

So, are we any closer to advocating a protective role of fibre in colorectal neoplasia? Certainly, the interventional studies fail to demonstrate any clear protective effect of fibre supplementation in patients who have an established neoplasia risk, and a habitual Western diet. Particularly in view of the findings of the most recent trial, which found an enhanced risk from fibre supplementation, such a course of action cannot be recommended.

It should be kept in mind, however, that these trials have not truly addressed the effect of a long-term diet that habitually contains unprocessed foods rich in fibre and other potentially beneficial nutrients. The epidemiological data, despite their inherent flaws, may provide the most reliable information on this, and suggest some benefit in terms of colorectal neoplasia. Additionally, dietary fibre has protective effects in vascular disease, hypertension and hypercholestraemia, which need to be considered in any dietary recommendation.

Future Directions

Limitations abound in attempts to determine fibre's role in colorectal neoplasia. To reiterate, small numbers studied, imprecise quantification of dietary intake, fibre subtype and compliance, confounding variables and ethical restraints plague prospective researchers.

The current literature involves interventional studies in those patients who are already at high risk. In such targeted populations, it is difficult to draw conclusions regarding fibre alone. Further subgroup analysis may identify more susceptible groups but this requires elucidation of the mechanism of action of fibre on the colonic mucosa. If and when colonic carcinogens are identified, the effects of dietary fibre on these substances can also be addressed. It appears that the most immediate source for enhancing our understanding in these areas are *in vitro* studies, with extrapolation to *in vivo* animal studies.

References

1. Burkitt DP. Related-disease-related cause? *Lancet* 1969; 2: 1229–31.
2. Kaaks R and Riboli E. Colorectal cancer and intake of dietary fibre: a summary of the epidemiological evidence, *Eur J Clin Nutr* 1995; 49 (Suppl 3): S10–7.
3. Harris PJ and Ferguson LR. Dietary fibre: its composition and role in protection against colorectal cancer, *Mutat Res* 1993; 290: 97–110
4. Burkitt DP, Walker AR and Painter NS. Effect of dietary fibre on stools and the transit-times, and its role in the causation of disease, *Lancet* 1972; 2: 1408–12.
5. Kritchevsky D. Cereal fibres and colorectal cancer: a search for mechanisms, *Eur J Cancer Prev* 1998; 7: S33–9.
6. Lupton JR and Turner ND. Potential protective mechanism of wheat bran fiber, *Am J Med* 1999; 106: 24S–7S.
7. Lipkin M, Reddy B, Newmark H and Lamprecht SA. Dietary factors in human colorectal cancer, *Annu Rev Nutr* 1999; 19: 545–86.
8. Velaquez OC, Lederer HM and Rombeau JL. Butyrate and the colonocyte: production, absorption, metabolism, and therapeutic implications, *Adv Exp Med Biol* 1997; 427: 123–34.
9. McBain JA, Eastman A, Nobel CS and Mueller GC. Apoptotic death in adenocarcinoma cell lines induced by butyrate and other histone deacetylase inhibitors, *Biochem Pharmacol* 1997; 53: 1357–68.
10. Marchetti C, Migliorati G, Moraca R *et al*. Deoxycholic acid and SCFA-induced apoptosis in the human tumor cell-line HT-29 and possible mechanisms, *Cancer Lett* 1997; 114: 97–9.
11. Hague A, Elder DJ, Hicks DJ and Paraskeva C. Apoptosis in colorectal tumour cells: induction of short chain fatty acids butyrate, propionate and acetate and by the bile salt deoxycholate, *Int J Cancer* 1995; 4: 359–64.
12. Archer S, Meng S, Wu J, Johnson J, Tang R and Hodin R. Butyrate inhibits colon carcinoma cell growth through two distinct pathways, *Surgery* 1998; 124: 248–53.
13. Sowa Y and Sakai T. Butyrate as a model for "gene-regulating chemoprevention and chemotherapy", *Biofactors* 2000; 12(1–4): 283–7.
14. McKeown-Eyssen GE and Bright-See E. Dietary factors in colon cancer: international relationships, *Nutr Cancer Inst* 1984; 6: 160–70.

15. Liu K, Stamler J, Moss D, Garside D, Persky V and Soltero I. Dietary cholesterol, fat, fibre, and colon-cancer mortality: analysis of international data, *Lancet* 1979; 2: 782–5.
16. Irving D and Drasar BS. Fibre and cancer of the colon, *Br J Cancer* 1973; 28: 462–3.
17. Armstrong B and Doll R. Environmental factors and cancer incidence and mortality in different countries, with special reference to dietary practices, *Int J Cancer* 1975; 15: 617–31.
18. McKeown-Eyssen GE and Bright-See E. Dietary factors in colon cancer; international relationships: an update, *Nutr Cancer* 1985; 7: 251–3.
19. Levi F, Pasche C, Lucchini F and La Vecchia C. Dietary fibre and the risk of colorectal cancer, *Eur J Cancer* 2001; 37(16): 2091–6.
20. Breuer-Katchinski B, Nemes K, Marr A, Rump B, Leiendecker N, Breuer N, Goebell H *et al.* Colorectal adenomas and diet, *Digestive Disease and Sciences* 2001; 46: 86–95.
21. Ghadiran P, Lacroix A, Maisoneuve P *et al.* Nutritional factors and colon carcinoma: a case control study involving French Canadians in Montreal, Quebec, Canada, *Cancer* 1997; 80: 858–64.
22. Slattery ML, Potter JD, Coates A *et al.* Plant foods and colon cancer: an assessment of specific foods and their related nutrients (United States), *Cancer Causes Control* 1997; 8: 575–90.
23. Almendingen K, Trygg K, Larsen S, Hofstad B and Vatn MH. Dietary factors and colorectal polyps: a case-control study, *Eur J Cancer Prev* 1995; 4: 239–46.
24. Kampman E, Verhoeven D, Sloots L and Van't Veer P. Vegetable and animal products as determinants of colon cancer risk in Dutch men and women, *Cancer Causes Control* 1995; 6: 225–34.
25. Kono S, Imanishi K, Shinchi K and Yanai F. Relationship of diet to small and large adenomas of the sigmoid colon, *Jpn J Cancer Res* 1993; 84: 13–19.
26. Little J, Logan RF, Hawtin PG, Hardcastle JD and Turner ID. Colorectal adenomas and diet: a case-control study of subjects participating in the Nottingham faecal occult blood screening programme, *Br J Cancer* 1993; 67: 177–84.
27. Neugut AI, Garbowski GC, Lee WC *et al.* Dietary risk factors for the incidence and recurrence for colorectal adenomatous polyps: a case-control study, *Ann Intern Med* 1993; 118: 91–5.
28. Sandler RS, Lyles CM, Peipins LA, Mc Auliffe CA, Woosley JT and Kupper LL. Diet and risk of colorectal adenomas:

macronutrients, cholesterol and fiber, *J Natl Cancer Inst* 1993; 85: 884–91.

29. Steinmetz KA and Potter JD. Food-group consumption and colon cancer in the Adelaide Case-Control Study, *Int J Cancer* 1993; 53: 711–9.

30. Zaridze D, Filipchenko V, Kustov V, Serdyuk V and Duffy S. Diet and colorectal cancer: results of two case-control studies in Russia, *Eur J Cancer* 1992; 29A: 112–15.

31. Arbman G, Axelson O, Ericsson-Begodski AB, Fredriksson M, Nilsson E and Sjodahl R. Cereal fiber, calcium, and colorectal cancer, *Cancer* 1992; 69: 2042–8.

32. Iscovich JM, L'Abbe KA, Castellato R *et al*. Colon cancer in Argentina. I. Risk from intake of dietary items, *Int J Cancer* 1992; 51: 851–7.

33. Iscovich JM, L'Abbe KA, Castellato R *et al*. Colon cancer in Argentina. II. Risk from fibre, fat and nutrients, *Int J Cancer* 1992; 51: 858–61.

34. Hu JF, Liu YY, Yu YK, Zhao TZ, Liu SD and Wang QQ. Diet and cancer of the colon and rectum: a case-control study in China, *Int J Epidemiol* 1991; 20: 362–7.

35. Benito E, Obrador A, Stiggelbout A *et al*. A population-based case-control study of colorectal cancer in Majorca. I. Dietary factors, *Int J Cancer* 1990; 45: 69–76.

36. Benito E, Stiggelbout A, Bosch FX *et al*. Nutritional factors in colorectal cancer risk: a case-control study in Majorca, *Int J Cancer* 1991; 49: 161–7.

37. Freudenhein JL, Graham S, Horvath PJ, Marshall JR, Haughey BP and Wilkinson G. Risks associated with source of fiber and fiber components in cancer of the colon and rectum, *Cancer Res* 1990; 50: 3295–300.

38. Gerhardsson de Verdier M, Hagman U, Steineck G, Rieger A and Norell SE. Diet, body mass and colorectal cancer: a case-referent study in Stockholm, *Int J Cancer* 1990; 46: 832–8.

39. Whittlemore AS, Wu-Williams AH, Lee M *et al*. Diet, physical activity, and colorectal cancer among Chinese in North America and China, *J Natl Cancer Inst* 1990; 82: 915–26.

40. Trock B, Lanza E and Greenwald P. Dietary fiber, vegetables, and colon cancer: critical review and meta-analyses of the epidemiologic evidence, *J Natl Cancer Inst* 1990; 82: 650–61.

41. Howe GR, Bento E, Castellato R *et al*. Dietary intake of fiber and decreased risk of cancers of the colon and rectum: evidence from the combined analyses of 13 case-control studies, *J Natl Cancer Inst* 1992; 84: 1887–96.

42. Fuchs CS, Giovanucci EL, Colditz GA *et al*. Dietary fiber and the risk of colorectal cancer and adenoma in women, *N Engl J Med* 1999; 340: 169–76.

43. Kato I, Akhmedkhanov A, Koenig K, Toniolo PG, Shore RE and Riboli E. Prospective study of diet and female colorectal cancer: the New York University Women's Health Study, *Nutr Cancer* 1997; 28: 276–81.

44. Gaard M, Tretli S and Loken EB. Dietary factors and the risk of colon cancer: a prospective study of 50,535 young Norwegian men and women, *Eur J Cancer Prev* 1996; 5: 445–54.

45. Giovanucci E, Rimm EB, Stampfer M, Colditz GA, Ascherio A and Willet WC. Intake of fat, meat, and fiber in relation to risk of colon cancer in men, *Cancer Res* 1994; 54: 2390–7.

46. Goldbohm RA, Van den Brandt PA, Van't Veer P, Dorant E, Sturmans F and Hermus RJ. Prospective study on alcohol consumption and the risk of cancer of the colon and rectum in the Netherlands, *Cancer Causes Control* 1994; 5: 95–104.

47. Steinmetz KA, Kushi LH, Bostick RM, Folsom AR and Potter JD. Vegetables, fruit and colon cancer in the Iowa Women's Health Study, *Am J Epidemiol* 1994; 139: 1–15.

48. Giovanucci E, Stampfer MJ, Colditz G, Rimm EB and Willett WC. Relationship of diet to risk of colorectal adenoma in men, *J Natl Cancer Inst* 1992; 84: 91–8.

49. Shibata A, Paganini-Hill A, Ross RK and Henderson BE. Intake of vegetables, fruits, beta-carotene, vitamin C and vitamin supplements and cancer incidence among the elderly: a prospective study, *Br J Cancer* 1992; 66: 673–9.

50. Thun MJ, Calle EE, Namboodiri MM *et al*. Risk factors for fatal colon cancer in a large prospective study, *J Natl Cancer Inst* 1992; 84: 1491–500.

51. Willett WC, Stampfer MJ, Colditz GA, Rosner BA and Speizer FE. Relation of meat, fat and fiber intake to the risk of colon cancer in a prospective study among women (*see comments*), *N Engl J Med* 1990; 323: 1664–72.

52. Schatzkin A, Lanza E, Corle D *et al*. Lack of effect of a low-fat, high-fiber diet on the recurrence of colorectal adenomas: Polyp Prevention Trial Study Group, *N Engl J Med* 2000; 342: 1149–55.

53. Alberts DS, Martinez ME, Roe DJ *et al*. Lack of effect of a high-fiber cereal supplements on the recurrence of colorectal adenomas: Phoenix

Colon Cancer Prevention Physicians' Network (*see comments*), *N Engl J Med* 2000; 342: 1156–62.

54. Bonithon-Kopp C, Kronborg O, Giacosa A, Rath U and Faivre J. Calcium and fibre supplementation in prevention of colorectal adenoma recurrence: a randomised intervention trial, European Cancer Prevention Organisation Study Group, *Lancet* 2000 14; 356(9238): 1300–6.

55. MacLennan R, Macrae F, Bain C *et al.* Randomized trial of intake of fat, fiber, and beta carotene to prevent colorectal adenomas: the Australian Polyp Prevention Prevention Project, *J Natl Cancer Inst* 1995; 87: 1760–6.

56. McKeown-Eyssen GE, Bright-See E, Bruce WR *et al.* A randomized trial of a low fat high fibre diet in the recurrence of colorectal polyps: Toronto Polyp Prevention Group, *J Clin Epidemiol* 1994; 47: 525–36.

57. DeCosse JJ, Miller HH and Lesser ML. Effect of wheat fiber and vitamins C and E on rectal polyps in patients with familial adenomatous polyposis, *J Natl Cancer Inst* 1989; 81: 1290–7.

58. Compher CW, Frankel WL, Tazelaar J *et al.* Wheat bran decreased aberrant crypt foci, preserves normal proliferation, and increases intraluminal butyrate levels in experimental colon cancer, *JPEN J Parenter Enteral Nutr* 1999; 23: 269–78.

59. Barrett JE, Klopfenstein CF and Leipold HW. Protective effects of cruciferous seed meals and hulls against colon cancer in mice, *Cancer Lett* 1998; 127: 83–8.

60. Harris PJ and Ferguson LR. Dietary fibre: its composition and role in protection against colorectal cancer, *Mutat Res* 1993; 290: 97–110.

61. Madar Z, Gurevich P, Ben-Hur H *et al.* Effects of dietary fiber on the rat intestinal mucosa exposed to low doses of a carcinogen, *Anticancer Res* 1998; 18: 3521–6.

62. Cameron IL, Hardman WE and Heitman DW. The nonfermentable dietary fiber lignin alters putative colon cancer risk factors but does not protect against DMH-induced colon cancer in rats, *Nutr Cancer* 1997; 28: 170–6.

63. Cassand P, Maziere S, Champ M, Meflah K, Bornet F and Narbonne JF. Effects of resistant starch- and vitamin A-supplemented diets on the promotion of precursor lesions of colon cancer in rats, *Nutr Cancer* 1997; 27: 53–9.

64. Ishizuka S and Takanori K. Inhibitory effect of dietary wheat bran on formation of aberrant crypt foci in rat colon induced by a single

injection of 1,2-dimethylhydrazine, *Biosi Biotechnol Biochem* 1996; 60: 2084–5.

65. Sakamoto J, Nakaji S, Sugawara K, Iwane S and Munakata A. Comparison of resistant starch with cellulose diet on 1,2-dimethylhydrazine-induced colonic carcinogenesis in rats, *Gastroenterology* 1996; 110: 116–20.

66. Weaver GA, Tangel C, Krause JA *et al.* Dietary guar gum alters colonic microbial fermentation in azoxymethane-treated rats, *J Nutr* 1996; 126: 1979–91.

67. Young GP, McIntyre A, Albert V, Folino M, Muir JG and Gibson PR. Wheat bran suppresses potato starch-potentiated colorectal tumorigenesis at the aberrant crypt stage in a rat model, *Gastroenterology* 1996; 110: 508–14.

68. Alabaster O, Tang Z, Frost A and Shivapurkar N. Effect of beta-carotene and wheat bran fiber on colonic aberrant crypt and tumor formation in rats exposed to azothymethane and high dietary fat, *Carcinogenesis* 1995; 16: 127–32.

69. Hardman WE and Cameron IL. Site specific reduction of colon cancer incidence, without a concomitant reduction in cryptal cell proliferation, in 1,2-dimethylhydrazine treated rats by diets containing 10% pectin with 5% or 20% corn oil, *Carcinogenesis* 1995, 16: 1425–31.

70. Alabaster O, Tang ZC, Frost A and Shivapurkar N. Potential synergism between wheat bran and psyllium: enhanced inhibition of colon cancer, *Cancer Lett* 1993; 75: 53–8.

71. McIntyre A and Gibson PR. Young GP, Butyrate production against large bowel cancer in a rat model, *Gut* 1993; 34: 361–91.

72. Heitman DW, Ord VA, Hunter KE and Cameron IL. Effect of dietary cellulose on cell proliferation and progression of 1,2-dimethylhydrazine-induced colon carcinogenesis in rats, *Cancer Res* 1989; 49: 5581–5.

73. Thorup I, Meyer O and Kristiansen E. Effect of a dietary fiber (beet fiber) on dimethylhydrazine-induced colon cancer in Wistar rats, *Nutr Cancer* 1992; 17: 251–61.

74. Tang CL, Ling BC, Fielding M, Tjandra JJ and Gibson PR. Cecal intubation model in the rat that facilitates selective in vivo study of colonic epithelial biology: preliminary report, *Dis Colon Rectum* 1998; 41: 1500–5.

Managing Anal Incontinence

HM Quah

Introduction

Anal continence is a complex function requiring an intact central nervous system and peripheral nervous system and a smooth muscle as well as striated muscle system. Disturbances in any of these mechanisms can result in incontinence. Anal incontinence can be described as the passage of faeces, mucus or flatus without the patient's knowledge or without voluntary contraction, or both.

Causes of Incontinence

From a management point of view, the causes of anal incontinence can be classified into trauma, colorectal disease, neurological conditions and miscellaneous conditions.

Trauma

Surgical trauma to the anal sphincters from fistula surgery and internal sphincterotomy may result in anal incontinence. Low anterior resection and pull-through operations can also result in incontinence. In the former operation, a decreased reservoir capacity of the neo-rectum and dilatation of the anus during either a transanal hand-sewn anastomosis or insertion of a staple gun may be responsible for the nocturnal leakage of faeces and urge incontinence that is observed.[1]

Obstetric trauma from third- or fourth-degree tears of the anal sphincter during normal vaginal delivery or forceps delivery can result in incontinence. Additionally, in the multiparous case, a component of pudendal neuropathy may contribute to incontinence. Also, an anovaginal or recto-vaginal fistula may be the reason for faecal incontinence following childbirth.

Accidental trauma from impalement or degloving injuries following road traffic accidents can cause disruption of the anal sphincter mechanism. Contamination of the extrarectal spaces can lead to sepsis, complicating surgical treatment.

Colorectal Disease

The incontinence of faeces and flatus may be due to the presence of an anorectal disease such as a fistula-in-ano. Rectal prolapse can cause anal dilatation and the associated chronic straining can result in pudendal nerve injury. Idiopathic inflammatory disease, rectal cancer, infective and parasitic infestation can result in diarrhoea that may overwhelm even a normal sphincter mechanism.

Neurological Disease

A neurological disease that affects either the central or peripheral nervous system may cause impaired bowel control. The most common cause of neuropathy is diabetes mellitus. The autonomic neuropathy that results may produce diarrhoea and the associated pudendal neuropathy may produce sphincter impairment. Systemic sclerosis and myopathies are less common causes of anal incontinence.

Miscellaneous

Laxative abuse and faecal impaction with resulting overflow incontinence is a common problem among the elderly. Faecal impaction from immobility and as a side effect of medication is common in this age group. Encoporesis or psychogenic soiling is usually observed in children. It is a term used when faecal incontinence is not caused by organic factors. Psychological factors such as excessive parental attention to toilet training, desire for attention or fear of the toilet have been implicated in the causation of encoporesis.

Evaluation

History

When one is evaluating anal incontinence, it is important to determine whether the cause is traumatic, neurological or due to an underlying colorectal disease. Occasionally, the patient may have incontinence due to a combination of causes. Patients who have sphincter injury due to trauma usually have good results from reconstructive procedures. Patients with neurological disease, in general, are better given medical treatment. In those with incontinence as a result of colorectal disease, treatment of the underlying problem (e.g. rectal prolapse) will often improve the patient's condition.

During history taking, information regarding bowel function, the degree of incontinence, and the presence of neurological symptoms as well as an obstetric history (for female patients) should be included.

Physical examination

Inspection of the perineum may reveal evidence of scars or defects in the sphincter mechanism. A patulous anus may be the result of anal sphincter or neurological impairment. Perineal descent is also an indication of the latter. Mucosal ectropion or rectal prolapse may be observed when the patient strains.

Palpation of the anal canal can give one the impression of resting anal pressure. Asking the patient to contract his sphincter will give one an idea of the extent of squeeze pressures. Palpation will also enable the examiner to determine the presence of any defect in the sphincter mechanisms. Sensory testing by touch or pinprick should elicit a contraction reflex.

Anorectal physiology

In relation to incontinence, the basic parameters that should be studied include anal manometry, rectal sensation and pudendal nerve terminal motor latency. Anorectal manometry evaluates the threshold for perception of rectal distension, resting anal pressure, maximum anal squeeze pressure, and duration of squeeze. There are no specific values that can discriminate patients with faecal incontinence from those that are continent, but incontinent patients as a whole tend to have lower squeeze pressures. Information from physiological studies may provide baseline measurements for serial follow-up. And detection of impaired rectal sensation (in diabetics, for example) is important, as biofeedback training for faecal incontinence may be beneficial.

Pudendal nerve terminal motor latency (PNTML) measures conduction function of the pudendal nerve, which innervates the external anal sphincter. PNTML is prolonged as a result of nerve injury. Some workers have reported poorer surgical results when sphincter repair for a childbirth sphincter defect was performed in the presence of significantly prolonged PNTML, compared to when there were normal measurements.[2,3] However, more recent reports showed that only late results are affected by the status of PNTML, suggesting that other associated factors, such as poor tissue condition, may be more important in affecting the results.[4,5] Endoanal ultrasound can enable the internal and external anal sphincter mechanism to be mapped out and is especially useful in obstetric injuries.

Treatment

Medical therapy

Constipation with faecal impaction and overflow incontinence accounts for an important proportion of cases of incontinence among institutionalized elderly patients. A regimen of bowel regulation may be the optimal method of management. The recommended treatment is a combination of a daily osmotic laxative and a habit-training programme that requires the patient to evacuate at scheduled intervals.

If faecal incontinence is due to diarrhoea, its cause needs to be identified and treated. But if the cause of diarrhoea is not found or cannot be treated, then antimotility agents should be used. Commonly, patients who are incontinent to loose stools can improve substantially or regain full control of their bowel movements when the stool consistency is firm. Agents such as loperamide or diphenoxylate may be used to change stool consistency enough to prevent leakage or "accidents".

Biofeedback

The patients thought to be most suitable for treatment with biofeedback are those with weakness of the external sphincter caused by injury to the pudendal nerve, or with impaired rectal sensation because of injury to the afferent nerve pathway. Patients are trained to detect rectal distension and respond by an immediate and sustained contraction of the pelvic floor muscle while avoiding the contraction of the abdominal wall muscles. This is commonly done using pressure sensors in the anal canal with a rectal balloon. Biofeedback has an overall success rate of approximately 70%. Biofeedback training is safe and painless but labour-intensive. It does not preclude future alternative treatment if it fails.

Surgical treatment

Surgical treatment in the form of a repair achieves the best results in incontinence arising from traumatic injuries. In patients with a neurological component, some form of pelvic floor repair may achieve restoration of continence. For patients with complete denervation or extensive muscle loss, encirclement procedures may be the only solution.

Anterior sphincteroplasty

Anterior sphincteroplasty is the procedure of choice for the repair of traumatic and obstetric anal sphincter injuries.

Routine preoperative care includes bowel preparation and prophylactic antibiotics. This repair is performed with an overlap of the divided ends of the muscles.[6] The mobilized scarred ends of the muscles are sutured with two rows of horizontal mattress sutures placed in the preserved scar tissue. The sutures are then tied to achieve a snug repair that should feel tight to the fifth digit. Significant improvement rates ranged from 70 to 90%.[7-10] Common causes of failure are postoperative sepsis, fistula formation and pelvic neuropathy. A significant factor in long-term failure may be abnormal pudendal nerve terminal motor latency, as previously discussed. Diverting stomas should probably not be used routinely. They may be reserved for reoperation cases and those that are exceptionally demanding technically.

Postanal repair

The postanal repair was first described by Parks[11] for patients with anal incontinence and an intact but poorly functioning anal sphincter. The operation achieves the effect of tightening the anorectal angle and lengthening the anal canal. Patients who benefit most from the repair are those with neurogenic incontinence, including those with pudendal neuropathy and persistent incontinence after a rectal prolapse repair. Parks reported a success rate of 83% but more recent studies have failed to duplicate this. The repair gives short-term benefits in up to 83% of patients but long-term effects last only in up to 28% of patients,[12-14] as neurogenic damage continues.

Encirclement procedures

Muscle transfers have recently been reintroduced as a means of encircling the anal sphincter to achieve continence. Baeten has described the use of an electrostimulated gracilis muscle to wrap round the anal sphincter muscle to achieve continence.[15] The purpose of electrostimulation is to convert fast-twitch, easily fatigable skeletal muscle to slow-twitch muscles that are resistant to fatigue, approximating normal external sphincter muscles. Good results have been reported in up to 78% of patients who had dynamic graciloplasty for incontinence.[16-20]

Another encirclement procedure that is of interest is the use of an implantable artificial anal sphincter; it is a modified version of the artificial urinary sphincter. The artificial anal sphincter includes a cuff, which surrounds and occludes the anal canal, connected to a pressure-regulating balloon implanted in the abdominal wall. A control pump is placed in the labia or scrotum, which controls the transfer of fluid to and from the cuff. The cuff pressure can thus be regulated during normal activity, and released during defecation. Three current published reports show a success rate of around 73%.[21–23] Complications result from infection and the extrusion of the device.

Conclusion

Faecal incontinence is a socially debilitating condition for the patient. Successful treatment of faecal incontinence depends on an accurate diagnosis of the underlying problem. This includes a detailed history and physical examination, anorectal physiology and ultrasound studies. Subsequent management by medication, biofeedback or surgery then depends upon the underlying cause. With the recent and coming advances in diagnosis and treatment, no patient should remain incontinent or contend with a permanent stoma.

References

1. Ho YH, Tsang C, Tang CL, Nyam DCNK, Eu KW and Seow-Choen F. Anal sphincter injuries from stapling instruments introduced transanally: randomized, controlled study with endoanal ultrasound and anorectal manometry, *Dis Colon Rectum* 2000; 43: 169–73.
2. Gilliland R, Altomare DF, Moreira H, Oliveira L, Gilliland JE and Wexner SD. Pudendal neuropathy is predictive of failure following anterior overlapping sphincteroplasty, *Dis Colon Rectum* 1998; 41: 1516–22.
3. Laurberg S, Swash M and Henry MM. Delayed external sphincter repair for obstetric tear, *Br J Surg* 1988; 75: 786–8.
4. Engel AF, Kamm MA, Sultan AH, Bartram CI and Nicholls RJ. Anterior anal sphincter repair in patients with obstetric trauma, *Br J Surg* 1994; 81: 1231–4.

5. Ternent CA, Shashidharan M, Blatchford GJ, Christensen MA, Thorson AG and Sentovich SM. Transanal ultrasound and anorectal physiology findings affecting continence after sphincteroplasty, *Dis Colon Rectum* 1997; 40: 462–7.

6. Parks AG and McPartlin JF. Late repair of injuries of the anal sphincter, *Proc R Soc Med* 1971; 64: 1187–9.

7. Fleshman JW, Dreznik Z, Fry RD and Kodner IJ. Anal sphincter repair for obstetric injury: manometric evaluation of functional results, *Dis Colon Rectum* 1991; 34: 1061–7.

8. Oliveira L, Pfeifer J and Wexner SD. Physiological and clinical outcome of anterior sphincteroplasty, *Br J Surg* 1996; 83: 502–5.

9. Sitzler PJ and Thomson JP. Overlap repair of damaged anal sphincter: a single surgeon's series, *Dis Colon Rectum* 1996; 39: 1356–60.

10. Young CJ, Mathur MN, Eyers AA and Solomon MJ. Successful overlapping anal sphincter repair: relationship to patient age, neuropathy, and colostomy formation, *Dis Colon Rectum* 1998; 41: 344–9.

11. Parks AG. Royal Society of Medicine, Section of Proctology; Meeting, 27 November 1974. President's Address. Anorectal incontinence, *Proc R Soc Med* 1975; 68: 681–90.

12. Jameson JS, Speakman CT, Darzi A, Chia YW and Henry MM. Audit of postanal repair in the treatment of fecal incontinence, *Dis Colon Rectum* 1994; 37: 369–72.

13. Setti-Carraro P, Kamm MA and Nicholls RJ. Long-term results of postanal repair for neurogenic faecal incontinence, *Br J Surg* 1994; 81: 140–4.

14. Engel AF, van Baal SJ and Brummelkamp WH. Late results of postanal repair for idiopathic faecal incontinence, *Eur J Surg* 1994; 160: 637–40.

15. Konsten J, Baeten CG, Spaans F, Havenith MG and Soeters PB. Follow-up of anal dynamic graciloplasty for fecal continence, *World J Surg* 1993; 17: 404–8.

16. Baeten CG, Geerdes BP, Adang EM, Heineman E, Konsten J, Engel GL *et al.* Anal dynamic graciloplasty in the treatment of intractable fecal incontinence, *N Engl J Med* 1995; 332: 1600–5.

17. Geerdes BP, Heineman E, Konsten J, Soeters PB and Baeten CG. Dynamic graciloplasty: complications and management, *Dis Colon Rectum* 1996; 39: 912–17.

18. Baeten CG, Bailey HR, Bakka A, Belliveau P, Berg E, Buie WD *et al.* Safety and efficacy of dynamic graciloplasty for fecal incontinence:

report of a prospective, multicenter trial. Dynamic Graciloplasty Therapy Study Group, *Dis Colon Rectum* 2000; 43: 743–51.

19. Madoff RD, Rosen HR, Baeten CG, LaFontaine LJ, Cavina E, Devesa M *et al*. Safety and efficacy of dynamic muscle plasty for anal incontinence: lessons from a prospective, multicenter trial, *Gastroenterology* 1999; 116: 549–56.

20. Mavrantonis C, Billotti VL and Wexner SD. Stimulated graciloplasty for treatment of intractable fecal incontinence: critical influence of the method of stimulation, *Dis Colon Rectum* 1999; 42: 497–504.

21. Christiansen J, Rasmussen OO and Lindorff L. Long-term results of artificial anal sphincter implantation for severe anal incontinence, *Ann Surg* 1999; 230: 45–8.

22. Wong WD, Jensen LL, Bartolo DC and Rothenberger DA. Artificial anal sphincter, *Dis Colon Rectum* 1996; 39: 1345–51.

23. Lehur PA, Michot F, Denis P, Grise P, Leborgne J, Teniere P *et al*. Results of artificial sphincter in severe anal incontinence: report of 14 consecutive implantations, *Dis Colon Rectum* 1996; 39: 1352–5.

CHAPTER 44

Recurrent and Extensive Anal Condylomas

KS Ho

Introduction

Anal condylomas or anal warts are caused by the human papilloma virus. This is a DNA virus with many different genotypes. Genotypes 6 and 11 are responsible for over 90% of cases of anal warts.[1] Some patients are infected with genotypes 16 and 18, which are associated with intraepithelial neoplasia and cervical cancer.[2] It is sexually transmitted and up to 90% of patients practise anal receptive intercourse. It has a propensity for the perianal skin and squamous epithelium and transitional zone of the anal canal. Its incidence in Singapore remains unknown, as it is not a reportable disease.

Histologically, viral warts show marked acanthosis with hyperplasia of the prickle cells. The upper prickle layer may become vacuolated, and there may be an underlying chronic inflammatory cell infiltrate. Morphologically, small, discrete, elevated lesions are seen which vary from pink to grey in colour. These lesions may coalesce into large polypoidal lesions.

Signs and Symptoms

Patients usually present with perianal lumps. They may also present with symptoms of pruritis ani, bleeding, discharge or pain.

Management

Anal warts have a propensity to recur. This is because, in addition to the visibly present anal warts at the perianal skin, up to 84% have concurrent anal warts and may be hidden from view within the anal canal.[3] It is thus mandatory to perform a proctoscopy to exclude intra-anal disease.

Secondly, anal warts are sexually transmitted and failure to treat the sexual partners may result in repeat contact and infection.

Thirdly, more extensive disease may occur in patients who are in an immunocompromised state. These include HIV-positive patients as well as patients on immunosuppressants after organ transplant.

Therapy

There are multiple treatment modalities available. Local therapy includes surgical destruction or topical application. Systemic treatment involves the use of interferon.

Two commonly used topical applications are podophyllin and bichloroacetic acid. Bichloro- and tricholoroacetic acids are keratolytics and also act as a cauterant. They can be applied to both skin and anal canal lesions. They require repeated applications and have a recurrence rate of about 25%.[4]

Podophyllin paint acts as a cytotoxic agent. It is not suitable for anal canal lesions, as it may result in anal stenosis and fistula formation.[5] It is also poorly absorbed by highly keratinized warts. Prolonged use may result in dysplastic changes in the skin. In addition, repeated applications are required and it also has a lower efficacy (20–40%) and higher recurrence rate than surgical excision.[6]

5-fluorouracil is available as a topical cream. It is applied daily for 10 weeks. It may cause erosive dermatitis and mucositis. It has a success rate of about 50–75% and may also be used for the prevention of recurrence.[7]

Liquid nitrogen is used in cryotherapy. It is applied directly onto the lesion, resulting in local destruction. The width and depth of treatment have to be well controlled. Repeated treatment is often required.

Surgery

Surgery is the gold standard for treatment of anal warts. It has the highest eradication rate and the lowest recurrence rate.

Surgical techniques for excision include scissors excision, diathermy excision and laser vaporization.

There is no advantage to laser treatment over electocautery. The degree of pain is similar in the two types of treatment, and use of laser requires specialized equipment and increases costs.[8]

Fulgaration of anal warts may result in release of infectious papillomaviruses in the vapour. Theorectically, this may be inhaled and result in respiratory tract papillomas.

Sharp scissors excision of anal warts is the preferred mode of excision. This is the only technique that provides for tissue diagnosis to exclude malignancy in suspicious lesions. It may be performed under local, regional or general anaesthesia, though regional or general anaesthesia is preferred for more extensive and multiple lesions. Diathermy may be used for haemostasis at the base of the lesion after excision. This method also prevents the release of papillomavirus into the surrounding air.

Immunotherapy

Interferon has been used in the treatment of anal warts. It may be used either topically or as a form of systemic treatment.

Results of topical application are poor, and studies have shown no difference in results when compared with controls. Interferon has also been used as intralesional injections. This shows better clearance rates, though it requires repeated treatment sessions and is not able to treat subclinical infections.[9]

Systemic interferon treats all infected tissues. However, there is a high rate of side effects, including flu-like symptoms, gastrointestinal upsets, abnormal liver function, leucopenia and thrombocytopenia.[10] The response rate reported varies from 14 to 82%.

Another novel technique for treatment of anal warts was described in 1977.[11] It involves the development of a vaccine using tissues from excised warts. This is then injected weekly for six weeks. This achieved results of 84%. However, it is not effective in immunosuppressed patients.[12,13]

Special Considerations

Immunocompromised patients form a special group of patients with anal warts. Anal warts are more common in these patients compared with the general population. They are also more aggressive, likely to recur and more dysplastic. These patients often need repeat treatments.

Immunotherapy with interferon is not suitable for transplant patients, as it may increase the risk of transplant rejection. In AIDS patients, surgery may result in poor wound healing. Topical 5-FU is the primary treatment of choice in such patients.

Conclusion

Recurrent anal warts are sexually transmitted. Treatment entails complete eradication of all clinical infection, including that within the anal canal. Surgery may be required. Treatment of sexual contacts is also required, to prevent reinfection.

References

1. Koutsky L. Epidemiology of gental human papillomavirus infection, *Am J Med* 1997; 102: 3–8.
2. Gross G, Ikenberg H, Gissmann L and Hagendorn M. Papillomavirus infection of the anogenital region: correlation between histology, clinical picture, and virus type, *J Invest Dermatol* 1985; 85: 147–52.
3. Sohn N and Robilotti JG. The gay bowel syndrome: a review of colonic and rectal conditions in 200 male homosexuals, *Am J Gastroenterol* 1977; 67: 478–83.

4. Swerdlow DB and Salvati EP. Condyloma acuminatum, *Dis Colon Rectum* 1971; 14: 226–31.
5. Wexner SD. Managing common anorectal sexually transmitted diseases, *Infect Surg* 1990; 9–48.
6. Jensen SL. Comparison of podophyllin application with simple surgical excision in clearnace and recurrence of perianal condyloma acuminatum, *Lancet* 1985; 2: 1146–8.
7. Congilosi SM and Madoff RD. Current therapy for recurrent and extensive anal warts, *Dis Colon Rectum* 1995; 38: 1101–7.
8. Billingham RP and Lewis FG. Laser versus electrical cautery in the treament of condylomata acuminata of the anus, *Surg Gynecol Obstet* 1982; 155: 865–7.
9. Baron S, Tyring SK, Fleischmann WR Jr, Coppenhauer DH, Niesel DW, Stanton GJ *et al*. Intralesional interferon: current recommendations, *JAMA* 1991; 266: 1375–83.
10. Olmos L, Vilata J, Rodriguez PA, Lloret A, Ojeda A and Calderon MD. Double-blind randomized clinical trial on the effect of interferon-beta in the treatment of condylomata acuminata, *Int J STD AIDS* 1994; 5: 182–5.
11. Abcarian H, Smith D and Sharon N. The immunotherapy of anal condyloma acuminatum, *Dis Colon Rectum* 1976; 19: 237–44.
12. Abcarian H and Sharon N. The effectiveness of immunotherapy in the treatment of anal condyloma acuminatum, *J Surg Res* 1977; 231–6.
13. Abcarian H and Sharon N. Long-term effectiveness of immunotherapy of anal condyloma acuminatum, *Dis Colon Rectum* 1982; 25: 648–51.

CHAPTER 45

Bowel Dysfunction After Anterior Resection

KS Ho

Introduction

With advances in surgical technique and instrumentation, only about 10% of rectal cancers require an abdominoperineal resection. Preservation of anal function decreases the physical and psychological morbidity associated with a stoma.

However, the re-establishment of gastrointestinal continuity may result in incontinence, urgency and frequency of stools.

Pathophysiology of Bowel Dysfunction

Many patients do not complain about bowel dysfunction unless directly questioned about it. This may be due to patients' accepting the dysfunction as being an unavoidable side effect of surgery. Surgeons may also be more concerned about recurrence than functional problems. This may lead to an underestimation of bowel dysfunction.

Factors that influence bowel function include site and length of colorectal resection, time since operation, anastomotic leakage, locoregional recurrences and adjuvant chemoradiotherapy.

A survey of 315 patients was conducted in this department, comparing the long-term bowel function after right hemicolectomy, extended right hemicolectomy, sigmoid colectomy and anterior resection.[1] We found that 32% of patients after anterior resection had some form of incontinence that affected their lifestyle, compared to 11.5% of patients for all other types of resection. Defecatory problems also occurred more frequently (25% after sigmoid colectomy; 28.4% after anterior resection) compared to others (15.4%). In addition, more than half of the patients had three or more bowel movements a day after anterior resection.

Three major factors contribute to the poor bowel function after anterior resection: sphincter damage, sensory loss and a reduced rectal reservoir.[2] Furthermore, loss of colonic length results in more rapid transit and a more liquid effluent reaching the anus, which places further stress on the anal sphincter.

It has been well documented that the introduction of the stapling device used can result in sphincter damage and a drop in sphincter pressures.[3,4] This damage is usually limited to the internal sphincter, and corresponds to a drop in the mean resting pressure. In addition, the nerve supply to the internal anal sphincter may be damaged during wide radial clearance of the mesorectum during surgery.[5] On the other hand, external sphincter injuries are less common, and their nerve supply, via the pudendal nerve, is also unlikely to get damaged during surgery. The damage to the internal sphincter may be aggravated during mucosectomy,[6] when the sphincter may be intentionally or unintentionally excised.

Anal sensation is important for distinguishing between flatus, liquid and solid stools. This is an important role of the anal transition zone, and helps maintain continence. Theoretically, preservation of the anal transition zone improves sensation and continence. However, studies that compared the stapled pouch (where the anal transition zone is preserved) with hand-sewn pouches with mucosectomy are not in total agreement over this point.[7–9]

The role of the rectoanal inhibitory reflex (RAIR) is also in dispute. It is well known that the RAIR pathway is interrupted with rectal excision and reanastomosis. However, this recovers with time, probably from recovery or reinnervation of the damaged nerves. One study showed that patients with normal continence are more likely to have RAIR.[10] However, another study found that only 25% of patients are incontinent after anterior resection, even though more than 80% of patients have lost the RAIR.[11] It is likely that RAIR assists in maintaining continence in suboptimal sphincter pressures, but it is not absolutely essential for continence.

The height of the anastomosis is another major factor affecting bowel function. It has been shown that bowel function is more likely to be impaired with anastomoses within 4.5 cm of the anal verge.[12] The amount of rectum retained corresponded to the eventual reservoir function. However, preservation of an adequate length of rectum may be limited by oncological or vascular considerations.

Adjuvant chemoradiation has also been reported to affect bowel function, resulting in increased stool frequency, clustering, incontinence and nocturnal bowel movements.[13,14] In a small prospective randomized study comparing pouch surgery alone, and pouch surgery with preoperative and postoperative radiation, we found that there were slightly more incontinent episodes in patients with preoperative radiotherapy, while there was no difference between surgery alone and the postoperative radiotherapy group. However, the rectal sensation to barostat ramp distension was also impaired in the postoperative radiotherapy group.[15]

Techniques to Improve Bowel Function

Direct anal spincter damage can be minimized by avoiding digital anal dilatation, using a small proctoscope for rectal washout, and using an appropriate-size stapling device. Meticulous surgical technique aids in preserving both the sympathetic and parasympathetic nerves during division of the inferior mesenteric artery as well as during mesorectal excision.

Using a double-stapling technique for anastomosis also avoids a mucosectomy and further damage to the internal sphincter. In addition, it avoids damaging the anal transition zone.

Finally, and most importantly, preservation of a length of rectum helps to improve bowel function. However, this is not always possible, for oncological or vascular reasons. Rectal compliance can then be increased by formation of a colonic pouch.

Colonic Pouch

It was initially believed that colonic pouches improved function by increasing the rectal reservoir capacity.[16] It is now known that the pouch functions more like a "pressure sump" to dissipate high intraluminal pressure waves within the noncompliant colon.[17]

The superiority of a pouch-anal anastomosis at one year postop compared to a straight coloanal anastomosis has been shown in randomized clinical trials.[18–21] Most trials showed that the frequency of stools and the use of antidiarrhoeal medication were decreased with the construction of a J-pouch, though improvements of other symptoms such as urgency or incontinence were present but less obvious.[2] Some reports also showed that patients with pouches may have evacuation difficulties, with the proportion of such patients increasing with time after surgery.

It has been shown that there was no functional difference between pouches of different lengths, but that evacuation problems occurred more often in the larger pouch.[22,23] There was also no difference in function between a sigmoid J-pouch and a descending colon J-pouch.[24]

It is known that the J-pouch improved functions in the short term. Most reports also showed that function in the straight coloanal anastomosis approximated that of pouch-anal anastomosis after 1–2 years and not much difference existed between the two groups in terms of bowel frequency and antidiarrhoeal medication requirements by this time.[21,25,26] However, the short-term superior results of the J-pouch are enough justification for its use, as most patients requiring a J-pouch are elderly or have rectal cancer, and life expectancy is limited. As such, the quality of life during the early postoperative period is important to the patient.

Another added benefit of the J-pouch is a reduced anastomotic leak rate, due possibly to better blood supply to the site of anastomosis.[20,25,27]

Short pouches 5–6 cm long using the sigmoid colon are preferred. These are usually constructed with a linear cutting stapler introduced through a colotomy at the apex of the "J". The distal end is then closed using either a linear stapler or sutures. The double-stapling technique is usually used for the pouch-anal anastomosis.

Alternatives to the J Pouch

Bern's pouch (transverse coloplasty)

This was first described by Z'graggen *et al.* in 1997.[28] The technique is similar to that of a pyloroplasty, in which a 4 cm longitudinal incision is made a short distance from the distal end of the colon, and then sutured transversely. The authors believed that there should be less evacuation difficulties, as the countercurrent force resulting in negation of propulsion was less than that of the antiperistaltic J-limb. It also led to a directional change in the propulsive forces in the anterior part of the pouch only. Our experience with Bern's pouch showed a propensity to anastomotic leakage, especially anteriorly.

Harder's pouch (ileocaecal interposition graft)

Von Flue and Harder first described the use of an ileocaecal interposition graft for pouch-anal reconstruction, in 1994.[29,30] This involved the isolation of the terminal ileum, caecum and ascending colon, which was then rotated into the pelvis and interpositioned between the colon and the anus. The authors believed that this technique avoided loss of intrinsic and extrinsic autonomic nerve supply to the left colon as it was not mobilized. The reported results were excellent. However, this was only from one centre. The procedure is also complex, requiring three anastomoses.

Management of Excessive Stool Frequency

The majority of patients with excessive stool frequency and incontinence can be managed with antidiarrhoeal medication and stool-bulking agents. With time, most will improve. However, the quality of life in some will be impacted by these problems.

Patients with excessive stool frequency of more than six times a day may benefit from biofeedback. Biofeedback therapy over a period of four weeks reduced the daily stool frequency and incontinent episodes.[31,32] Each therapy consisted of four sessions of one hour of biofeedback, over a period of four weeks. Following therapy, the weekly incontinent episodes were reduced and the antidiarrhoeal medication requirements were also reduced.[31,32]

Conclusion

Excessive stool frequency and incontinence may be distressing and reduces the quality of life of patients after anterior resection. Using a colonic J-pouch reduces the frequency of stools for up to two years. Patients with intractable excessive stool frequency in spite of a pouch benefit from biofeedback.

References

1. Ho YH, Low D and Goh HS. Bowel function survey after segmental colorectal resections, *Dis Colon Rectum* 1996; 39: 307–10.
2. Brown SR and Seow-Choen F. Preservation of rectal function after low anterior resection with formation of a neorectum, *Semin Surg Oncol* 2000, 19: 376–85.
3. Ho YH, Tsang C, Tang CL, Nyam D, Eu KW and Seow-Choen F. Anal sphincter injuries from stapling instruments introduced transanally: randomized, controlled study with endoanal ultrasound and anorectal manometry, *Dis Colon Rectum* 2000; 43: 169–73.
4. Lewis WG, Martin IG, Williamson MER, Stephenson BM, Holdsworth PJ, Finan PJ and Johnston D. Why do some patients experience poor functional results after anterior resection of the rectum for carcinoma? *Dis Colon Rectum* 1995; 38: 259–63.
5. Havenga K, DeRuiter MC, Enker WE and Welvart K. Anatomical basis of autonomic nerve-preserving total mesorectal excision for rectal cancer, *Br J Surg* 1996; 83: 384–8.
6. Gamagami R, Istvan G, Cabarrot P, Liagre A, Chiotasso P and Lazorthes F. Fecal continence following partial resection of the anal canal in distal rectal cancer: long term results after coloanal anastomosis, *Surg* 2000; 127: 291–5.
7. Johnston D, Holdsworth PJ, Nasmyth DG, Neal DE, Primrose JN, Womack N and Axon AT. Preservation of the entire anal canal in consecutive proctocolectomy for ulcerative colitis: a pilot study comparing end-to-end ileo-anal anastomosis without mucosal resection with mucosal proctectomy and endo-anal anastomosis, *Br J Surg* 1987; 74: 940–4.
8. Sugerman HJ and Newsome HH. Stapled ileo-anal anastomosis without a temporary ileostomy, *Am J Surg* 1994; 167: 58–65.

9. Reilly WT, Pemberton JH, Wolff BG, Nivatvongs S, Devine RM, Litchy WJ and McIntyre PB. Randomized prospective trial comparing ileal pouch-anal anastomosis performed by excising the anal mucosa to ileal pouch-anal anastomosis performed by preserving the anal mucosa, *Ann Surg* 1997; 225: 666–77.

10. Miller R, Bartolo DC, Cervero F and Mortensen NJ. Anorectal sampling: a comparison of normal and incontinent patients, *Br J Surg* 1988; 75: 44–7.

11. O'Riordain MG, Molloy RG,Gillen P, Horgan A and Kirwan WD. Rectoanal inhibitory reflex following low stapled anterior resection of the rectum, *Dis Colon Rectum* 1992; 35: 874–8.

12. Ho YH, Wong J and Goh HS. Level of anastomosis and anoretal manometry in predicting function following anterior resection for adenocarcinoma, *Int J Colorec Dis* 1993; 8: 170–4.

13. Dahlberg M, Glimelius B, Graf W and Pahlman L. Preoperative irradiation affects functional results after surgery for rectal cancer, *Dis Colon Rectum* 1998; 41: 543–51.

14. Graf W, Ekstrom K, Glimelius B and Pahlman L. A pilot study of the factors influencing bowel function after colorectal anastomosis, *Dis Colon Recum* 1996; 39: 744–9.

15. Ho YH, Lee KS, Eu KW and Seow-Choen F. Effects of adjuvant radiotherapy on bowel function and anorectal physiology after low anterior resection for rectal cancer, *Tech Coloproctol* 2000; 4: 13–16.

16. Lazorthes F, Fages P, Chiotasso P, Lemozy J and Bloom E. Resection of the rectum with construction of a colonic reservoir and colo-anal anastomosis for carcinoma of the rectum, *Br J Surg* 1986; 73: 136–8.

17. Williams N and Seow-Choen F. Physiological and functional outcome following ultra-low anterior resection with colon pouch-anal anastomosis, *Br J Surg* 1998; 85: 1029–35.

18. Seow-Choen F and Goh HS. Prospective randomized trial comparing J colonic pouch-anal anastomosis and straight coloanal reconstruction, *Br J Surg* 1995; 82: 608–10.

19. Ho YH, Tan M and Seow-Choen F. Prospective randomized controlled study of clinical function and anorectal physiology after low anterior resection: comparison of straight and colonic J pouch anastomosis, *Br J Surg* 1996; 83: 978–80.

20. Hallböök O, Pâhlman L, Krog M, Wexner SD and Sjodahl R. Randomized comparison of straight and colonic J pouch anastomosis after low anterior resection, *Ann Surg* 1996; 224: 58–65.

21. Ho YH, Seow-Choen F and Tan M. Colonic J-pouch function at six months versus straight coloanal anastomosis at two years: randomized controlled trial, *World J Surg* 2001; 25: 876–81.

22. Hida J, Yasutomi M, Fujimoto K, Okuno K, Ieda S, Machidera N *et al.* Functional outcome after low anterior resection with low anastomosis for rectal cancer using the colonic J-pouch: prospective randomized study for determination of optimum pouch size, *Dis Colon Rectum* 1996; 39: 986–91.

23. Lazorthes F, Gamagami R, Chiotasso P, Istvan G and Muhammad S. Prosepctive randomized study comparing clinical results between small and large colonic J-pouch following coloanal anastomosis, *Dis Colon Rectum* 1997; 40: 1409–13.

24. Heah SM, Seow-Choen F, Eu KW, Ho YH and Tang CL. Prospective, randomized trial comparing sigmoid vs descending colonic J-pouch after total rectal excision, *Dis Colon Rectum* 2002; 45: 322–8.

25. Joo JS, Latulippe JF, Alabaz O, Weiss EG, Nojueras JJ and Wexner SD. Long-term functional evaluation of straight coloanal anastomosis and colonic J-pouch: is the functional superiority of the colonic J-pouch sustained? *Dis Colon Rectum* 1998; 41: 740–6.

26. Lazorthes F, Chiotasso P, Gamagami R, Istvan G and Chevreau P. Late clinical outcome in a randomised prospective comparison of colonic J pouch and straight coloanal anastomosis, *Br J Surg* 1997; 84: 1449–51.

27. Hallböök O, Johansson K and Sjödahl R. Laser doppler blood flow measurement in rectal resection for carcinoma—comparison between the straight and colonic J pouch construction, *Br J Surg* 1996; 83: 389–92.

28. Z'graggen K, Maurer CA, Mettler D, Stoupis C, Wildi S and Buchler MW. A novel colon pouch and its comparison with a straight coloanal and colon J-pouch-anal anastomosis: preliminary results in pigs, *Surgery* 1999; 125: 105–12.

29. Von Flue M and Harder F. A new technique for pouch-anal reconstruction after total meorectal excision, *Dis Colon Rectum* 1994; 37: 1160–2.

30. Von Flue M, Degen LP, Beglinger C *et al.* Ileocaeal reservoir reconstruction with physiologic function after total mesorectal cancer excision, *Ann Surg* 1996; 224: 204–12.

31. Ho YH, Chiang JM, Tan M and Low JY. Biofeedback therapy for excessive stool frequency and incontinence following anterior resection or total colectomy, *Dis Colon Rectum* 1996; 39: 1289–92.

32. Ho YH and Tan M. Biofeedback therapy for bowel dysfunction following low anterior resection, *Ann Acad Med Singapore* 1997; 26: 299–302.

Duplicated Colon and Rectum

KS Ho

Introduction

Duplication of the colon and of the rectum are rare congenital conditions that are more often seen by the paediatric surgeon than by the adult surgeon. They are also known as enteric cysts, enterogenous cysts or neurenteric cysts. Such duplication accounted for between 4 and 18% of all gastrointestinal duplications.[1,2] A PubMed search from 1968 to 2001 revealed only 18 publications regarding this condition, of which there are 15 case reports of 18 patients. Three large series of gastrointestinal duplications with a total of 73 cases of colon and rectal duplications were reported from 1876 to 2000.[3–5]

Embryogenesis

The pathogenesis of duplication is a "pinching off" of the gastrointestinal tract into the form of a diverticulum during the eighth to ninth week of gestation.[6] This leads to a separate tract that may or may not communicate with the normal GI tract. Another form is a complete division of the budding GI tract at the fifth week, leading to "caudal twinning" of the hindgut.

Signs and Symptoms

The majority of duplications present in childhood, of which 40% present by 1 month of age and 67% by 1 year. About 17% remain asymptomatic and present in later childhood or even adulthood.[3]

Most cases, however, present at birth with an anomaly of the perineum. This is usually in the form of a urogenital anomaly suggestive of a hindgut disorder. Such anomalies include double phallus, bladder exstrophy or anorectal deformities.

Other modes of presentation include rectal bleeding, rectal prolapse, perineal mass, perineal fistula, abdominal pain and constipation. In those that remain asymptomatic, presentation may be as an incidental finding or in adults over 30 years of age after undergoing malignant transformation.

Pathology

Ladd and Gross first defined the nature of gastrointestinal duplication in 1940.[7] The lesion must be in continuity or closely adherent to the gastrointestinal tract; it must have a smooth muscle wall and the mucosa must have one or more cell types that are consistent with that of the gastrointestinal tract.

Duplications are usually described as spherical or tubular. Spherical duplications account for about 75% of all duplications. They are less likely to communicate with the normal GI tract (20%) compared to the tubular form (68%).[3] Duplications usually share a blood supply and lie within the same mesentery as the normal tract, though the former may occasionally have its own mesentery and blood supply. They may also have a common smooth muscle wall with the normal GI tract.

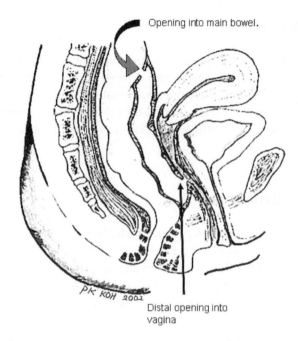

Opening into main bowel.

Distal opening into
vagina

Figure 1. Duplicated rectum with proximal communication and distal fistulous opening into the vagina.

The duplication may also take one of several forms. It may present as a cyst that is adherent close to the normal GI tract or its mesentery, with no communication with the normal tract. It may also present as a tubular duplication, with proximal communication with the GI tract, while distally ending as either a blind pouch or a fistulous communication with the vagina or bladder (Fig. 1). Less frequently, it presents as a "twinning", where there are two normal tracts, which may end at two separate functioning anuses. More than 50% of duplications have some form of fistulous communication with the normal gut.

Associated Anomalies

GI duplications are associated with other congenital defects in up to 80% of cases. For hindgut duplications, there may be associated urogenital anomalies such as bladder duplication or exstrophy, urethral duplication, double phallus or vagina. There could also be associated vertebral anomalies, with vertebral dysraphism being the most common. For midgut duplications, malrotation and intestinal atresia may be present as well.

Management

Management of patients has to be individualized. All communications between the duplication and the normal GI tract and/or urogenital tract should be delineated before surgery is undertaken. It is also important to identify all other associated anomalies. In cases where the duplication is found during an emergency surgery, associated bowel atresia has to be excluded. It may not be possible to identify the fistulous communications in such cases and it may be better to defunction the bowel and complete the surgery at a later stage after full investigations.

Treatment may require a multidisciplinary approach involving the colorectal surgeon, urologist, and plastic and reconstructive surgeon. In addition, as the patients usually present young, staged operations may be required.

In some cases of complete twinning of the hindgut, there may be two sets of normal-looking colon and rectum, each ending in a normal functioning anus. This is compatible with normal function and surgery is for cosmesis. However, the possibility of malignant change in the future cannot be ruled out, though data regarding this is sparse.

The type of surgery performed depends on the site and length of the duplication, its communication and its vascular supply.

Complete excision is usually possible for cystic lesions. Long tubular duplications with a common vascular supply may pose a problem for resection, as it is important to avoid devascularizing normal bowel, which may result in short gut syndrome. In such circumstances, it may be necessary to perform a partial excision with stripping of the remnant mucosa. The fistulous opening is then closed carefully. Other options include dividing the septum in between the two lumens or performing a long side-to-side anastomosis, converting the two sides into a common channel.

The mortality and morbidity for excision of colorectal duplications are less than for thoracic GI duplications. The main problem lies in vascular damage resulting in short gut syndrome.

There have been reports of malignant changes in the duplication, assumed to be due to the "unstable mucosa" within the duplicated tract. However, there is too little data to confirm or refute this theory.

Conclusion

Colon and rectum duplications are rare, congenital conditions that are usually seen in the paediatric or neonatal population. Management should be according to the underlying anomalies and needs to be individualized.

Acknowledgement

I would like to thank Dr Koh Poh Koon for his contribution to the medical illustration.

References

1. Bond SJ and Groff DB. Gastrointestinal duplications. In: O'Neill JA, Rowe MI, Grosfeld JL et al. (eds.), *Pediatric Surgery*. St Louis, MO, Mosby Year Book, 1998, pp. 1257–67.
2. Gopal SC, Gangopadhyay AN, Gupta DK, Sinha CK, Sahoo SP and Sharma LB. A unique presentation of atypical complete duplication of terminal ileum, colon, rectum, and urinary bladder, *J Pediatr Surg* 1997; 32(8): 1250–1.
3. Stringer MD, Spitz L, Abel R, Kiely E, Drake DP, Agrawal M, Stark Y and Brereton RJ. Management of alimentary tract duplication in children, *Br J Surg* 1995; 82: 74–8.
4. Holcomb GW 3rd, Gheissari A, O'Neill JA Jr, Shorter NA and Bishop HC. Surgical management of alimentary tract duplications, *Ann Surg* 1989; 209(2): 167–74.
5. Yousefzadeh DK, Bickers GH, Jackson JH Jr and Benton C. Tubular colonic duplication—review of 1876–1981 literature, *Pediatr Radiol* 1983; 13(2): 65–71.
6. Prasil P, Nguyen LT and Laberge JM. Delayed presentation of a congenital recto-vaginal fistula associated with a recto-sigmoid tubular duplication and spinal cord and vertebral anomalies, *J Pediatr Surg* 2000; 35(5): 733–5.
7. Ladd WE and Gross RE. Surgical treatment of duplication of the alimentary tract: enterogenous cysts, enteric cysts, or ileum duplex, *Surg Gynecol Obstet* 1940; 70: 295–307.

CHAPTER 47

Rectoceles and Constipation

C Barben

Introduction

The rectovaginal septum tends to weaken with age and parturition, allowing the rectum to protrude into the vagina during evacuation, and this outpouching is termed a rectocele. Rectoceles do occur in men, but are much less common. The influence of childbirth is strong, with most patients being multiparous. Rectoceles can be classified into high, mid and low (see Fig. 1).

In high rectoceles, there is disruption of the upper third of the vaginal wall, and an association with other abnormalities, such as eneteroceles, cystoceles and uterine prolapse. Midlevel rectoceles are the most common, and are caused by loss of pelvic floor support, influenced by parturition. Low level rectoceles are usually the consequence of perineal body defects, as a result of childbirth.

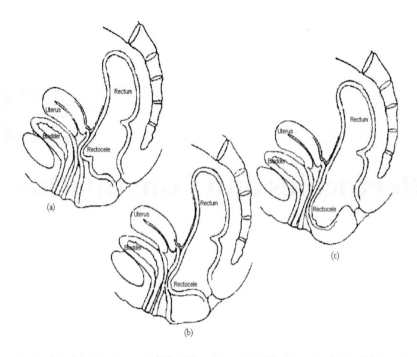

Figure 1. Sagittal section of the pelvis showing the (a) high, (b) mid and (c) low rectoceles.

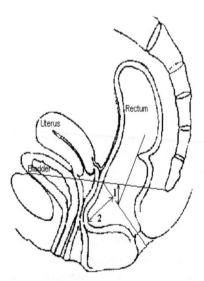

Figure 2. Measurements taken during cinedefecography include (1) perineal descent and (2) rectocele diameter.

So what is the relevance of a rectocele? It has been suggested that up to 80% of females may present with asymptomatic rectoceles. Rectoceles less than 2 cm in diameter are usually accepted as a normal finding. One suggestion for the pathophysiology of rectoceles is that they are caused by paradoxical puborectalis contraction rather than being a primary phenomenon. This may account for disappointing surgical results in some patients.

Investigation

The diagnosis of a rectocele is, like any other condition, made by taking an adequate history and performing a thorough physical examination. A rectocele may cause mild to severe anorectal symptoms, which are usually associated with constipation, a sense of incomplete evacuation, the need for prolonged straining or difficult evacuation. This may necessitate vaginal or rectal digitation, or perineal support, to assure a rectal evacuation. Patients may also notice the sensation of a bulge into the vagina. Physical examination may be performed with the patient prone or supine with the use of the squatting position if necessary, with bearing down, to determine if a cystocele or other pelvic disorder is associated with the rectocele. Although physical examination is sensitive in two thirds of cases, it does not quantify size, and cannot measure emptying ability.

Cinedefecography is the most useful test for diagnosing recotceles.[1] Defecography is performed by introducing 100–250 ml of barium paste into the rectum, with a further 20–50 ml of liquid barium to assist in using a double contrast method. This is performed with the patient lying left lateral on the X-ray table. Subsequently, the X-ray table is positioned upright so that the patient is seated in a lateral position over a plastic radiolucent commode filled with water. The fluoroscopic monitor is connected to a video to allow recording of the procedure. Images are taken at rest, and during the squeeze and push phases. The procedure is performed with synchronous anal manometry and EMG studies.

Barium trapping in rectoceles has been used as a criterion to indicate surgery. The volume of retention depends on methodological variables, such as the amount of barium injected and the technique used to measure the volume. A retrospective study showed no difference in evacuation time, evacuation completeness rectal pressure, or the need for digitation between the patients without a rectocele, those with a rectocele, and those with a rectocele and greater than 10% barium retention.[2] Dynamic pelvic magnetic resonance imaging has been used to assist in the diagnosis of rectoceles. There are suggestions that it may be of use in those patients who have complex pelvic disorders,[3] but it is unlikely that its use will become routine.[4]

There are also other considerations. A full colonoscopy should be performed to exclude organic causes of constipation. If this is normal, colonic inertia should be excluded by transit marker studies, and the patient's thyroid function should also be checked. Finally, other associated anorectal conditions should be excluded, such as rectal intussusception and paradoxical puborectalis contraction, as undertaking rectocele repair in patients with these conditions is associated with a poorer outcome.

Treatment

The treatment options for rectoceles fall into three broad categories: conservative, biofeedback and surgery. All patients should undergo a period of conservative management before surgery is offered and this includes a high fibre diet (25–35 g per day), and ingestion of two to three litres of noncaffeinated, nonalcoholic fluids per day. If symptoms persist after this, further treatment may be considered.

It has been suggested that the symptoms associated with a rectocele may be due to a disturbance of rectoanal co-ordination, which may be suitable for treatment with biofeedback.[5] Most studies show symptomatic improvement in about 50% of patients who complete the therapy, and this may be of use as a first line therapy.[6]

Having decided that a patient may warrant an operation, which patients will be suitable for surgical intervention? By looking at the results from surgical repair, it can be seen that not all patients with rectoceles will benefit, and some preoperative symptoms are associated with a better outcome. The rectocele should be at least 4 cm on defecography, and should also demonstrate incomplete evacuation. Symptoms should have been present for a long time, despite a trial of increased fibre and fluid intake, and the need for digitation preoperatively is associated with a better outcome from surgery.[7] It has been suggested in a paper from Block that most rectoceles are of no clinical consequence,[8] but selecting the appropriate rectoceles to operate on can give success rates of over 80%.[9] Other studies have shown that the need for perineal or vaginal digitation is associated with a better outcome. A previous hysterectomy, a large rectal area on defecography and the preoperative use of enemas are all associated with a poor surgical outcome.[10]

The methods available for dealing with rectoceles operatively are the transvaginal repair, the transperineal repair and the transanal repair.

The transvaginal repair includes redundant vaginal wall resection and puborectalis plication. The patient is placed in the lithotomy position, retractors are placed in the vagina to expose the rectocele, and a finger in the rectum can be used to confirm the extent of the defect. The submucosal plane is then infiltrated with dilute adrenaline solution. Using diathermy, a transverse or anchor-shaped incision is created, and flaps are elevated in the submucosal plane. This dissection continues to the extent of the rectocele defect. The defect can then be closed in a vertical or horizontal manner with interrupted Vicryl sutures. A finger placed in the rectum can confirm the adequacy of the repair. After excising redundant mucosa, the mucosa is closed with absorbable sutures. Some series have noted an incidence of rectovaginal fistulas, vaginal narrowing and postoperative dyspareunia.

The transperineal repair is less commonly used. After the patient is placed in the prone jackknife position, the buttocks are taped apart. A U-shaped perineal incision is used. The dissection is undertaken to beyond the limit of the rectocele, after which a section of the redundant posterior vaginal wall is resected. The defect is closed with a running, absorbable suture, and the space between the vaginal and rectal walls is closed. A levator plication is then executed with two or three single sutures. The American proponents of this technique claim that it has a high success rate with low complications, although it is not widely used.

The transanal approach is the one that most people are familiar with. Again, the procedure is performed in the prone jackknife position with the buttocks taped apart. After cleaning, the extent of the rectocele is confirmed, and the submucosal plane is infiltrated with dilute adrenaline solution. A vertical, horizontal or elliptical incision can be used, and mucosal flaps are raised with sharp and blunt dissection. The main difficulty is in keeping the dissection in the submucosal plane. The defect, once demonstrated, is repaired with interrupted vicryl, and any redundant mucosa is excised. The mucosa is closed with absorbable sutures. Lately a promising new technique of rectocele repair using the PPH01 haemorrhoidectomy has been tried. We are evaluating this procedure in the department.

Table 1. Results from a variety of series of rectocele repairs.

Author	Patients	Technique	Success Rate (%)
Sullivan (1968)	151	Transrectal	79.5
Khubchandani (1983)	59	Transrectal	79.6
Sehapayak (1985)	355	Transrectal	84.5
Arnold (1990)	35	Transrectal	80
Sarles (1991)	39	Transrectal	95
Janssen (1994)	76	Transrectal	92
Redding (1965)	20	Transvaginal	100
Pitchford (1967)	44	Transvaginal	Ns
Arnold (1990)	29	Transvaginal	80
Mellgren (1995)	25	Transvaginal	88
Khubchandani (1997)	123	Transrectal	82
Ho (1998)	21	Transrectal	100

Table 1 shows the results from various series of transanal and transvaginal repair. As has been said previously, a success rate of around 80% can be expected. The complication rate from these series ranged from 0 to 35%.

There are potential problems with the transrectal repair, as demonstrated by the last of the studies in Table 1. In this series, although all patients were fully continent both before and after surgery, postoperative anal manometry revealed significant reductions in resting and squeeze pressures.[11] Patients are, therefore, at risk of incontinence after transanal rectocele repair.

Summary

In summary, the rectocele is a commonly discovered phenomenon in patients undergoing investigation for constipation, especially in multiparous women. The indications for repair are controversial, but careful selection of patients can give satisfactory results in almost all patients.

References

1. Janssen LW and van Dijke CF. Selection criteria for anterior rectal wall repair in symptomatic rectocele and anterior rectal wall prolapse, *Dis Colon Rectum* 1994; 37(11): 1100–7.
2. Halligan S and Bartram CI. Is barium trapping in rectoceles significant? *Dis Colon Rectum* 1995; 38(7): 764–8.

3. Rentsch M, Paetzel C, Lenhart M, Feuerbach S, Jauch KW and Furst A. Dynamic magnetic resonance imaging defecography: a diagnostic alternative in the assessment of pelvic floor disorders in proctology, *Dis Colon Rectum* 2001; 44(7): 999–1007.

4. Matsuoka H, Wexner SD, Desai MB, Nakamura T, Nogueras JJ, Weiss EG, Adami C and Billotti VL. A comparison between dynamic pelvic magnetic resonance imaging and videoproctography in patients with constipation, *Dis Colon Rectum* 2001; 44(4): 571–6.

5. Fucini C, Ronchi O and Elbetti C. Electromyography of the pelvic floor musculature in the assessment of obstructed defecation symptoms, *Dis Colon Rectum* 2001; 44(8): 1168–75.

6. Mimura T, Roy AJ, Storrie JB and Kamm MA. Treatment of impaired defecation associated with rectocele by behavorial retraining (biofeedback), *Dis Colon Rectum* 2000; 43(9): 1267–72.

7. Rosato GO. In *Fundamentals of Anorectal Surgery*, Beck D and Wexner S (eds.). Saunders, London, 1998.

8. Block IR. Transrectal repair of rectocele using obliterative suture, *Dis Colon Rectum* 1986; 29(11): 707–11.

9. Sehapayak S. Transrectal repair of rectocele: an extended armamentarium of colorectal surgeons: a report of 355 cases, *Dis Colon Rectum* 1985; 28(6): 422–33.

10. Karlbom U, Graf W, Nilsson S and Pahlman L. Does surgical repair of a rectocele improve rectal emptying? *Dis Colon Rectum* 1996; 39(11): 1296–302.

11. Ho YH, Ang M, Nyam D, Tan M and Seow-Choen F. Transanal approach to rectocele repair may compromise anal sphincter pressures, *Dis Colon Rectum* 1998; 41(3): 354–8.

Difficult Abdominal Closure: Alternative Strategies

PG Skaife

Abstract

In surgery, we are occasionally faced with the prospect of not being able to close the abdomen following laparotomy. Abdominal wall closure may be rendered impossible by trauma, infection, and local tissue necrosis from radiation or following tumour resection. A staged approach to closure or reconstruction may then become necessary when the musculofascial layers are injured or absent.

At operation, there are three basic reasons why an abdominal wound cannot be closed:

1. Physical inability to bring the wound edges together;
2. Tissues not able to take suture placement;
3. Ongoing intra-abdominal sepsis preventing abdominal closure.

Methods to address this problem have been tried with varying success, this fact suggesting that none are completely satisfactory.

Introduction

An abdomen that presents difficulty in closing is encountered by most surgeons on occasions, requiring a change of technique to achieve approximation of wound edges. Technical considerations in closing the abdomen are the points of greatest interest to surgeons. Wound dehiscence within the first few days of surgery is undoubtedly a technical error—the responsibility lying squarely on the shoulders of the surgeon. Knot slipping and suture breaking is unusual in experienced hands. For laparotomy closure, continuous closure with a nonabsorbable suture gives the lowest incidence of hernia,[1] and the suture-length-to-wound-length ratio should be 4:1.[2] These ideal principles may not always be possible in practical terms and lead to a compromised closure.

Objective criteria have been listed that identify a wound which is at risk for dehiscence, therefore requiring special attention to closure.[3] This occurs in the following circumstances:

1. Large size wound ($>40 \, cm^2$)
2. Absence of stable skin coverage
3. Recurrence of defect after previous closure
4. Systemic compromisation (see table)
5. Compromised local tissue
6. Concomitant intra-abdominal complications

Pathophysiology of Wound Healing

There are three stages of wound healing:

Stage 1

The inflammatory stage follows the traumatic initiation of the wound. Within the cavity of the wound there is deposition of inflammatory cells. This lasts for five days and during this time there is no tensile strength within the wound. The integrity of wound closure is dependent entirely upon the suture closure. Failure of the wound at this stage may be deemed a technical failure by the operator.

Stage 2

This is the fibroplastic stage. There is deposition of collagen across the wound defect, haphazardly arranged at first and becoming arranged gradually across the lines of wound stress to produce an increase in intrinsic strength. This stage lasts for around 10 days.

Stage 3

The maturation stage lasts for anything up to 12 months and involves the resorption of old and mal-arranged collagen.

It follows that impairment of any of the above stages will cause the wound to fail. From a surgical standpoint, the first two stages are the most relevant.

Alternative Closure Techniques

The consequence of early wound failure is a burst abdomen and this is associated with considerable morbidity and mortality. The two major pathophysiological causes for this are wound ischaemia and wound infection. Primary wound closure involving placement of sutures that are too tight will cause local ischaemia of the musculofascial tissue and the resulting necrosis will cause the sutures to cut through the tissue, leading to a burst abdomen. During a difficult closure where wound tension is appreciated by the surgeon, methods have been described to reduce the tension:

Lateral relaxing incisions. Generally, lateral abdominal fascial incisions, unilaterally or bilaterally, are made lateral to the rectus muscle. The aponeurosis remains attached to its muscle belly superiorly and inferiorly. The site below the incision is protected from herniation by the deeper muscular tissues. Meanwhile, the medial edge of the aponeurosis is lax and facilitates its approximation to the midline wound.

Deep tension suture placement. This involves the use of a nonabsorbable suture on a large needle to produce interrupted, wide bites of all layers of tissue. The purpose is that the wound edges are approximated with the tension being distributed between all tissue layers (muscle, aponeurosis, subcutaneous tissue and skin). This permits a mass closure of the medial fascial layer with reduced tension.[4] Sutures are generally left in place for at least 14 days when tensile strength within the wound should be sufficient to maintain integrity.

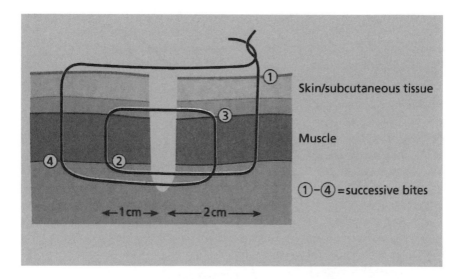

Figure 1. Double-loop deep tension technique.

Double-loop deep tension technique. A novel approach incorporating the principles of tension distribution has been described. This is performed using a nonabsorbable suture and possesses the advantage of reducing the width of wound closure (Fig. 1).

Double near and far Prolene suture closure. This technique for reducing tension in the wound was originally described for the repair of incisional hernia[5] but has recently been described in the closure of laparostomy wounds.[6] Again, the technique distributes the tension across a wider area along the axis of the wound using a single tissue plane (Fig. 2).

Prosthetic Mesh

The demonstration of a tension-free repair of hernia has made the imposition of prosthetic mesh[2] an attractive proposition when tension from wound closure is likely. This is particularly so if the musculofacial tissue at the wound edge is of poor quality or there has been tissue loss. Prosthetic meshes used for repair include polypropylene (Marlex), PTFE (Goretex), Dacron (Silastic) and Polyglycolic (Vicryl). The placement of mesh to bridge abdominal wall defects is an effective means of restoring continuity. A number of small series have been reported outlining the benefits and pitfalls of

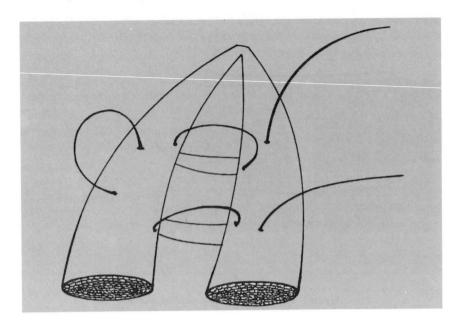

Figure 2. Double near and far Prolene closure technique.

its use. One of the most common and difficult complications to manage is the development of an enterocutaneous fistula, with the resultant fluid loss and electrolyte alterations. The use of an absorbable polypropylene synthetic mesh was thought to address this problem. However, fistulation rates are not significantly different from nonabsorbable mesh.[8] In addition, once the mesh is resorbed, an incisional hernia occurs.

A study of mesh closure using prolene mesh involving 26 patients with intra-abdominal catastrophe from trauma had mesh placement has been described.[9] This series demonstrated a fistulation rate approaching 40%. This unacceptable high incidence is consistent with other reports.[10,11] A single series of incisional hernia repairs using intraperitoneal or extraperitoneal placement of polypropylene mesh in 33 cases[3] demonstrated no fistulous complications. Fistulation is thought to occur due to the proinflammatory nature of the mesh, causing adherence of underlying bowel. This is combined with the abrasive nature of the mesh causing serosal injury. Abscess formation between intestine and mesh occurs and fistulation results. It must be stressed that fistulous complications seem to be a rare problem when the imposition of mesh is used in an elective setting for the repair of incisional hernia, when direct contact of the mesh with intestine can be avoided. A new product incorporating Prolene mesh, combined with a hyaluronidase coating to prevent adherence of intestinal content (Sepramesh, Johnson & Johnson), may address this problem but, as yet, no reports of its use are available.

Laparostomy

Occasionally the abdomen cannot be closed or simply should not be closed. Laparostomy is the technique of leaving the abdomen open following laparotomy that can be adopted in acute situations, or in the management of ongoing, chronic infection. It has usually been employed in the presence of ongoing intra-abdominal sepsis, resulting from infected pancreatic necrosis, but has also been described for sepsis of colonic origin.[12] Delayed fascial closure is often practised following "damage control" strategies in major trauma, and severe intra-abdominal sepsis. In acute trauma to the abdomen, oedema of intestine, mesentry and retroperitoneal tissues can make closure difficult, while aggressive fluid replacement involved in early resuscitation may compound this. Attempts at abdominal closure under these circumstances may result in abdominal compartment syndrome and cause acute respiratory embarrassment, and so laparostomy may be employed as a temporizing method until this oedematous situation resolves (Table 1). Measures must be taken to prevent desiccation of exposed intestine for the duration of the laparostomy wound. Skin closure alone with towel clips allows enteric cover[13] and provides a sufficient hydrostatic pressure to reduce oedema, allowing later closure. A second method to prevent intestinal exposure is abdominal containment.[14] Here, a clear polyurethane bag, identical to that in which intravenous fluids are

Table 1. Benefits and pitfalls of laparostomy.

Advantages	Disadvantages
Prevents repeat and progressively more difficult closure[16]	Requires prolonged hospitalization
Permits re-exploration in ITU setting	Intensive, expert nursing care required for wound management
Allows effective drainange of multiple fistulas	Fluid and electrolyte imbalances, protein loss
Closure by granulation possible	Potential of intestinal dessication, evisceration and fistulation

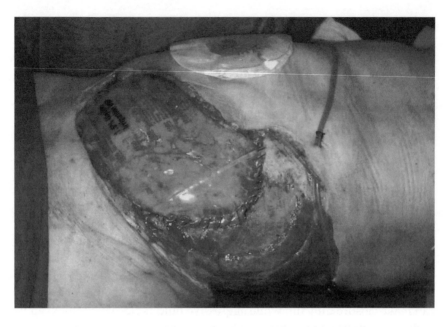

Figure 3. Bogota bag used in abdominal sepsis to contain intestines.

delivered, is sutured to the wound edges. The so-called Bogota bag provides an "annex" to the abdominal cavity and permits free expansion of the intra-abdominal content, so preventing a rise in abdominal pressure. Such a bag is demonstrated in Fig. 3.

Definitive closure of the abdomen can be undertaken around two weeks later by fascial closure, split-skin grafting over granulation tissue or the imposition of mesh.[15]

In the presence of intra-abdominal sepsis, there is an increased chance of wound dehiscence, and it may be preferable to accept a purposeful laparostomy wound. It may be used in preference to on-demand or "second look" laparotomy, where there is the recurrent chance of injury to intestine, and tissues become increasingly friable and difficult to close.

A method of temporary closure allowing repeated and easy access to the abdominal cavity has been developed by employing a zipper device. This is sutured to the skin surrounding the abdominal defect. It may be opened and closed at will (Fig. 4).

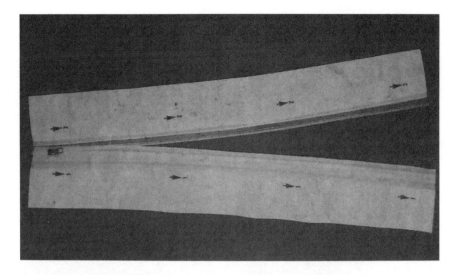

Figure 4. Abdominal zipper allowing easy repeated access to the abdomen.

Autologous Graft Closure

If it is anticipated that tissue loss will occur and result in a difficult closure, as a result of abdominal wall resection for tumour or necrosis, then an autologous graft can be harvested in the same procedure (Fig. 5). This may consist of fascia with or without cutaneous cover. The latter method has the advantage if skin loss is associated with a fascial defect where sensate skin is used to cover the defect. This is necessary in the abdominal waistline area, as this area is subject to pressure from clothing. This method has been successfully employed in the same procedure as abdominal wall resection.[17]

Summary

To address the problem of difficult abdominal wall closure following laparotomy, the matters to be addressed include:

- The underlying pathology;
- The setting of acute emergency surgery or elective;
- The sterile or grossly infected abdominal cavity.

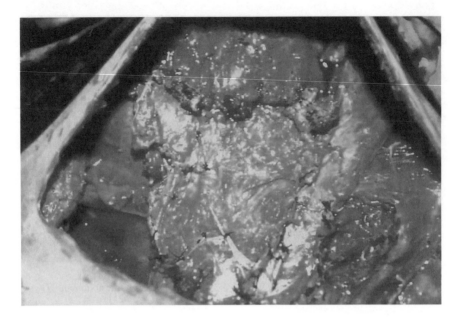

Figure 5. Fascial graph from tensor fascia lata of thigh to close abdominal wall defect.

Simple physical tension on the wound during closure should be appreciated by the operator and the techniques described to reduce tension may be employed. Planned resection of the abdominal wall is best managed by one of the autologous flap repairs. In the emergency situation where gross contamination or visceral oedema may lead to compartment syndrome, one of the techniques of laparostomy or open containment may be employed. On the basis of the evidence available, mesh closure of large abdominal defects cannot be recommended.

References

1. Hodgson NC, Malthaner RA and Ostbye T. The search for an ideal method of abdominal fascial closure: a meta-analysis, *Ann Surg* 2000; 231(3): 436–22.
2. Jenkins SD, Klamer TW, Parteka JJ and Condon RE. A comparison of prosthetic materials used to repair abdominal wall defects, *Surgery* 1983; 94: 392–8.

3. Mathes SJ, Steinwald PM, Foster RD, Hofmman WY and Anthony JP. Complex abdominal wall reconstruction: a comparison of flap and mesh closure, *Ann Surg* 2000; 586–96.

4. Lansdown MR and McMahon MJ. Use of deep tension sutures and buttress plates for frequent relaparotomy, *Br J Surg* 1989; 76(4): 400.

5. Hughes LE. Leading Article: incisional hernia, *Asian Journal of Surgery* 1990; 13: 69–72.

6. A-Malik R and Scott NA. Double near and far prolene suture closure: a technique for abdominal wall closure after laparostomy, *Br J Surg* 2001; 88: 147–7.

7. Goris JA. Ogilvie's method applied to infected wound disruption, *Arch Surg* 1980; 115(9): 1103–7.

8. Green MA, Mullins RJ, Malangoni MA *et al*. Laparotomy wound closure with absorbable polyglycolic acid mesh, *Surg Gynecol Obstet* 1993; 176: 213–18.

9. Fansler RF, Taheri P, Cullinane C, Sabates B and Flint LM. Polypropylene mesh closure of the complicated abdominal wound, *Am J Surg* 1995; 170: 15–8.

10. Voyles CR, Richardson JD, Bland KI *et al*. Emergency abdominal wall reconstruction with polypropylene mesh, *Ann Surg* 1981; 194: 219–23.

11. Boyd WC. Use of Marlex mesh in acute loss of abdominal wall due to infection, *Surg Gynecol Obstet* 1977; 144: 251–2.

12. Bailey CMH, Thomson-Fawcett MW, Kettlewell MGH, Garrard C and Mortensen NJM. Laparostomy for severe intra-abdominal infection complicating colorectal disease, *Dis Colon Rectum* 2000; 43: 25–30.

13. Smith PC, Tweddell JS and Bessey BQ. Alternative approaches to abdominal wound closurein severely injured patients with massive visceral oedema, *J Trauma* 1992; 32: 16–20.

14. Ghimenton F, Thomson SR, Muckart DJ and Burrows R. Abdominal content containment: practicalities and outcome, *Br J Surg* 2000; 87: 106–9.

15. Howard CA and Turner WW. Successful treatment of early, postoperative, necrotizing infection of the abdominal wall, *Crit Care Med* 1989; 17: 586–7.

16. Schein M. Planned reoperations and open management in critical intra-abdominal infections: prospective experience in 52 cases, *World J Surg* 1991; 15: 537–45.

17. Koshy CE, Kumar MV and Evans J. Lower abdominal wall reconstruction using the anterior thigh fasciocutaneous flap, *Br J Plast Surg* 1999; 52(8): 667–9.

CHAPTER 49

Modern Management of Adhesions

SM Heah

Introduction

Adhesion formation after peritoneal surgery is a major cause of postoperative bowel obstruction, infertility in women and chronic pelvic pain.[1] After an adhesive small bowel obstruction, recurrence rates are high: 53% after an initial episode and over 85% after the second, third or later episodes.[2] Colorectal surgery is the most common procedure performed in the abdomen and it is the most common reason for reoperation for adhesive intestinal obstruction.[2] It has been shown that 3% of all laparotomies are for adhesion-induced intestinal obstruction.[3] For the year 1994 in the United States alone, there were 303 836 hospitalizations during which adhesiolysis was performed. This accounted for 846 415 inpatient days and an estimated US$1.3 billion in expenditures.[4] Understanding the aetiology of adhesion allows us to target strategies in order to minimize its formation. This involves minimizing surgical trauma by using smaller wounds such as those in laparoscopic surgery and the introduction of bioresorbable mechanical barriers.

Morphogenesis of Adhesion Formation

Adhesions form when two peritoneal surfaces are apposed after surgery. Adhesion formation begins with a fibrin matrix occurring typically during coagulation in the presence of suppressed fibrinolysis.[5] Surgical injury of tissue reduces blood flow, producing ischaemia leading to local persistence of the fibrin matrix. This matrix is gradually replaced by vascular granulation tissue containing macrophages, fibroblasts and giant cells. The clots, being slow to achieve complete organization, consist of erythrocytes separated by strands or condensed masses of fibrin which are covered with two to three layers of flattened cells and contain a patchy infiltrate of mononuclear cells. Eventually, a fibrous band forms, containing small nodules of calcification. The adhesions are often covered by mesothelium and contain blood vessels and connective tissue fibres, including elastin.

The minimum postoperative interval required for the use of an impermeable barrier to prevent adhesion formation has been established. Harris *et al*.[6] investigated the removal of a silastic sheet at 6, 12, 18, 24, 30, 36, 72 and 96 hours after peritoneal injury and found that the incidence of adhesion formation dropped from 100 to 0% during the first 36 hours.

Methods to Reduce Adhesions

Effect of cauterization

Cauterization of peritoneal surfaces causes more tissue damage, which promotes adhesions.[7] Three weeks after using cautery at surgery, there are abundant polymorphonuclear leukocytes and minimal fibroblasts or collagen formation at the tissue site and delayed wound healing. There is excessive carbonization in the wound surfaces, which leads to giant cell formation and foreign body granulomas. Sharp dissection by scissors does not induce carbonization or necrosis and may minimize adhesion formation compared to cautery.

Blood

The role of blood in the peritoneal cavity in the formation of adhesions has been studied. Jackson found that 100 ml of free blood and well-formed clots took 8 days to be absorbed from the peritoneal cavity.[8] Addition of fresh blood and clots without peritoneal injury induces adhesions.[9] This is further enhanced if the peritoneal surface is incised. The same effects are seen with serosal damage. Clotted blood constitutes a fibrinous network upon which fibroblasts proliferate, resulting in adhesions.[10] Therefore, washing away blood clots prior to closure of the abdominal wound may minimize adhesions.

Laparoscopic surgery

Laparoscopic surgery has been shown to decrease adhesions when compared to conventional surgery.[11] This may be due to minimal handling and smaller incisions, thereby minimizing trauma to the visceral and parietal peritoneum. In using a porcine model, Reissman *et al.*[12] reported significantly reduced adhesion formation when laparoscopic anterior resection was performed, compared to deliberately abraded loops of ileum. Laparoscopic surgery has also been shown to reduce adhesion formation when used in peritonitis compared to open surgery.[13] In the same study,[13] when performing laparoscopic surgery, the use of helium was found to result in less adhesions when compared to the use of carbon dioxide. It was postulated that the bacterial inhibiting properties of helium cause a reduction in inflammation and damage to the mesothelial cells, thereby minimizing collagen deposits and ultimately adhesions to form. However, we have noticed that the left iliac fossa incision used in our department for rectal surgery dramatically reduces adhesions compared to the long line incision as well.

Mechanical barriers

This is the latest innovation being used to prevent adhesions. Studies have shown that by placing an absorbable barrier oxidized regenerated cellulose (INTERCEED® [TC7] Absorbable Adhesion Barrier, Ethicon Inc., Somerville, NJ, USA), expanded polytetrafluoroethylene (Preclude® Surgical Membrane, W.L. Gore and Assoc., Flagstaff, AZ, USA) or hyaluronic acid/carboxymethylcellulose (Seprafilm® Surgical Membrane, Genzyme

Corp., Cambridge, MA, USA) between injury sites or addition of a viscous solution (dextran, Hyskon® Solution, Pharmacia Inc., Piscataway, NJ, USA; hyaluronic acid, Sepracoat®, Genzyme Corp.) into the peritoneal cavity during or after surgery can reduce postoperative adhesion formation.[14] Although gel formulations have the theoretical advantage of reducing adhesion formation throughout the peritoneal cavity, Hyskon® in clinical settings has been shown to result in ascites due to its oncotic properties,[15] as well as being ineffective in pelvic surgery resulting from gravitational pooling in the cul-de-sac.[16]

Hyaluronic acid is a linear polysaccharide with repeating disaccharide units composed of sodium D-glucuronate and N-acetyl-D-glucosamine. It is a major component of many body tissues and fluids, providing mechanically protective as well as physically supportive roles. Intergel™ (Lifecore Biomedical Inc., Chaska, MN) is a new antiadhesive gel preparation containing hyaluronic acid. Hyaluronic acid has been shown to possess antiadhesive properties and other beneficial effects on wound healing.[17] Cross-linkage of the carboxylate groups on the hyaluronic acid molecules by chelation with ferric (Fe^{3+}) ions results in a viscous lubricating gel preparation. Instillation into the peritoneal cavity following abdominal surgery minimizes tissue apposition during the critical period of the fibrin formation and mesothelial regeneration. Lymphatic drainage is the major route of elimination from the peritoneal cavity, with a half-life of approximately 51 hours.[18] Hyaluronic-acid-based gels have been shown to reduce adhesion formation in animal studies.[19] A randomized controlled trial was recently conducted at the Colorectal Department, Singapore General Hospital, to evaluate the role of Intergel as an antiadhesive agent following open colorectal surgery. Initially aiming to recruit 700 patients, the study was discontinued after accrual of only 32 patients due to several adverse effects. These results are currently being assessed. However, randomized controlled trials involving Intergel following pelvic gynaecological, surgery showed significant (59%) reduction in adhesions.[20] No serious side effects or serious adverse events were noted in these trials. Gynaecological procedures are generally of a "clean" nature. In contrast, colorectal surgery usually involves the opening of bowel at some stage in constructing the anastomosis. The risk of releasing bacteria-laden enteric contents into the peritoneal cavity, which initiates intra-abdominal sepsis, thereby predisposing to anastomotic dehiscence, is ever-present. Ordinarily, this will not pose problems clinically, but the effect of gel instillates on the incidence of intra-abdominal sepsis following bowel resection is unknown in humans.

There is evidence that iron-containing solutions can markedly increase the virulence of several different bacterial species, and certain strains have evolved the ability to scavenge free iron from their environment.[21] Therefore, until evidence points to the contrary, gel instillates into the peritoneal cavity should not be used in surgery involving enterotomy or colostomy. Nevertheless, it can be safely used in gynaecological surgery or after adhesiolysis without any bowel resection or enterotomy.

Seprafilm® is a bioresorbable membrane composed of sodium hyaluronate and carboxymethylcellulose. When these two substances combine, they form a transparent, thin, adherent and absorbable membrane. This forms a physical barrier by providing temporary separation of serosal tissues during the initial postoperative healing phase and, in so doing, prevents adhesions from forming.[22] It has been shown to significantly reduce adhesions at the sites of application.[23] A total of 183 patients with either ulcerative colitis or familial adenomatous polyposis coli undergoing restorative panproctocolectomy with ileal pouch-anal anastomosis and defunctioning ileostomy were prospectively randomized into either receiving Seprafilm placed under the midline wound or not (control group).[23] A laparoscope was used to assess 175 patients at ileostomy closure 12 weeks later. Significant differences in favour of the treated group were found with regard to "no adhesions" (51% vs 6%), "mean incision length percentage involved with adhesion" (23% vs 63%) and presence of "dense adhesions" (15% vs 58%). There was no significant difference in adverse events between the two groups.[23] The authors justifiably concluded that Seprafilm was safe and effective for use in large bowel surgery. Perhaps more significantly, its use during open bowel contaminated surgery has been shown to be both safe and efficacious in preventing adhesions.[24] The study[24] showed decreased incidence of adhesion formation in rabbits which underwent repaired or unrepaired myotomy among those covered by Seprafilm. Septic complications such as leak rates and phlegmon formation were not different in the treated or control groups. Recently, Seprafilm-induced peritoneal inflammation has been reported.[25] The patient had undergone completion proctectomy for ulcerative colitis and Seprafilm was placed beneath the midline wound prior to closure. On the fourth postoperative day, the patient was reoperated for intestinal obstruction when it was discovered that the membrane had diffusely melted over the surrounding small intestine and caused a dense inflammatory reaction. Biopsies taken showed intense foreign body reaction which confirmed an acute inflammatory response to Seprafilm.

Postoperatively, the patient was treated with steroids and antibiotics and recovered uneventfully. Surgeons need to be aware of this possibility.

Salum *et al.*[26] reported on the impact of limited selective placement of Seprafilm (under the fascial layer, around ileostomy and in the pelvis) in preventing adhesions. Comparing 259 treated patients with 179 untreated, well-matched controls, they found no differences in the bowel obstruction and the adhesiolysis rate between the two groups. Complications were also similar. The effective placement of Seprafilm requires drying the intended area of application. The flimsy membrane should not be allowed to come into contact with any wet surfaces, because it will otherwise shrivel away and be ineffective. This is so because the membrane must stay long enough between the tissues (36 hours) to prevent adhesion formation in the immediate postoperative period. Placement of Seprafilm in the pelvis is probably ineffective, as there is often a pool of "wash fluid" there which tends to dislodge the membrane from its intended site of action. However, its placement under laparotomy wounds is effective provided steps are carefully taken to ensure that it stays there, i.e. drying the surfaces before application.

In another series of yet-unpublished data, the Colorectal Department at the Singapore General Hospital prospectively randomized 120 patients with ileostomy after low anterior resection. Sixty patients had Seprafilm wrapped around the ileostomy and an equal number had no Seprafilm® applied. For patients with closure of ileostomy at 3 weeks, there was significant reduction in adhesions around the stoma in the Seprafim group. However, if the stoma was closed at 6 weeks or beyond, no differences in terms of adhesions were noted. Morbidity was similar in the two groups. Therefore the use of Seprafilm around temporary stomas is effective and allows safe early closure of stomas.

Summary

Adhesions are formed by peritoneal injury during laparotomy. There is relative ischaemia in the damaged tissues immediately postoperatively, resulting in impaired fibrinolysis and a relative increase in fibrin matrix deposition. Simple methods to minimize adhesion formation include using sharp scissors dissection instead of cauterization, gentle handling of intestinal loops, and washing away blood before closing the abdomen. Laparoscopic surgery to minimize trauma should be undertaken whenever the expertise is available and within the constraints of cost. Modern methods of preventing adhesions involve the use of bioresorbable barriers in the form of gel instillates (Intergel) or membranes (Seprafilm). Intergel is effective and safe in laparotomies that do not involve contamination or enterotomies, i.e. gynaecological surgery or adhesiolysis without enterotomies. Seprafilm can effectively prevent adhesion formation when placed under incisional wounds and around stomas. It does not cause increased septic complications when used in open bowel surgery.

References

1. Ellis H. The magnitude of adhesion-related problems. In: diZerega GS (ed.), *Peritoneal surgery*. Springer-Verlag, New York, 2000, pp. 297–306.
2. Barkan H, Webster S and Ozeran S. Factors predicting the recurrence of adhesive small bowel obstruction, *Am J Surg* 1995; 170: 361–5.
3. Menzies D and Ellis H. Intestinal obstruction from adhesions: how big is the problem? *Am Roy Coll Surg Engl* 1990; 71: 60.
4. Beck DE, Opelka FG, Bailey HR, Rauh SM and Pashos CL. Incidence of small-bowel obstruction and adhesiolysis after open colorectal and general surgery, *Dis Colon Rectum* 1999; 42: 241–8.
5. diZerega GS. *Use of Adhesion Barriers in Pelvic Reconstructive and Gynecology Surgery*. Springer-Verlag, New York, 2000, pp. 379–9.
6. Harris ES, Morgan RF and Rodeheaver GT. Analysis of kinetics of peritoneal adhesion formation in the rat and evaluation of potential antiadhesive agents, *Surgery* 1995; 117: 663–9.
7. diZerega GS and Campeau JD. Peritoneal repair and post-surgical adhesion formation, *Hum Repro Update* 2001; 7(6): 547–55.
8. Jackson BB. Observations on intraperitoneal adhesions: an experimental study, *Surgery* 1958; 44: 507–18.
9. Ryan GB, Grobety J and Majno G. Postoperative peritoneal adhesions: a study of the mechanisms, *Am J Pathol* 1978; 65: 117–48.
10. Pfeiffer CJ, Pfeiffer DC and Misra HP. Enteric serosal surface in the piglet: a scanning and transmission electron microscopic study of the mesothelium, *J Submicrosc Cytol* 1987; 19: 237–46.
11. Jorgensen JO, Lalak NJ and Hunt DR. Is laparoscopy associated with a lower rate of postoperative adhesions than laparotomy? A comparative study in the rabbit, *Aust N Z J Surg* 1995; 65: 342–4.
12. Reissman P, Teoh TA, Skinner K, Burns JW and Wexner SD. Adhesion formation after laparoscopic anterior resection in a porcine model: a pilot study, *Surg Laparosc Endosc* 1996; 6(2): 136–9.

13. Jacobi CA, Sterzel A, Braumann C, Halle E *et al*. The impact of conventional and laparoscopic colon resection (CO_2 or helium) on intraperitoneal adhesion formation in a rat peritonitis model, *Surg Endosc* 2001; 15: 380–6.

14. Lundorff P, Geldorp HV, Tronstad SE, Lalos O *et al*. Reduction of postsurgical adhesions with ferric hyaluronate gel: a European study, *Hum Repro* 2001; 16(9): 1982–8.

15. Gauwerky JF, Heinrich D and Kubli F. Complications of intraperitoneal dextran application for prevention of adhesions, *Biol Res Pregnancy Peritatol* 1986; 7: 93–7.

16. diZerega GS. Contemporary adhesion prevention. *Fertil Steril* 1994; 61: 219–35.

17. King SR, Hickerson WL, Proctor KG and Newsome AM. Beneficial actions of exogenous hyaluronic acid on wound healing, *Surgery* 1991; 109: 76–84.

18. Johns DB, Rodgers KE, Donahue WD, Kiorpes TC and diZerega GS. Reduction of adhesion formation by postoperative administration of ionically cross-linked hyaluronic acid, *Fertil Steril* 1997; 68(1): 37–42.

19. Sawada T, Tsukada K, Hasegawa K and Ohashi Y *et al*. Cross-linked hyaluronate hydrogel prevents adhesion formation and reformation in mouse uterine horn model, *Hum Repro* 2001; 16(2): 353–6.

20. Johns DB, Keyport GM, Hoehler F and diZerega GS. Reduction of postsurgical adhesions with Intergel adhesion prevention solution: a multicenter study of safety and efficacy after conservative gynecologic surgery, *Fertil Steril* 2001; 76(3): 595–604.

21. Torres AG and Payne SM. Haem iron-transport system in enterohaemorrhagic *Escherichia coli* 0157 : H7, *Mol Microbiol* 1997; 23: 825–33.

22. Burns JW, Colt MJ, Burgees LS and Skinner KC. Preclinical evaluation of Seprafilm bioresorbable membrane, *Eur J Surg Suppl* 1997; 577: 40–8.

23. Becker JM, Dayton MT, Fazio VW *et al*. Sodium hyaluronate-based bioresorbable membrane in the prevention of postoperative abdominal adhesions: a prospective randomized, double blinded multicenter study, *J Am Coll Surg* 1996; 183: 297–306.

24. Moreira H Jr, Wexner SD, Yamaguchi T, Pikarsky AJ *et al*. Use of bioresorbable membrane (sodium hyaluronate + carboxymethylcellulose) after controlled bowel injuries in a rabbit model, *Dis Colon Rectum* 2000; 43: 182–7.

25. Klingler PJ, Floch NR, Seelig MH, Branton SA *et al*. Seprafilm®-induced peritoneal inflammation: a previously unknown complication: report of a case, *Dis Colon Rectum* 1999; 42: 1639–43.